ALSO BY THOMAS K. SHOTWELL

Books:

The Complete Handbook of Approved New Animal Drug Applications in the United States
(Published by Shotwell & Carr, Inc., 1980)

Workbook and Laboratory Guide to the World of Plants
(Published by The Allen College, 1965)

The Ecology of Antibiotic Usage
(Published by Salsbury Laboratories, Inc., 1967)

FDA: The Formative Years: 1956-1967
(Published by Shotwell & Carr, Inc., 1992)

Veterinary Practitioner's Guide to Approved New Animal Drugs
(Published by Shotwell & Carr, Inc., 1988)

Important Papers:

The Fragility of the Scientific Revolution
(In: Biotechnology and Applied Biochemistry)

Information Flow in an Industrial Research Laboratory--A Case Study
(In: IEEE Transactions on Engineering Management)

An Essay on Beauty
(In: Zygon, Journal of Religion and Science)

Regulating Agricultural Technology
(In: Proceedings, Annual Meeting of the American Society of Agricultural Consultants)

Superbugs:

E. coli, Salmonella, Staphylococcus and More!

DOES SUPER FARMING CAUSE SUPER INFECTIONS?

Thomas K. Shotwell

Biontogeny Publications
P.O. Box 457
Bridgeport, Texas 76426

First Edition January 2009

Printed in the United States of America

Superbugs: *E. coli, Salmonella, Staphylococcus* and More!
Does Super Farming Cause Super Infections?

Library of Congress Control Number 2008912172

Includes bibliographic references and index

1. Antibiotics 2. Bacteriology 3. Medicine 4. Agriculture

ISBN: 1-4392-1298-8
ISBN-13:9781439212981

Visit www.biontogeny.com to order additional copies.

DEDICATION

This book is dedicated to the memory of John Stuart Skinner, publisher of the **American Farmer**, a weekly agricultural newspaper published from April 2, 1819, until March 7, 1834. Skinner labored as the editor for many years to promulgate new and better methods of farming.

CONTENTS

ELEVEN IMPORTANT WORDS
AS USED IN THIS BOOK

As in most affairs, words often have overlapping or vague meanings. Science is not always a tidy enterprise because we must use carefully chosen words to communicate but as time passes and more is learned about the subject those carefully chosen words often become less and less useful. Occasionally the terminology customarily used by the scientific community to refer to something specific becomes too broad or vague to permit clear discussion of the subjects presently at hand. The following definitions will assist the reader to understand how some key words are used in this book.

Antibacterial: Any substance or mixture of substances having some useful ability to significantly interfere with the growth or reproduction of at least one species of bacteria. Antibacterials may be produced by fermentation, fermentation plus chemical modification, or may be produced entirely by chemical synthesis. Includes bactericides, bacteriostats, antibiotics, anti-infectives, disinfectants, and sanitizers.

Antibiotic: Any substance or mixture of substances produced by the growth of microorganisms and which has the ability to significantly interfere with the growth or reproduction of at least one species of bacteria. Antibiotics may or may not be chemically modified before use and some antibiotics, for example chloramphenicol, are synthesized entirely.

Anticoccidials: Any substance or mixture of substances having the ability to significantly interfere with the growth or reproduction of at least one species of coccidia, a protozoa that infects the digestive tract. Includes coccidiostats and coccidiocides. Some anticoccidials are also antibacterial and thus are also antibiotics.

Anti-infective: Any substance or mixture of substances intended for use in the prevention or control of infection by disease-causing microorganisms. Includes all antimicrobials, antibacterials and antibiotics and is frequently used to refer to topically applied products.

Antimicrobial: Any substance or mixture of substances having the ability to significantly interfere with the growth or reproduction of microscopic organisms. Includes antivirals, antibacterials, antifungals, and antiprotozoals.

Antiviral: Any substance or mixture of substances having the ability to significantly interfere with the growth or reproduction of viruses.

Bactericide: Any antibacterial which has the ability to kill bacteria.

Bacteriostat: Any antibacterial which inhibits growth or reproduction of bacteria but does not kill them.

Coccidiocide: Any anticoccidial that kills coccidia.

Coccidiostat: Any anticoccidial that inhibits the growth or reproduction of coccidia but does not kill them.

Superbug: Any strain of *Staphylococcus aureus* resistant to methicillin. Often referred to as "MRSA" (methicillin resistant *Staphylococcus aureus*). Sometimes used to refer to any strain of pathogenic bacteria having the ability to resist the usual effects of several antibiotics

PROLOGUE: SCIENTISTS PANIC

Forty years ago, rumor held that infectious antibiotic resistance in bacteria was spreading like wildfire across America in a pandemic that could make all bacteria resistant to all known antibiotics within a few years—or possibly even a few months. A one-day meeting of bacteriologists was organized to address the impending crisis, and T. Watanabe, a Japanese scientist, was scheduled to reveal how "infectious antibiotic resistance" was spread rapidly from one infected bacterium to others.

Most of the attendees knew that Joshua Lederberg had received the Nobel Prize in 1958 for his discovery that bacteria could mate and exchange genes, but the rumor of a sudden pandemic spread of antibiotic resistance was alarming, and as Watanabe took the podium a chilling silence fell over the audience of about 200 in anticipation of the new data about to be disclosed. When he completed his presentation, the moderator recognized the audience was in turmoil and declared a 10-minute break to give the bacteriologists time to talk among themselves and calm down for the next presentation. As I remember it, everyone in attendance, including the speakers, rushed to the back of the room and into the lobby area where we broke into groups of two to five or six to tell each other what we thought we had heard and to argue about the credibility of Watanabe's report.

Bacteria have chromosomes just as humans, and, like humans, they are known to evolve new attributes through errors made in DNA replication followed by natural selection. With each succeeding generation, the DNA splits and duplicates itself. Some bacteria can reproduce by cell division in as little as eight minutes while others reproduce more slowly, some doubling their numbers once per year or even less often, depending in large part on the suitability of the environment, especially the availability of nutrients such as carbohydrates and amino acids. One way the rapidity with which beneficial coding errors are made in bacterial chromosomes can be measured is by growing bacteria in nutrient media spiked with marginal levels of antibiotics, just enough to kill most but not all the bacteria, then growing the survivors in media with slightly higher levels of the same antibiotic and repeating the procedure many times. But such a procedure also selects for already existing variability in the pool of genes represented in the particular species of bacteria being cultured. Soon the rate of increase in antibiotic resistance falls to almost zero indicating that errors in the duplication of DNA are rare and usually not at all beneficial for resisting antibiotics. Because we knew this, Watanabe's report was stunning.

Watanabe announced he had isolated a strain of bacteria that was not only resistant but that could somehow almost instantly transfer a DNA copy of its resistance genes to non-resistant bacteria of the same or even of a different species and even of a different genus such as from *Escherichia coli*, a common and rarely pathogenic resident of the human digestive tract, to potentially dangerous pathogens such as *Campylobacter jejuni*. He and his associates had shown such transfers occur almost immediately between enteric bacteria in culture media as well as in the mouse intestine.

The roar arising from so many scientists talking excitedly in the lobby made re-convening the meeting almost impossible, so the moderator waited and finally after about 20 minutes pleaded that all participants return to the meeting room so as to allow the next paper to be read. That paper just added fuel to the fire, and another break became necessary. Throughout the day, almost every paper presented resulted in feverish discussions about "infectious" antibiotic resistance.

What Watanabe and others revealed that day was that some strains of antibiotic-resistant bacteria are able to duplicate a coil of extra-chromosomal DNA and transfer that small amount of genetic material coded for specific antibiotic resistance to other non–antibiotic-resistant bacteria by means of a small tunnel that serves as a conduit for the DNA. This meant one could mix antibiotic-resistant and non–antibiotic-resistant bacteria into antibiotic treated media, and practically all the bacteria would become resistant quickly.

Other speakers presented data showing bacteria often exchange small amounts of extra-chromosomal genetic material coding for a number of properties other than antibiotic resistance. Quickly the attendees realized bacteria exist which are antibiotic-resistant but cannot transfer that resistance to other bacteria other than through normal reproduction involving duplication of entire chromosomes, bacteria which can exchange small amounts of extra-chromosomal DNA not including antibiotic resistance, and bacteria that are antibiotic-resistant and can transfer their extra-chromosomal, antibiotic-resistant genes to other non–antibiotic-resistant bacteria within minutes. In fact, some bacteria with resistance to several antibiotics were transferring the entire resistance package.

It all sounded as if the miracle of curing deadly infectious diseases with antibiotics such as penicillin, streptomycin, and neomycin was certain to be short lived. No wonder the bacteriologists were excited, almost delirious, over the reports that day. We have since learned that their concerns were well founded, but the fear that antibiotics would quickly cease to have value was not.

The following chapters describe how antibiotic resistance occurs, where it occurs, what has been proposed to reduce it, and show the broad scope of our activities which involve antibacterial uses that almost certainly contribute to problems at hospitals and clinics. In the last 60 years, we have learned the following:

1. Although conclusive scientific data is not yet broadly available to support decisions about the safety of using currently approved antibiotics in animals, producers of poultry, swine, and cattle are now cautiously reducing the use of antibiotics with an eye on humane treatment of animals, economic impacts, and safety to consumers.

2. Microorganisms have used antibiotics to inhibit or kill their competitors for millions of years.

3. Antibiotic resistance is now encountered in health care facilities more often than in the past, and the steadily increasing incidence of resistance is due to our use of antibiotics and other antibacterials in humans, plants, animals, and industry to control bacteria.

4. Methicillin-resistant *Staphylococcus aureus* (MRSA or "superbugs") were first reported by a hospital in Great Britain in 1961, one year after methicillin was first used.

5. The United States Centers for Disease Control and Prevention (CDC) estimated that 94,360 Americans developed serious MRSA infections in 2005; however, most but not all strains of these and other antibiotic-resistant bacteria encountered in treating humans were traceable to human health care facilities, including hospices and nursing homes.

6. MRSA was associated only with hospitals and other health care facilities for several years after it was first reported.

7. MRSA has recently been identified almost everywhere we have looked for it (for example, in or on water, soil, dogs, chickens, hogs, horses, and humans), but we do not know whether it has been there all along or not.

8. MRSA infections are normally contracted by direct physical contact, not by food and not through the air. Most people who are carriers do not get sick.

9. Although subtherapeutic use of antibiotics in food-producing animals to prevent and/or to control disease in groups of animals or to improve growth and feed efficiency has been the subject of great

controversy since the 1960s, not one case of problems in treating humans with antibiotics has been traced to the subtherapeutic use of any antibiotic in animals. The opposition to subtherapeutic use is based on the assumption that long-term, low-level use will result in high levels of resistance so as to compromise human therapy and on the conviction that subtherapeutic use of antibacterials is purely for economic gain.

10. The United States Food and Drug Administration (FDA) has approved many antibiotics for subtherapeutic use in animals. In fact, there are hundreds of such approvals—as documented in Appendix C of this book.

11. At the urging of activists, Senators Edward Kennedy, Olympia Snowe, Jack Reed, and Sherrod Brown and Representative Louise Slaughter proposed legislation in 2007 to ban all non-therapeutic uses of antibiotics in animals if those antibiotics are considered to be essential for protecting human health. A copy of this proposed legislation is included in Appendix D. Their proposed legislation defines non-therapeutic use as "use in the absence of any clinical sign of disease in the animal for growth promotion, feed efficiency, weight gain, routine disease prevention, or other routine purpose." It also defines "essential for protecting human health" to include all penicillins, tetracyclines, macrolides, lincosamides, streptogramins, aminoglycosides, and sulfonamides or any other drug or derivative of a drug that is used in humans or intended for use in humans to treat or prevent disease or infection caused by microorganisms. In Appendix C of this book, these uses of those antibiotics have been underlined (although identification is uncertain in some cases) to document which antibiotic products the legislators apparently propose to ban. All currently approved uses of antibacterials in animals (approximately 1300) are included in Appendix C to provide perspective. The underlining shows the proposed legislation would ban several hundred of these; however, close examination of the

underlined items reveals the legislation cannot be rationally applied to many of them, suggesting the legislation was put forward not with the expectation it would be passed into law but rather to place pressure on the FDA and the pharmaceutical industry to dedicate more resources to the antibiotic resistance problem.

12. The controversy over antibiotic use in agriculture is fueled by activists in the medical community, in the animal rights community, in the anti-industrial community, and in the vegetarian community. Most or all of these activists have hidden agendas. Many scientists are concerned about antibiotic resistance, but the controversy has now moved from scientific to political. The activist groups seem to include: Center for a Livable Future, Center for Science in the Public Interest, Environmental Defense, Food Animals Concerns Trust, Global Resources Action Center for the Environment, Humane Society of the United States, Institute for Agriculture and Trade Policy, National Catholic Rural Life Conference, Natural Resources Defense Council, Physicians for Social Responsibility, Sierra Club, Union of Concerned Scientists, Waterkeeper Alliance, Safe Tables Our Priority, and several others.

13. Some of the reduction in antibiotic use in animals in the United States has resulted from threats made by activist organizations against retail food suppliers such as McDonalds.

14. Since 1960, only one animal drug (a water additive for sick chickens and turkeys) has been withdrawn from the market by the FDA on the grounds that it contributed to antibiotic resistance problems in human patients. Additionally, FDA proposed and later withdrew a requirement that one entire class of antibiotics, the cephalosporins, be categorically limited to use by licensed veterinarians only according to the approved labeling on the grounds that off-label use may contribute to resistance problems. Laymen have always been denied off-label use.

15. Creating fear about antibiotic-resistant bacteria spreading at the hospital and being present on food is extremely easy. Both are subjects which the general public understands poorly and that journalists easily dramatize.

16. Restricting antibiotic use without scientific data to support the need for or the safety of such restrictions can be dangerous both in terms of cost and in terms of lives lost. American agriculture produces an abundance of food and fiber. Banning antibiotics from agricultural use would cause horrific food shortages almost immediately.

17. Reasonable estimates indicate the United States uses more tons of antibacterials for sanitizing and disinfecting than antibiotics for treating humans and animals combined. Most of these antibacterials are known to be contributors to antibiotic resistance problems, but we do not have studies to determine whether their contributions to human health problems are negligible or serious.

18. Almost everyone proposing restrictions on the uses of antibiotics and antibacterials does so on the grounds that in the absence of scientific certainty of safety we should not permit such technologies to be used—regardless of whether or not the responsible governmental agencies have declared such uses to be safe. This position is known as "The Precautionary Principle" and is not science-based. It holds that any theoretical risk is an unacceptable risk. All European restrictions on the use of antibiotics in animals have been based on this well-recognized political weapon, not on science.

19. European restrictions on antibiotic uses in animals put into effect in 1998 and 1999 have resulted in no significant improvement in treating sick humans.

20. Discussions regarding the relationship between antibiotic use in animals and human health problems are typically about as rational and about as productive as discussions between left-wing democrats and right-wing republicans regarding climate change or military activities in the Middle East. Unfortunately, many otherwise excellent scientific papers in this area reveal this same polarization in the design of studies, the choice of words, and the interpretation of results.

21. The trickle of new antibiotics coming to market is the heart of the problem, but we cannot expect enough new antibiotics until adequate economic incentives for the pharmaceutical industry are in place. Then superbugs will probably just become a memory. But it is more likely that entirely new technologies to control bacterial will play a larger role.

Obviously, a lot has been learned, and a lot remains. Activists have put significant pressure on the FDA to withdraw approvals for the marketing of several antibiotics for use in animals as well as all antibiotics used for disease prevention, disease control, and for growth and feed efficiency; however, the agency is required by the Food, Drug, and Cosmetic Act to base such decisions on science, not intuition, political emphasis, or activist demands. The agency does not always avoid mistakes in this area (for example, review the history of FDA approval of "Plan B" for morning-after birth control), but it should. The way to change the decision-making process on a national basis from science-based to something else is by new legislation. Those who do not like the present Food, Drug, and Cosmetic Act requirements can always ask their elected representatives to change the law. Changing the law is not easy when the subject is highly controversial.

Writing a book intended both for interested scientists and the educated general public presents special challenges and risks. To make the book more readable, references have been placed at the end of each chapter rather than as footnotes. This is helpful to most readers but requires others keep one hand on the current page and one on the page(s) bearing references. There is also the risk of seeming superficial to some readers and of being too technical for others. Every effort has been made to make the following chapters interesting and understandable, but some readers may want to skip over chapters that explain the details of antibiotic resistance.

Finally, in Appendix A the table of antibacterials and their uses in humans, animals, and/or as disinfectants provides a surprising, if not shocking, new perspective on what we use to control bacteria and deserves more attention and further elaboration. Appendix C, an exhaustive itemization of approvals issued by the FDA for application of antimicrobials to animals, can serve as a basic reference for persons concerned with the use of antibiotics in veterinary medicine.

CHAPTER I
ZAUBERKUGELN!
The Impossible Dream

Americans were just learning how to serve as a Quaker-dominated British colony when a Dutchman with no university degree and no scientific training put various objects, including drops of water from a rain barrel and plaque scraped from his teeth and the teeth of several other people, under a single-lens microscope he had constructed, and thereby became the first human to observe a menagerie of squirming, darting, and spinning animalcules, or as he called them, "wee beasties," present in all imaginable shapes and sizes. He did this during the last 20 years of the seventeenth century. He was actually a cloth merchant named Antoni van Leeuwenhoek. Those animalcules were the first bacteria seen by any human. The views he had seen through his lenses were so surprising, even shocking, that he kept his early observations secret for a long time—until he could feel sure they were not illusions. Even then the first paper he sent to the Royal Society of London was denied publication, apparently on the grounds that it was just preposterous.

Let's be very clear at the start. Humanity has no chance of conquering bacterial diseases in the foreseeable future. Notwithstanding the U.S. Surgeon General's comment, reported in 1967, that we would soon close

1

the book on infectious diseases, those wee beasties are now clearly seem to have the upper hand (Stewart 1967). The war will not soon be won because microbes outnumber humans by more than a billion to one, reproduce far more profusely, and change their DNA very fast indeed. For example, bacteria are small, about one-fiftieth the size of a human cell, but all bacteria on earth have a total weight estimated to be 10,000 times the total combined weight of all humans on earth. Although no one has yet been able to count the number of cells in a human body, the total count is currently estimated at perhaps 100 trillion cells; however, 90 percent of them are not human cells (Hooper, et al. 1998). Our bodies and our lives are so completely intertwined with and dependent on the bacteria in or on our bodies that the scientific community is beginning to think of humans as superorganisms, that is, colonies of many species. These not-human cells are bacteria, protozoa, and fungi, and they occupy our bodies as guests, some of which are essential, some sort of friendly, and, occasionally, some which are not friendly at all. Under ideal conditions, some bacteria reproduce as frequently as once every eight minutes, and they can thereby rapidly adapt and evolve. We humans went through 50,000 generations over a period of one million years during which time we evolved from the earliest hunter/gatherers to the beginning of the agricultural revolution, about 500 generations ago (McKeown 1988, 31). Even if bacteria reproduce only once per hour, they go through generations far more rapidly than we do at our sluggish one generation every 20 years. Their opportunities for genetic diversity would seem to be far greater than ours in such time frames. The major protection we have is that bacteria apparently cannot escape the ecological niches they occupy because, it seems, any movement toward a new niche, a smaller size, or any movement toward a larger size, such as the protozoa, and any movement toward multicellularity, such as most fungi, will be immediately met by fierce competition from organisms that made that transition long ago and are now marvelously adapted to exploiting their niches. And all the niches seem to be occupied. Only when some sort of cataclysmic event opens up niches do organisms radiate out into new niches where food and space are not being used. When the dinosaurs disappeared, many species began to take over the space and food supplies left unused. Biologists agree that had the dinosaurs not disappeared there would probably be no humans today on planet earth.

Each species of bacteria becomes specialized in making a living by doing things that result in growth, reproduction, and, usually, movement by at least a few members to another suitable site. An estimated 100,000 species of bacteria reside successfully within the human digestive tract, and almost all are either helpful or at least not harmful enough to cause concern. A few aggressive species take a lot more than we can provide without serious damage and are considered "disease-causing" species. Some of these, such as *Escherichia coli*, are apparently harmless in general except for "strains" that have become aggressive and therefore cause disease in humans, although not necessarily in other animals. A strain is a subpopulation of a species that clearly belongs to the designated species but differs enough to be identified as outside the species' main stream.

Looking back to see how microbes came to be such a formidable force, we see the "Cenancestor" and the "Archea" are names assigned by scientists to the common ancestors of all life on earth. Genetic studies have shown one or both of them almost certainly gave rise to all protozoa, fungi, and bacteria and through them to all plants and animals. Most people are surprised to learn that the most successful form of life on earth today is the bacterium. In fact, if all bacteria were stacked at the surface of the planet, we would all be swimming in a five-foot deep global ocean of bacteria. Thus, if we are to understand antibiotic resistance, we must first understand that we live within that ocean of bacteria and our bodies are deeply involved in and dependent upon its presence.

According to William Whitman, a microbiologist at the University of Georgia, the number of true bacteria and related organisms is estimated to be 5×10^{30}. They weigh roughly one gigaton! Bacteria are able to live almost everywhere. They thrive in flower gardens, decomposing corpses, solid ice, hot springs, hot desert soil, above the tops of mountains, at the bottom of the sea, and more than 100 meters below the surface of the earth deep inside solid rock. Today's bacteria enjoy the benefits of numerous remarkable technologies, including electric motors (an oar-like appendage attached to a disk rotating in a magnetic field) to facilitate movement and breathing, the capacity for stockpiling uranium in their colonies (perhaps to generate heat), a vast range of digestive abilities, a language called "quorum sensing" or "Bacterial Esperanto" that allows them to sense when their population at a given location passes a critical point, and above all, the ability to exchange packets of DNA with each other, to name just a few. We should not, therefore, be surprised when we encounter bacteria with elegant and wonderfully complex defenses, feeding styles, and novel genetic mechanisms. With a billion competing bacteria in every teaspoon of ordinary topsoil inexorably reproducing and competing for food, water, and space for 3.8 billion years, the result has been to push the limits of what can be done within a tiny cell. We have learned a lot about bacteria, but we have a long way to go. The typical little bacterium appears to be more complex and more sophisticated than an automobile, a locomotive, or even a space shuttle. In fact, it seems far more complex than Big Blue or any other computer yet designed by humans. This book is about the ability of various species of bacteria to overcome the effects of ancient and modern antibacterials, including the ability to spread resistance in response to antibacterial use, and including the virtual certainty that we will not soon (and possibly never) win our war with bacteria that cause disease. Above all, this book is about the importance of sanitation, hygiene, and prudent management of antibacterial use.

Learning that bacteria exist was terribly important, and knowing what trouble they can cause was equally important. But how to discover what bacteria actually do was and in large part still is quite a puzzle. In the eighteenth and nineteenth centuries, the wheels of science were turning slowly, at least by our twenty-first century clocks. About 60 years after Leeuwenhoek first saw his animalcules, John Needham demonstrated that cooking food prevented those animalcules from just appearing suddenly and spoiling the food (1745), but the idea that bacteria and a lot of other beasts were spontaneously created hung around until Louis Pasteur finally laid the idea to rest by showing bacteria were getting into food from the air (1859). Within a year, Joseph Lister used that knowledge of the microscopic world to prevent infections in hospital patients. When he graduated from London and Edinburgh Universities, he took a job at the Glasgow Royal Infirmary. While studying blood in injuries and surgical wounds at the infirmary, he noticed a lot of infections that could not be blamed on dirty rooms. He decided spraying carbolic acid on surgical instruments, wounds, and surgical dressings might help to prevent infections, but the idea was greeted with scorn from the surgeons. When the results of Lister's carbolic acid applications were tabulated in 1860, the treatment was shown to have greatly reduced mortality in the patients. The medical community finally came to recognize Lister as a hero, a man who had saved many, many lives. He was made a baron by Queen Victoria in 1897.

Next came Robert Koch, a man who practiced medicine for a while and then in 1870 served in the Franco-Prussian war. From 1872 to 1880, he served as a district medical officer where he conducted research on *Bacillus anthracis*, a puzzling and sometimes deadly species of bacteria thought to cause disease. This species was able to hibernate inside tough, tiny capsules called spores and there remain dormant but viable and dangerous for years or perhaps even centuries. Koch learned how to cultivate the bacteria in the laboratory and reported its ability to hibernate. Both animals and humans were affected by it, and Koch proved the disease was caused by, and only by, that species of bacteria. While doing that work, he also set up criteria (called "Koch's postulates") whereby other scientists could prove the cause of various diseases. Publication of his work in 1876 made him famous. Koch subsequently studied cholera, tuberculosis, rinderpest, malaria, blackwater fever, "surra" of cattle and horses, plague, East Coast fever of cattle in Africa, *Babesia*, *Trypanosoma*, and tick-borne spirochaetosis. In 1905 he received the Nobel Prize for

Physiology or Medicine. With his work, everyone in the scientific community learned the cause of many diseases really was Leeuwenhoek's animalcules. The obvious next step was to find something that would poison those animalcules and not humans or other animals.

In the early 1900s, a few scientists got the idea that some chemicals might be synthesized that would be safe to give to humans while being highly toxic to these little beasties. Unfortunately, most scientists were persuaded that idea was an impossible dream. Anything able to kill the wee beasties, they were convinced, would surely also kill us if we swallowed it. After all, poisons were poisons.

Paul Ehrlich (1854–1915) was known to his colleagues as the man with blue, yellow, red, and green fingers and a box of cigars under his arm. Aniline dyes, discovered by W.H. Perkins in 1853, somehow became Ehrlich's obsession. Their ability to selectively stain animal tissues and microorganisms led him into a frenetic career involving the ability of various dyes and other chemicals to selectively affect living things, especially the immune system and disease-causing microorganisms. He called these unique chemicals "zauberkugeln" (German for "magic bullets") because they moved relatively harmlessly through the human body and killed or crippled disease-causing microorganisms. His conviction that chemicals could be synthesized to attack many diseases led him to the discovery of Salvorsan, the first effective treatment for syphilis, as well as to the discovery of treatments for malaria and sleeping sickness.

Ehrlich's vision of magic bullets was novel and contrary to the widespread conviction that any substances able to kill bacteria, fungi, and protozoa would surely kill humans and other animals as well. But the idea of magic bullets did infect a few other people, particularly Heinrich Horlein, head of the pharmaceutical research program at Friedrich Bayer & Company in Germany. In 1927 Horlein hired Gerhard Domagk, a bright young physician, as well as two chemists and other supporting personnel, to pursue the idea of magic bullets. He provided laboratory facilities and assigned them the task of synthesizing new chemicals and testing them against bacteria that cause disease. Five years and hundreds of chemicals later, they found one. It turned out to be sulfanilamide, the first really effective antibiotic (Hager 2006, 94).

Sulfanilamide was a commodity on which the patent had expired long before Domagk's work began. When news of its antibacterial activity spread, many firms in Europe and the United States quickly began producing the drug. By October 1937 the United States alone was producing more than 10 tons of sulfanilamide per week by one estimate. By 1942 that total had risen to more than 32 tons per week, and the amount produced worldwide was probably two or three times that much. By 1943 the United States was producing 86.5 tons of various sulfa drugs weekly, some of which were being stockpiled, but most of which were used. All sulfonamides were available without prescription at the local drugstore, thereby leading to a vast amount of misuse, that is, use other than in accordance with the labeling and often for conditions where the drug would not have worked in any case—such as the common cold. Sulfanilamide was effective against *Streptococcus* bacteria, but the population of *susceptible Streptococcus* encountered in hospitals dwindled. The percent of the resistant population encountered increased slowly but surely to take over wherever the sensitive bacteria had previously been seen. In the 1930s most *Streptococcus* populations, about 90 percent, were controlled, but in the early 1940s that dropped to 45 or 50 percent, enough to alarm physicians across the world. But then "yellow magic" came to the rescue of the first magic bullet. That yellow magic was penicillin.

A French medical student, Ernest Duchesne, discovered penicillin in 1896, but its usefulness was not obvious, and techniques for isolating and using penicillin were unknown. He dropped it. Then in the fall of 1928, Alexander Fleming, a Scottish physician, noticed bacteria dissolving around a colony of mold which he thought was penicillin. He recorded the observation and, recognizing it held some potential for medicine, published his findings in *The British Journal of Experimental Pathology* in June 1929. But neither Fleming nor the scientific community at large saw any apparent way the witches' brew mold broth (it seemed to them like something right out of William Shakespeare) Fleming had produced could ever be pumped into humans in sufficient quantities to provide a medical benefit. Their calculations showed mild infections would require gallons of broth and severe infections would require tank car loads to be injected (Ratliff 1945, 44). The best way and probably the only way, they thought, was to synthesize new chemicals and test them for antibacterial activity.

For nearly 10 years, Fleming focused on other things and lost interest in working on penicillin because it seemed unstable and too difficult to extract from the mold broth. But Howard Florey, Ernst Chain, and Norman Heatley at Oxford continued to see the promise of penicillin and to work toward its development. They were hampered in their attempts to get funded at Oxford due to the prevailing opinion that brewing up a mold broth to treat disease was foolish. They received just enough money from the Rockefeller Foundation in the United States to keep going. They were able to concentrate the active component just barely enough to be useful in treating patients orally and by injection. But their best efforts indicated a single dose of penicillin would cost thousands of dollars unless improvements could be made in growing and extracting penicillin. Florey laced his pockets with penicillin spores so that he would be able to restart his work if the Germans successfully invaded England. As the war progressed he and Chain then went to America because America was the only friendly country with pharmaceutical firms like Pfizer and Merck that had the capital and the scientific personnel needed to continue and expand their work.

Chain wanted to patent their invention, but Florey, being in the mainstream of British science, would have none of that—on ethical grounds. He felt their invention belonged to humanity. When they arrived in America, they disclosed everything they knew to the scientists at Pfizer and Merck. The Americans quickly obtained the necessary funding and soon found new ways to grow the mold, and later, by isolating new strains of penicillin (one from a cantaloupe), found new ways to grow more penicillin in every ounce of broth. By developing techniques that allowed the mold to grow deep in the broth as well as on its surface and new ways to extract the penicillin itself, in the first five months of 1943 some 400 million units of penicillin were produced. That amount was enough to treat about 180 people orally or by injection. By the end of the year, an additional 20.5 billion units had been produced.

In a June 26, 1945, interview published in *The New York Times* (page 21), Fleming expressed concern about careless and inappropriate use of penicillin selecting and propagating resistant bacteria; however, other scientists involved in the discovery and development of penicillin seem not to have dwelled at much length in their various publications about how bacteria have undoubtedly encountered penicillin many times over many millennia and, because of that, evolved ways to negate its lethal effects. But that is an inescapable conclusion for any scientist reasonably well versed in the principles of biological evolution. *Penicillium notatum*, the mold that produces penicillin, was very likely present long before humans emerged (Cano and Borucki 1997), and it obviously found certain bacteria to be competitors for food and space. This point did not go entirely unnoticed. J.D. Ratliff wrote in 1945: "In the end it may turn out that the greatest single job that penicillin has done is in refocusing attention on the constant warfare that goes on in nature. Penicillin is but a single example of how one micro-organism, a mold, fights other micro-organisms, bacteria" (Ratliff 1945, 167).

The reason penicillin was so dramatically effective against an array of disease-causing bacteria and so ineffective against others may be due to some bacteria species having encountered *P. notatum* rarely and others having encountered it often. Most of the bacteria controlled by penicillin did not and do not normally flourish in the same environments occupied by *P. notatum*. The disease-causing bacteria and disease-causing fungi that concern us specialize in living on man and other animals while *P. notatum* is more specialized in living on plants, like the cantaloupe from which it was isolated in the early 1940s, like potatoes as was noticed when potato dextrose was added to broth to enhance penicillin growth, and like many types of bread, but not often on meat or meat products.

By June of 1943, penicillin production in large fermentation tanks was in full swing in the hands of Abbott, Merck, Pfizer, Squibb, and Winthrop. By June of 1944, enough penicillin was available to meet the needs of all allied military forces, civilian needs, and to establish 1,000 depot hospitals where it could be and was being stockpiled (Ratliff 1945, 102). But, as production expanded, the separation of liquids containing penicillin from the mass of solids in the fermentation tanks resulted in great piles of solids called "biomass" that daily grew in size until they were more like low mountains. Soon spontaneous combustion set in, and difficult fires at pharmaceutical disposal sites became a problem. Records, if any, of the number of such fires, their dates, and locations, are lost or are buried in the archives of pharmaceutical firms and fire departments.

After some heavy head scratching, pharmaceutical firms began offering the nutrient-rich biomass to the animal feed industry at no charge. Just pay the freight! The antibiotic content was nil, or at least below the detection limit, and university professors soon published studies showing increased growth and improved efficiency of feed utilization when a few pounds of this biomass was added to a ton of feed for pigs, chickens, or turkeys. Initially "unidentified growth factors," "protein sparing," and other mechanisms were imagined to be responsible for the benefits, but when the antibiotic detection limit was lowered due to enhanced analytical techniques the hidden antibiotic, although far below therapeutic levels, was suddenly visible and recognized as a possible source of the improved performance—as well as a potential source of antibiotic resistance (Stokstad and Jukes 1951).

The discovery and development of streptomycin was similar to the stories of sulfanilamide and penicillin. Selman Waksman of Rutger's University began studying the microbiology of soils in 1915. He knew tuberculosis bacteria were destroyed when placed in soil and speculated that reason was the warfare between microorganisms. Twenty-four years later when the news about penicillin was announced, he was persuaded that he could get better results with the *Actinomycetes* (bacteria that look a lot like mold) he was studying in soils. In 1940 he isolated a new "antibiotic" (a word he coined for antibacterials found in nature), but it was highly toxic to mammals. Finally in 1943 he isolated streptomycin then worked toward purifying it and determining which diseases it could control. One of the most important was tuberculosis, but streptomycin was excellent for many other bacterial infections as well.

Waksman received the Nobel Prize in 1952 for his discovery of streptomycin. He worked with the Mayo Clinic in Rochester, Minnesota, and with the drug company Merck to expedite moving this magic bullet into the hospital's medicine cabinet to save lives. And it did—by the thousands and hundreds of thousands. Now, with three new magic bullets identified, the discovery efforts moved into high gear in all the major drug companies around the world. Antibiotic after antibiotic was discovered, developed, and brought health to the sick and big bucks to the drug companies. Incidentally, it also brought some badly needed credibility to hospitals and physicians.

The federal government had no authority to approve or disapprove the introduction of new drugs for use in humans or animals until 1938 when the Food, Drug, and Cosmetic Act was passed. The new law required governmental review of the safety of new drugs prior to marketing. With the widespread, almost trouble-free deployment of sulfanilamide, penicillin, and streptomycin for human use, the federal government was as eager as veterinarians and farmers to get these wonder drugs into use in pets and farm animals. Approvals came in the 1940s and continued at a rapid pace for many years. For example, we know from the original governmental approval dates on currently approved animal drug products that penicillin was approved by 1950, tetracycline by 1951, and streptomycin by 1953. Polymyxin B and bacitracin were also approved by 1953, and erythromycin, chloramphenicol, and neomycin were approved by 1955.

The FDA has archives that include the original approval dates for all the antibiotic products no longer approved for marketing, but access to the FDA's huge archives is difficult—even for the FDA itself. Antibiotic resistance was encountered from time to time in hospitals and on farms and ranches, but it was manageable and did not appear to threaten humans or animals. The idea of banning antibiotic use in animals because it produced resistance was little more than a laughable matter for more than a decade.

Because magic bullets had been discovered in large numbers, many pharmaceutical firms turned away from the frantic search for antibiotics to an equally frantic search for other classes of magic bullets for treatment of other diseases, particularly magic bullets with more financial promise.

REFERENCES

Cano, Raul J. and Monica K. Borucki. 1997. *Ancient microorganisms*. U.S. Patent 5593883. January 14.

Hager, Thomas. 2006. *The demon under the microscope*. New York: Harmony Books.

Ratcliff, J.D.1945. *Yellow magic: The story of penicillin*. New York: Random House.

Hooper, Lora V., Lynn Bry, Per G. Falk, and Jeffrey I. Gordon. 1998. Host-microbial symbiosis in the mammalian intestine: Exploring an internal ecosystem. *Bio-Essays* 20:336-43.

McKeown, Thomas. 1988. *The origins of human disease*. Oxford: Basil Blackwell.

Stewart, William H. 1967. *A mandate for state action*. Presented at the Association of State and Territorial Health Officers, December 4, in Washington, D.C. (by the Surgeon General of the United States.) (Although often referenced, the quote has been questioned and has also been referred to as testimony to Congress in 1969 but seems not to be in the Congressional Record. Stewart himself is quoted as having said later that he did not remember making the comment.)

Stokstad, E.L.R. and T.H. Jukes. 1951. Growth promoting effect of aureomycin on turkey poults. *Poultry Science* 29:611-12. See also Moore, P.R., A. Evenson, E. Luckey, E. McCoy, C.A. Elvehjem, and E.B. Hart. 1946. Use of sulfasuxidine, streptothricin and streptomycin in nutritional studies with the chick. *J. Biol. Chem.* 165:437-41.

CHAPTER II
SEX AND SURVIVAL
How Bacteria Become Resistant

For generations we have been taught that bacteria reproduce asexually by simply replicating their chromosome and dividing into two cells. Well, our teachers were wrong. Sexual reproduction is the passage of hereditary material from one organism to another so that descendents receive some hereditary material from both. Many bacteria do just that. In some cases DNA floating in the environment is merely absorbed through the bacteria's cell wall and subsequently incorporated into the chromosome. Other times a tube forms between two bacteria to permit a packet of DNA to be passed from one bacterium to another where it replicates independent of the chromosome and a copy is subsequently passed along to offspring. In fact, there are many ways bacteria are able to enhance their hereditary recipes. What is more impressive is that some bacteria not only exchange DNA amongst themselves but also pass DNA to (and from) other species, even other genera. Identifying the number of bacterial gene pools and their connectivity remains difficult even today (Waples and Gaggiotti 2006). It is therefore little wonder that bacteria change so fast.

SUPERBUGS

When Charles Darwin's *The Origin of Species* was published in 1859, the book was read not just by scientists and theologians but also by polite, well-educated Victorian ladies. Legend holds that having read the book carefully one such lady said something to the effect of: "Mr. Darwin is obviously correct, but please don't tell anyone about it!" Darwin shocked Victorian England and most of the world because his explanation was profoundly simple and quickly became obvious to all except persons with obsessive commitments to traditional theological assertions about the origin of species. That so many humans still do not understand the origin of species is just plain shameful. A recent survey of physicians revealed 85 percent of them believe God intervenes from time to time to affect their patients' health. Even Pope Benedict has recently asserted that evolution is just a theory that cannot be proven.

The four simple generalizations Darwin set forth 150 years ago also reveal how bacteria evolve resistance to antibiotics today:

1. Living things produce more offspring than are needed to maintain a steady population.

2. Offspring vary in their attributes and are not always identical to each other or to their parents.

3. There is a limited amount of food and space for living things to utilize.

4. With constant population pressure, there is competition within and among species for food and space.

Obviously these four practically undeniable assertions about all living things lead to the conclusion that a struggle for existence exists in which the best adapted offspring tend to survive and flourish while less well adapted offspring tend to leave fewer or no descendants. This was called "natural selection," and it set us all on a new path for thinking about life, including bacteria. But Darwin did not understand the basis for variation and especially not for endless genetic variation. He, and every other rational person, could not avoid the conclusion that natural selection in any given species would slowly weed out attributes that were unneeded or counterproductive and slowly spread attributes that enhanced the ability to secure food and space. But how entirely new attributes might arise was simply unknown, and this became a serious concern in evolution theory.

In the 1850s while Darwin was still shuffling his papers and re-examining the specimens from his ocean voyages on *The Beagle* in preparation for publication of his book, an Austrian monk was methodically studying hereditary variations in garden plants. Gregor Mendel's work began in 1856, and his report of findings was read at two meetings (February 8 and March 8) in 1865 of the Natural History Society of Brunn in Bohemia and published in 1866. We know Mendel had read Darwin's book by the time of his own publication because he repeatedly makes reference to the "evolution" of life forms. Even if Mendel understood the importance of his findings for Darwinian evolution, he was almost certainly reluctant to publish or possibly forbidden to publish because of the swirling theological controversy pervading churches in the late 1800s. Unfortunately, Darwin never read Mendel's paper—even though Darwin's personal papers show he received a reprint of Mendel's report. After Darwin's death, the reprint was found with the pages "uncut," meaning it was not opened and could not have been read by Darwin. In fact, Mendel's work went practically unnoticed until 1900 when some scientists recognized its value and repeated Mendel's experiments. Before 1900, popular opinion held that mixing hereditary material was like mixing paint. Crossbreed garden peas bearing red flowers with garden peas bearing white flowers and the offspring bear pink flowers. Likewise, crossbreed tall peas with dwarf peas and all offspring are of medium height. Like mixing paint.

Mendel showed this was true, but he went a step further and crossed garden peas with pink flowers with other garden peas bearing pink flowers, and he got not all pinks but some red, some white, and some pink. This revelation that hereditary material was better viewed as particulate rather than as liquid quickly led to the field of genetics and, further, to a synthesis of genetics and Darwinian evolution in the first half of the twentieth century. Darwin had been vindicated because Mendel had shown us how heredity works.

In 1953 James D. Watson and Francis H.C. Crick revealed that the hereditary material, DNA, consisted of a double helix with amino acid cross-links that conferred hereditary traits. Before Watson and Crick we could see chromosomes, and we knew they carried the hereditary traits (genes) of the organism, but the structure of Mendel's hereditary particles remained a mystery until Watson and Crick published their work. Now we know the replication of the double helix is subject to occasional errors in the amino acid sequences that sometimes lead to novel attributes which, if they accumulate over long periods of time, can so completely change a group of organisms that they become a new species, one distinctly different from their remote ancestors. The speed with which the genome changes may seem glacial but it is inexorable. All it needs is a lot of time.

Thus in the late 1950s the scientific community seemed to have it all figured out. Mendel was right, Darwin was right, and Watson and Crick were right. The early work done on antibiotic resistance in bacteria was conducted under this assumption, but experiments soon showed the speed with which some bacteria could become resistant and pass that resistance along to descendents was far too rapid for Mendel and Darwin. In the 1940s and early 1950s, the only known source of new attributes in bacteria was genetic errors made during replication. Although many bacteria reproduce quickly, the chance production of the genes needed to produce new biochemically complex antibiotic resistance mechanisms in a few days seemed to violate all the known rules of probability. Mendel and Darwin were both threatened!

In the late 1950s and the 1960s, scientists discovered that while bacteria do play by Mendel's rules, they cheat. They employ a variety of techniques that allow rapid spread of inheritable antibiotic resistance and other attributes as well. The hereditary transmission of these newly acquired characteristics seemed to violate the principles of evolution and to validate Trofim Lysenko's and Ivan Vladimirovich Michurin's previously disqualified assertions that characteristics acquired during life are passed along to descendents, a vestige of Karl Marx's cold war ideology. Understanding how bacteria cheat genetically is critical to any inquiry regarding the spread of antibiotic resistance and equally critical to formulating a plan to manage such resistance. Most bacteria have a single circular chromosome with all hereditary information but no organized nucleus. Except for a small group called the *Mollicutes*, which includes pathogens such as the mycoplasmas, bacteria have a rigid cell wall. Inside that cell wall is a distinct cell membrane but no other readily visible structures (organelles); however, bacteria operate a vast array of molecular mechanisms too small to be seen through traditional light microscopes—including such things as the tiny electric motors mentioned earlier.

By the year 2000, bacteriologists and geneticists were overwhelmed with a wealth of new information because the genomes of many pathogenic bacteria were being or had been sequenced. Although we knew in the 1960s some bacteria were passing genetic material around, we now understand bacterial genomes are inherently amazingly dynamic within very short time frames, with large and small blocks of DNA being rapidly and routinely acquired or deleted (Mullany 2005). The speed of genetic change in bacteria is not glacial after all. The tiny packets of DNA we observed being exchanged between bacteria in the 1960s are still called plasmids, and they carry extra-chromosomal DNA that provides virulence genes, antibiotic resistance genes, and/or metabolic mechanism genes to allow their host to occupy diverse niches. Plasmids carry nonessential genes; that is, all the genes needed to produce a bacterium are on the chromosome whereas the plasmids carry genes that are nice to have in an emergency. Because the chromosomal DNA and the plasmid DNA exist independent of each other, they also evolve independently of each other. So the evolution of bacteria occurs on at least two levels. Although not all species of bacteria utilize plasmids, any effort to manage the problem of antibiotic resistance must take into consideration that many bacteria do employ these dual evolving sets of DNA. Following the evolution of chromosomal DNA is difficult, following the evolution of plasmid DNA is difficult, and simultaneously following the evolution of both increases the difficulty enormously. Other forms of DNA exchange have recently been identified, complicating our efforts to understand the evolution of bacteria.

Bacteria may get rid of antibiotics and other unneeded substances by pumping them out through the cell membrane and cell wall. Such "efflux pumps" apparently serve to remove a variety of substances from bacteria and are not a result of human antibiotic usage but have been around for a very long time. Similarly, bacteria may slow absorption of antibiotics with influx pumps that selectively control the movement of substances into the cell. Importantly, given that such pumping mechanisms exists, the number of fortuitous mutations needed to modify them to pump out or reduce absorption of specific antibiotics is a tiny fraction of the mutations needed to build the pump itself. In addition, antibiotics are toxic to specific bacteria because their chemical structure causes inhibition or degradation of one or more essential metabolic processes within those bacteria. Resistant bacteria sometimes produce substances that break the antibiotic molecule into inactive parts or bind to the antibiotic to render it harmless. Because bacteria are inherently enormously complex, random mutations that enhance or slightly modify existing metabolic reactions can rather easily result in antibiotic resistance. For example, according to the FDA, in *Campylobacter* a single point mutation conferring resistance to fluoroquinolone antibiotics is estimated to occur naturally in approximately one to five in 100 million bacteria (FDA 2005, 17). That pretty much says anyone with a *Campylobacter* infection will have some fluoroquinolone resistant bacteria. Fortunately, that population is usually, but not always, too small to make the infection unmanageable by the patient's natural defenses—unless the patient is immunocompromised. If so, the resistant *Campylobacter* can quickly multiply and populate the intestine—and maybe the hospital as well.

Another of the surprises that shocked the scientific community was the discovery that in some cases the DNA in a plasmid uncurls and inserts itself into the bacterium's chromosome where it becomes a routine part of the hereditary material. Plasmids that have this ability are called "episomes." And still another shock to the system was the discovery that loose DNA in the environment taken into the bacterium may subsequently be incorporated into the chromosome. Still other experiments suggest bacteria chronically exposed to a given antibiotic may undergo mutations to "uncover" resistance genes that were present all along but somehow silent, muted. Finally, bacteriophages are small, virus-like organisms that attach to bacteria and inject their DNA. Sometimes the injection includes DNA that helps the bacteria to resist antibiotics. These and other ways bacteria exchange DNA within a given species and across species and genera lines suggests we might do well to consider the evolution of bacteria to be a broad phenomenon that crosses all, or at least many, species lines, and most resistance genes predate any human use of antibiotics. In fact, so much inter-species and inter-genera transfer of DNA casts doubt on the idea of using binominal nomenclature in classifying bacteria and other microorganisms. The concept of "genus" and "species" loses much of its relevance.

Given all these genetic tricks, it would seem that all the bacteria on the planet should now be resistant to all commonly used antibiotics. That would be catastrophic. It was this fear that fueled the alarms sounded by Stuart B. Levy in both the first (1992) and second (2002) editions of

SUPERBUGS

The Antibiotic Paradox, books that frightened the medical community and continue to fuel emotional pleas to stop the use of antibiotics unless the attending physician is certain of the patient's need and probable benefit and to ban many uses of antibiotics, especially in "healthy" livestock and poultry. He presumably did not know that more than 80 percent of hospitalized patients with resistant bacteria got those resistant bacteria while in the hospital. If Levy's 1992 concerns had been justified, no antibiotic should now be effective in the treatment of any disease. Even in areas where his concerns were justified the bacteria have, as was earlier observed, a more dynamic genome than he envisioned. When antibiotic resistance is needed bacteria become resistant because only the survivors repopulate the area, and when it is not needed that resistance is discarded over time. How much time this process takes varies, but it does happen. The new survivors have lost their useless resistance genes and are sensitive to antibiotics. Studies showing chromosomal or plasmid antibiotic resistance to be stable over long periods of time usually omit competition from non-resistant bacteria and thereby give misleading conclusions. Recent studies (Lenski 1998) suggesting resistant bacteria adapt to carrying extra genes by further mutations of a compensatory nature are probably true but must be confirmed and their applicability to conditions existing outside the laboratory determined because the evidence that evolution gets rid of unneeded genes is overwhelming. Any pattern of sustained and consistent outlay of metabolic material, such as amino acids, for the perpetuation of complex antibiotic-resistant genes on chromosomes or in plasmids cries out for explanation if it is alleged to occur in the absence of antibiotics and in competition with bacteria not carrying such genes. Excess genes for antibiotic resistance are all cost and no benefit—like the genes for eyes in cave-dwelling fish. Beyond that, one must deal with the near certainty that antibiotics have been in use in nature for more than a billion years, and antibiotic resistance has obviously become a small part of the gene pool for many species and has not become universal. Little competition for amino acids exists in the media used to culture bacteria because the media contains an abundance of it. No competition, no natural selection, no evolution. An exception is those surprising plasmids that may be lost simply due to cell division. A bacterium may carry only one copy of a plasmid, so when it divides into two bacteria one of the two will be without a plasmid. In other cases bacteria may carry many copies of their plasmid(s) and thereby be likely to pass one or more along.

The bacterial population of any given space is termed the "microflora." In hospitals, nursing homes, hospices, and clinics where antibiotics are continuously used, much of the microflora of the premises becomes resistant, regardless of whether the bacteria cause disease, unless serious steps are taken to minimize the spread of resistance, and when antibiotics are not used on the premises that resistance is ultimately lost or at least returns to the natural background level. Our experience is that the process takes months or years and, alone, is not a practical solution. Still, in actively growing cultures, most of a given resistant *E. coli* population has been found to lose its resistance plasmids within 96 hours (Miller 2005), not weeks or months or years but in 96 hours. Such a rapid loss of resistance plasmids clearly does not occur with bacteria reproducing at a slower rate or in bacteria that have resistance on their chromosomes (Smith and Bidochka 1998).

More studies to document the rate of loss under representative conditions are needed. Funds for a study to document the decline of antibiotic resistance are obviously more difficult to obtain than funds to study the rate of increase. Good news is never as exciting as bad news. Frequently replicating even a small circle of DNA also has unquestionable metabolic costs. As Bonnie Bassler, a professor of molecular biology at Princeton University, has said, bacteria "don't have enough room in their genome to be stupid" (Holloway 2004). In a rapidly reproducing organism that cost becomes a burden when competing with other fast-growing organisms. It's a little like a foot race through an airport terminal when one party is carrying luggage and the other is not. If the plane is overbooked, the last to arrive will not board. Much more research to clearly identify and quantify the rate of gain and loss of antibiotic resistance in various bacteria is needed for pathogens as well as for other bacteria.

If passing DNA around is a clear sign of sex, then some apparently harmless bacteria are now known to be engaged in sexual activity that turns out to be quite unpleasant for humans. While bacteriologists were feverishly studying antibiotic resistance in disease-causing bacteria, other species of bacteria harmless to animals and humans were becoming resistant for all the same reasons pathogenic bacterial populations become resistant, that is, selective pressure due to repeated exposure to antibiotics. These resistant populations of friendly bacteria were initially viewed as irrelevant to the problem of resistant pathogens, but now we know they are unquestionably involved by passing their plasmids with genes for antibiotic resistance to unrelated pathogenic bacteria. So a patient may be diagnosed with an intestinal infection due to antibiotic-susceptible *Salmonella, Campylobacter, C. diff. (Colostridium difficile)*, or *E. coli*, but if an antibiotic is administered those bacteria may suddenly become resistant because the harmless bacteria handed off copies of their plasmid-borne DNA to the pathogens. Little wonder the scientists involved in the first studies of plasmids described the resistance as "infectious." It spreads from resistant to susceptible bacteria like a plague. They all become magic bullet-proof. To most life forms sex is about assuring diversity of descendents and thus the evolveability of the species, not the survival of the individual organism engaging in sexual activity. Bacteria are different!

Federal agencies and hospital administrators must also begin sustained efforts to deal with the development and spread of antibiotic resistance in health care facilities. Studies have already been done that demonstrate such programs are effective. The idea that antibiotics never act by killing 100 percent of the pathogen population in a sick patient has long been known but has not been much discussed. Sick people harbor billions of pathogens, at least a few of which are inherently resistant to whatever antibiotic is used—due to spontaneous mutations such as those seen in the *Campylobacter* species. Until sustained programs are put in place to deal with these simple but critical problems, there is little benefit to be derived from banning any agricultural, industrial, or domestic use of antibiotics.

Finally, any comprehensive program to control bacteria in health care facilities is dependent on the use of biocides (antiseptics, disinfectants, sanitizers, preservatives, and sterilants), but at present conclusive scientific information needed to allow their prudent use does not exist. We know these products are generally effective, but we also know their use can select for intrinsic or acquired antibiotic resistance—including transferable plasmids—and therefore adds a new dimension to antibiotic resistance problems (Sheldon 2005).

REFERENCES

Crawford, Lester M. 2005. (Docket No. 2000N-1571). Animal drugs, feeds, and related products; Enrofloxacin for poultry; Withdrawal of approval of new animal drug application. *Federal Register* 70: 44048-49. http://www.fda.gov/oc/antimicrobial/baytril.html (accessed August 4, 2005).

Holloway, Marguerite. 2004. Talking bacteria. *Scientific American 290 (2)*: 34–35.

Lenski, Richard E. 1998. Bacterial evolution and the cost of antibiotic resistance. *International Microbiology* 1:265–70.

Miller, Colin. 2005. Loss of antibiotic resistance in *Escherichia Coli* bacteria. http://homepages.bw.edu/~mbumbuli/biotech/colin/ (accessed July 18, 2005).

Mullany, Peter, ed. 2005. *The dynamic bacterial genome*. Cambridge: Cambridge University Press.

Sheldon, Albert T., Jr. 2005. Antiseptic "resistance": Real or perceived? *Clinical Infectious Diseases* 40: 1650–6. See also by the same author: 2005. Antiseptic resistance: What do we know and what does it mean? *Clin. Lab. Sci.* 18(3):181. http://findarticles.com/p/articles/mi_qa3890/is_200507/ai_n14825286 (accessed December 17, 2007).

Smith, M. Alex and Michael J. Bidochka. 1998. Bacterial fitness and plasmid loss: The importance of culture conditions and plasmid size. *Can. J. Microbiol.* 44:351–55.

Waples, Robin S. and Oscar Gaggiotti. 2006. What is a population? An empirical evaluation of some genetic methods for identifying the number of gene pools and their degree of connectivity. *Molecular Ecology* 15:1419–39.

CHAPTER III

WHERE SUPERBUGS ORIGINATE

Where Resistant Bacteria Come From

Alexander Fleming's 1945 acceptance lecture upon receipt of the Nobel Prize for the discovery of penicillin was brief, but the third sentence out of his mouth was, "To my generation of bacteriologists the inhibition of one microbe by another was commonplace." He continued, "We were all taught about these inhibitions and indeed it is seldom that an observant clinical bacteriologist can pass a week without seeing in the course of his ordinary work very definite instances of bacterial antagonism."

Fleming was telling us microbially-produced antibacterials and microbial resistance to those antibacterials was commonplace before penicillin. In fact, in that same lecture he warned that using less than a full therapeutic dose of penicillin would immediately lead to overgrowth of resistant pathogens. More recently the isolation and culturing of bacteria from the intestines of bees entombed in amber 25 to 40 million years ago told us unequivocally that microbially-produced antibacterials are not new, and by inference, neither is resistance (Cano and Borucki 1997). And ants, it seems, have been using microbially-produced antibacterials to protect their crops for 50 million years (Currie 2003).

As described in Chapter One, 22 years after Fleming's lecture a group of bacteriologists and other interested scientists called a special symposium to learn about rumors that antibiotic resistance had become "infective," thereby spreading like a disease and threatening a pandemic of resistant pathogens in hospitals and clinics. Watanabe carefully explained his research and caused something of a panic when his data showed us that resistance in one bacterium was passed to another in minutes.

Fast-forward 40 years to the present, and resistance has indeed become an increasingly serious but not yet critical problem. Many bacteriologists, recognizing DNA recipes for resistance genes are being passed around among bacteria rather freely, now speak of resistance as a worldwide "resistome" within the common pool of all bacterial genes, a play on the word "genome." Using antibacterials selects for resistance, and when anyone uses an antibacterial they destroy sensitive bacteria, open the door for overgrowth of resistant bacteria, and thereby tilt the population toward more resistance, adding a bit more "pollution" to that commons. Parallels can be drawn with "The Tragedy of the Commons," a paper published by Garrett Hardin in *Science* in 1968 to describe the consequences of our disposal of wastes into rivers, lakes, oceans, and the atmosphere, all the common property of everyone and the responsibility of no one. The net result, Hardin pointed out, is destruction of the commons unless coercion is used to stop it.

PLACING THE BLAME

Efforts to identify the sources of "superbugs" require that we define as precisely as possible what a superbug really is. The scientific community generally describes superbugs as any strain of *Staphylococcus aureus* that is resistant to customary dosages of methicillin and other more common antibiotics such as oxacillin, penicillin, nafcillin, and amoxicillin and the cephalosporins. Methicillin was a new antibiotic introduced for human use in Great Britain in 1960 and was thought to be a major new tool for long-term control of resistant staph infections; however, resistance turned up one year later in a British hospital. It subsequently began showing up everywhere, and the acronym MRSA was applied to methicillin-resistant *Staphylococcus aureus*. Research into the various sources of MRSA focused primarily on the quantity of antibiotics used in various applications on the premise that the amount used, not the type of use, was the key to the development of resistance. We only recently learned that the conditions of use (such as prolonged use in immunocompromised patients) are extremely important.

Unfortunately, at present the only measure available seems to be total pounds used per year, an admittedly crude measure because antibiotic potency, not weight, is the best measure, and antibiotics vary greatly in their potency. But weight seems to be our most practical measure. Community-associated MRSA (resistant strains found outside the hospital) were first discovered only a few years ago because apparently few researchers were looking for them outside the hospital before the year 2000. Consequently, recent attention has focused on the various non-human and non hospital uses of antibiotics, particularly those antibiotics commonly relied upon in therapeutic applications in human hospitals and clinics. This brought attention to use in veterinary medicine and agriculture, particularly to use in food-producing animals such as poultry, swine, cattle, and fish. Although methicillin itself has never been approved for use in animals in the United States, early estimates suggested as much or more of the other important antibiotics was being used in animals as in humans. The U.S. Food and Drug Administration reported 48.76 percent of all antibiotics produced in the U.S in 1975 was used for "nonmedicinal" applications. The basis for that estimate is unclear (FDA 1977). The reason for the high level of animal use, many assumed, was simply overuse in "factory farming" to control diseases that became rampant due to overcrowding. They were correct insofar as farmers, like physicians, operated to maximize the efficiency of their operations by using antibiotics to compensate for or mitigate problems that could sometimes have been prevented by better management and better sanitation.

Then, as if to add insult to injury, the use of tetracycline and strepto-mycin in powerful aerial sprays on fruit trees was brought to everyone's attention. Some other antibacterials were being used on various fruits and vegetables. About the same time reports in the scientific literature indicated the use of sanitizers and disinfectants in commercial establish-ments, homes, clinics, hospitals, farms, and the like could be selecting not only for resistance to the products being used but that those resistance mechanisms, such as efflux pumps, were often effective against several antibacterials. They may also select, we discovered, for bacteria having those "infective" small bits of DNA (plasmids) that spread like a disease and can carry recipes for resistance to disinfectants as well as many or all therapeutically valuable antibiotics (Suller and Russell 2002). Even resis-tance to pine oil can involve resistance to vancomycin (Price 2002). But the link between disinfectants and sanitizers and resistance to hospital use of therapeutically valuable antibiotics was also confusing (Suller and Russell 2000; Rutala 2006). Much more research was needed.

SHIFTING THE FOCUS

All this meant our focus had to broaden to include the use of *all antibac-terials* including sulfonamids, nitrofurans, coccidiostats, organic arseni-cals, antiseptics, sanitizers, disinfectants, and food additives, as well as the key antibiotics. Worry turned to fear and fear to anger in the minds of numerous physicians, bacteriologists, and other scientists. Stuart B. Levy, a physician at Tufts University who turned bacteriologist and then turned activist, published the first (1992) and second (2002) editions of *The Antibiotic Paradox* to call for immediate action. Journalists picked up on it, hospitals struggled with resistant bacteria, and a broad political movement to increase controls over any and all antibacterial product uses began developing.

Additionally, the CDC in Atlanta reported in 2005 that 1.6 million people resided in nursing homes, 250,000 of these had bacterial in-fections, and 27,000 of those had antibiotic-resistant infections (CDC

2005). Likewise, in the year 2000 CDC reported about one in every five hospitalized patients nationwide contracted an infection *while in the hospital* and 88,000 died each year as a result of infection during their visit there (CDC 2000). By 2005 the number increased to 94,000 deaths as a result of hospital-acquired infections (CDC 2007). Federal and state governments, the medical community, and the general public are now increasingly concerned about such numbers. Still, we seem not to be nearly as vocal in our concerns about hospital-caused deaths as we seem to be about the number of American troops dying each year in the Middle East—an average of less than 1000 per year. Some medical professionals have finally broken their silence and are demanding better hygiene practices by medical professionals (Collignon, Grayson, and Johnson 2007). When only half of all clinical staff and students observe the infection control procedures of their own institution, it is time for urgent corrective action. The prevailing attitude among physicians that antibiotic resistance is everyone else's problem is beginning to change, albeit slowly. At a few hospitals pharmacists and infectious-disease doctors (or even automated computerized systems) review antibiotic prescriptions and contact the doctors or even change the prescription when a poor choice of antibiotic is observed. In some hospitals doctors must answer several questions before any antibiotic prescription can be filled. These programs are clearly effective in reducing in-hospital antibiotic resistance, but the programs are not without problems because overriding the doctors' decisions and/or forcing them to answer to pharmacists does not sit well with most doctors. That is not the traditional pecking order (Landro 2008).

HUMAN USE

For a variety of reasons, hard data on the pounds of antibiotics used annually in human medicine is not publicly available, the main reason being that sales volumes are proprietary information to pharmaceutical companies. Revealing a company's sales volume would be valuable to competitors searching for the biggest markets to enter. Therefore, we have only estimates. The FDA has records of the total amount sold because it receives annual reports from every drug company of the amount of every drug sold. According to the Institute of Medicine antibiotic production was estimated to be 24.6 million pounds in 1980, 31.9 million pounds in 1983 and 44.4 million pounds in 1986. The Institute further estimated about 20 million pounds of the total, was used in animals and the remainder, about 24.7 million pounds, was used in humans; however, the Institute acknowledged there were problems with these estimates (IOM 1989, 61-77). Thus an estimate of 35 million pounds used in humans in 2007 seems reasonable, allowing for the continuing growth in antibiotic use during the 20 years from 1986 to 2006. Indeed, this estimate may be low because heavy use of various antibiotics in each patient with an infection due to resistant bacteria is difficult to estimate and the number of such patients has increased significantly. The heaviest uses appear to be in hospitals, nursing homes and hospices, and by outpatients at the local level. Over-the-counter sales of antibiotics to consumers, especially of therapeutically important antibiotics, in the U.S. seem negligible, consisting mostly of topical ointments containing neomycin, bacitracin and polymyxin.

As previously discussed, for several years MRSA was considered to be a sort of death angel wandering around hospitals from room to room and from patient to patient. That superbug problems are mostly produced and spread by hospitals (Hecker, et al. 2003; Steinman, et al. 2003) and other human health care facilities is not really controversial (Klevens, et al. 2007). The discharge from hospitals of patients with superbug infections obviously can contribute to spread of the bacteria to any persons who have contact the discharged patient; however, hospitals presently cannot long keep superbug patients because of the loss of payments by insurance and Medicare programs.

The contribution to the environmental resistome through disposal of solid medical waste and sewage is less well recognized. Disposal of most solid medical waste probably contributes little to the resistome because it is burned or buried; however, discharge of hospital waste through sewage treatment plants has apparently been a concern for a long time. A paper published in 1973 was an early warning about discharge from hospitals but little seems to have been done (Grabow and Prozesky 1973). Our municipal sewage treatment facilities are not specifically designed to destroy antibiotics, antibiotic-resistant bacteria, or antibiotic resistance DNA sequences, so it is not surprising that antibiotic residues and resistant bacteria are routinely found at fairly high levels in streams, lakes, and rivers where treated sewage is discharged. From there they obviously go into the general environment and occasionally pay a return visit to the hospital.

OTHER SOURCES OF RESISTANCE

Drug manufacturing firms, basic research facilities, regulatory agencies, and academic laboratories engaged in studying or teaching bacteriology obviously contribute to antibiotic resistance to some unknown degree. For example, not long ago the inherent difficulties in producing antibiotics by fermentation were such that the FDA required samples from every production batch be submitted for agency testing and certification prior to release of the batch for sale. Certification ended several years ago, but stories about what happened to the leftover samples retained by the FDA can still be heard now and then. On one occasion when complaints were circulating about FDA employees taking leftover samples home for use by family and friends, FDA administrators ordered all excess samples discarded, not taken home in briefcases. Naturally, until a directive came down to the contrary, a lot was simply flushed down the toilet, in fact enough to wipe out the desirable microflora of the local municipal sewage treatment plant. According to a veterinarian who was working at that time in the FDA's Center for Veterinary Medicine, investigations traced the antibiotics that killed the bacteria critical for sewage treatment back to the FDA itself (Loomis 2008). We assume this to be a problem only because we have so much more to learn about the sources of superbugs and their movement in the environment.

SUPERBUGS

Hospitals, clinics, hospices, and pharmacies have long flushed unusable antibiotics down the toilet but only recently has the issue been documented and its possible impact on the environment discussed (Halford 2008). Even soil-dwelling bacteria produce both antibiotics and express antibiotic resistance. Some bacteria are able not only to resist antibiotics but are also able to utilize antibiotics as a food source, even as their sole source of food (Dantas, et al. 2008). Soil is a vast and mostly unappreciated reservoir of countless bacteria and resistance genes and constitutes a readily available source of resistance plasmids and other mobile DNA sequences. A recent study of soil-derived bacteria revealed 480 bacteria carried almost 200 different antibacterial resistance profiles, including two strains with resistance to 15 of 21 drugs tested (D'Costa, McGrann, et al. 2006). Fertile soils contain large amounts of organic matter where fungi, protozoa, and bacteria thrive and compete with their own genetic weapons of war. A recent report of resistant bacteria being "disseminated" into the Arctic seems to be of concern; on examination, however, the absence of baseline data regarding the number and types of resistant genes existing there prior to the antibiotic era means the conclusion the authors and the journal's editors suggested (that the resistant bacteria found in the Arctic are a consequence of widespread drug use) is politically influenced. That conclusion may or may not be true, but the very title of the paper is cause for concern that political correctness seems to creep into even the best scientific reports on antibiotic resistance (Sjolund, et al. 2008).

AGRICULTURAL USES

There is great controversy about the size of the contribution from agricultural use of antibiotics. That controversy has been around for years, but in late 2007 several reports of MRSA superbugs found in domestic dogs, horses, poultry, and swine (and on the people around them) were published (Hanselman, et al. 2007; Khanna, et al. 2007). In 2008 MRSA was reportedly found on pork products in general distribution to consumers (Salvage, 2008). Thus the controversy has shifted because

MRSA was presumed to be moving from the hospital, clinic, and hospice to the community, and presumably to farmers. Dr. George Saperstein, Chairman of the Department of Environmental and Population Health at Tufts University Cummings School of Veterinary Medicine, recently observed: "Everybody assumes it goes just one way, but it really goes both ways. The question of the day is which way did it go? Did the pigs give it to the people? Did the people give it to the pigs?" (Smith, 2007). Either way, such movement is alarming, but as in the case of human uses, we have only estimates of the amount of antibiotics used in dogs and swine and in animals generally—for the same reason: sales information is proprietary.

How antibiotics are used in human medicine is fairly well known; however, few persons outside the general field of agriculture know how antibiotics are used on the farm. For example, the discovery of a few sick chickens in a flock of 10,000 results in immediate sacrifice and posting (autopsy) of most or all sick birds to remove them from the premises and to diagnose the disease so as to determine whether flock treatment of some sort may be needed. In other species individual sick animals are usually diagnosed and treated by the person(s) managing the operation. Dairymen, beef cattle producers, swine producers, poultry producers, and fish producers are far better educated and trained on the diagnosis and treatment of disease than one might expect. Failure to keep current on the use of antibiotics on the farm is usually disastrous, and such farm operators are soon out of the business. The FDA has been aware of this condition for a very long time and has approved many antibacterials for over-the-counter sales to treat farm animals.

The sometimes heard suggestion that veterinary prescriptions should be required for all antibiotic uses in agriculture never goes very far because there are not nearly enough veterinary practitioners and because farmers are skilled at what they do. Calling the veterinarian to visit and write a prescription is usually not practical or financially feasible, and also diagnosis and treatment of various farm animal diseases is so specialized that the farmer is likely to know better what to do with his animals than the community veterinarian who treats practically all species for all diseases. Of course some veterinarians do specialize in managing the health of specific types of farm animals, and when they do their knowledge of the best treatment in any given instance is likely to be superior to that of the farmer. However, these veterinarians usually become consulting veterinarians whose talents are spread over large geographic areas to educate and train farmers and other veterinarians. Not nearly enough veterinarians so specialized are available to prescribe needed antibiotics. In fact, many rural counties reportedly have not even a single veterinarian.

Diagnosis of the presence of certain diseases in one or more animals in a group of animals often triggers the need for antibiotic treatment to *control the spread* of the disease through the group. The dose needed is usually lower than a full therapeutic dose. In still other cases where there are no sick animals in a group but where there is epidemiological or historical information to indicate the animals are highly likely to develop a known disease, a still lower dose of an antibiotic or combinations of antibiotics may be used for disease *prevention*. Other uses include minimizing the effect of a pathogen on a certain organ or tissue such as abscessation of the mandibular, cervical, and cephalic lymph nodes or various liver infections. The most controversial is the use of very low doses in feeds (a few grams per ton) to increase the rate of weight gain and to reduce the amount of feed needed to produce each pound of weight gain. Given this variety of uses and given that the total amount of antibiotics used in animals each year is about the same as the amount used in humans each year while the total combined weight of all farm animals is ten times greater than the total weight of all humans, one must recognize that on a *per pound of body weight* basis we use about ten times more antibiotics per year in humans than is used in animals (COAH 2001). The Coalition on Animal Health, made up of the Animal Feed Industry Association, Animal Health Institute, National Cattlemen's Beef Association, National Chicken Council, and the National Pork Producers Council, pointed this out in a response to the launch of the "Keep Antibiotics Working" campaign in 2001. There are many reasons why humans use so much more antibiotics than animals, and critics should recognize that the allegation of unsanitary, crowded conditions on the farm as the root cause of "excessive" use of antibiotics by farmers is at best highly questionable.

Available estimates and surveys regarding the amount of antibiotics used annually in animals vary greatly and all have been severely criticized as inaccurate. One estimate sponsored by the Union of Concerned Scientists stated most of the use of antibiotics in the United States was in healthy animals. Specific amounts were estimated but the manner in which the estimates were developed has been disqualified. Subsequently, the Alliance for the Prudent Use of Antibiotics sponsored an advisory committee to evaluate priorities, sources, and methods for collecting animal antimicrobial use data for the United States; however, their report revealed that gathering reliable information will at best be extremely difficult and expensive (De Vincent and Viola 2006). The total for all animal-use antibiotics (including anticoccidials and organic arsenicals but excluding disinfectants and sanitizers) is probably about 30 million pounds per year in the United States (AHI 2007).

The amount used has been declining somewhat, allegedly due to improved nutrition, better breeding, more sophisticated farm management, and reduced use of antibiotics as feed additives for increased rate of weight gain and improved efficiency of feed utilization in broiler chickens, growing swine, and growing beef cattle. Unfortunately, discontinuing such use apparently triggers the need for more therapeutic use because more animals get sick. Also, activists threatened to picket fast-food chains about antibiotic use by their suppliers and thereby persuaded many of them to begin purchasing their meat, milk, and eggs from farms where antibiotic use was verifiably minimized. The first and most prominent of these was the "Global Policy on Antibiotic Use in Food Animals," a policy developed by McDonalds through consultation with a variety of experts, including physicians, suppliers, animal welfare scientists, veterinarians, retail representatives, and environmental experts (McDonalds 2003).

Adopted in June 2003, the global policy required human-use antibiotics not be used to promote growth, must always be used under the oversight of a veterinarian, and overall use must be minimized in several specific ways. Finally, farmers must maintain accurate records of all antibiotic administrations, certify their compliance with the policy in writing, and McDonalds must audit their suppliers to verify compliance. The policy is a great example of the importance of open discussion and sober consideration of the concerns expressed by all sides regarding the use of antibiotics. McDonalds celebrated their new policy as an important way to address public concern about the use of antibiotics in animals, and the organizations threatening the picketing celebrated what they felt was a major victory. Ironically, McDonalds suppliers of beef and poultry products were mostly in compliance with the policy even before McDonalds called the first meeting of experts to create the policy. The company's management may have known that to be the case; however; the activists probably did not or else they would not have been so concerned about antibiotic use and certainly would not have gone to such great lengths to demand other fast-food establishments and animal producers adopt the McDonalds policy or its equivalent.

Surprisingly, when all the cards were on the table, the various parties each found they could agree to the demands of the others. Even though little actually had to change, all parties celebrated a victory, even Stuart B. Levy, the most vocal advocate of reduced antibiotic use in animals! And the biggest burden on farmers and fast-food chains was documentation, certification, and auditing, not the risk of disastrous disease outbreaks. One lesson to be taken from this seems to be that fears about how antibiotics *might be used* in animals can become just as important as if those worst fears were true. Another lesson is that the McDonalds policy received considerable publicity and thereby helped activists persuade consumers that treating chickens with antibiotics was unsafe. One consequence of all this has been that Purdue Farms, Tyson Foods, and Sanderson Farms recently got into a lawsuit over who could truthfully label their chicken as "raised without antibiotics." A triumph for the activists!

As in the case of human medical waste, the treatment and disposition of animal waste (which, to at least some extent, can be considered medical waste) is a problem of larger and uncertain dimensions, albeit consisting of a different set of issues. Because the combined total body weight of all farm animals (poultry, swine, cattle, fish, etc.) is about 10 times that of all humans, the problems of waste disposal are also about 10 times as great. Anyone going to a store where fertilizer is sold knows composted animal manure is popular for flower and vegetable gardens. In fact most animal manure is composted and then applied to pasture or cropland as fertilizer. Studies have been conducted to determine how long such composting should continue in order to degrade antibiotics present in the fresh manure; however, very few studies seem to have been conducted to determine how many antibiotic-resistant bacteria and antibiotic resistance genes are present during or after the composting process.

In some cases, animal waste is collected and transferred to a lagoon where fermentation similar to municipal sewage treatment is employed prior to spreading the waste over pasture and/or cropland. Both composting and lagoons use microorganisms to digest and otherwise degrade the manure and any antibiotics present but this simultaneously sets up conditions of fierce microbial warfare in which microorganisms employ antibiotics as weapons against each other. These processes almost certainly create conditions similar to the decomposition of home-style compost piles or litter on forest floors. Forest floors have been one of the most productive sources of new antibiotics as well as for multiply resistant bacteria.

SANITIZERS AND DISINFECTANTS

Increasing public awareness of bacteria in homes, public places, on food, and in air and water has created a general climate of anxiety and a trend toward liberal use of sanitizers and disinfectants, including countertop sprays, toilet sprays, air treatments, antibacterial bath soaps, and an enormous array of related products. Many public schools, for example, have installed hand sanitizer dispensers in every classroom and restroom. In 2001 the U.S. Environmental Protection Agency (EPA) reported U.S. use of disinfectants, sanitizers, and other specialty biocides totaled 109 million pounds, plus some 244 million pounds of recreational and industrial water treatments *not* including chlorine and hypochlorites which are generally used in municipal and industrial water treatment systems (EPA 2001). The current use of these antibacterials is probably greater due to the trend toward increased use since 2001.

Dismissing the use of disinfectants and sanitizers as unimportant is no longer possible due to our improving knowledge of the direct connections between their use and antibiotic resistance. Even the use of chlorine and hypochlorites can no longer be considered irrelevant because we now know their use, as well as other stress factors such as ionizing radiation, causes genomic instability which in humans can lead to cancer and in bacteria to antibiotic resistance. Thus reasonable estimates of the use of these non-antibiotic antibacterials in the United States, 109 million pounds plus 244 million pounds (not including chlorine and hypochlorites), is more than five times greater than the reasonable estimates of the total use of antibiotic drugs in animals and humans combined (30 million pounds plus 35 million pounds). That is surely a cause for concern, but no one seems to have shown an interest in investigating this area.

HURDLE TECHNOLOGIES

In food production, processing, and distribution facilities, a series of antibacterial hurdles are placed between food production and food consumption. The intent is to reduce bacterial populations, especially human pathogen populations, to the lowest level feasible so as to deliver safe food to the consumer. Hurdle technology is the application of multiple physical, chemical, and biological factors at individually sublethal levels. This approach is intended to achieve pathogen inactivation through metabolic exhaustion or growth inhibition for a certain period of time, that is, until the product is consumed. For example, in food animal slaughter cetylpyridinium chloride, lactic acid, sodium hydroxide, ethanol, trisodium phosphate, acidified chlorine, and phosphoric acid may be added to cleaning or wash solutions to reduce contamination on hides. Steam, hot and chilled water, lactic and acetic acids, chlorine based compounds, trisodium phosphate, sodium chloride, hydrogen peroxide, ozonated water, peroxyacetic acid, benzoates, proprionates, sodium metasilicate, and sodium bisulfate may be used for carcass washing. Food preservatives are used to prevent spoilage and control pathogens. Common applications include antibacterials such as sodium nitrite, organic acids, risin, lysozyme, lactates, diacetate, natamycin, lactoferrin, acetoin, reuterin, and bacteriocins. The Institute of Food Technologists released a comprehensive expert report on antimicrobial resistance related to food technology in July 2006 but did not include estimates of quantities of antibacterials used per year (IFT 2006). We can speculate about the overall contribution to selection for superbugs, but estimating that contribution on the basis of pounds used per year is not currently feasible.

CONCLUSIONS

Widespread antibiotic resistance problems are mostly the result of human activity, the product of our intensive, worldwide use of antibiotics in treating humans. Because antibiotic and other antibacterial use is worldwide, resistant bacteria also arrive here from other countries, many of which have little or no control over the use of antibacterials. The continuous international movement of people, animals, and food brings super bacteria from afar, and we have a program to control, at least to some extent, the movement of people with multiply resistant tuberculosis. But we have practically none for people carrying that death angel of hospital wards, MRSA. As most travelers know, there is also very little control over the movement of people with gastrointestinal diseases caused by resistant bacteria.

Superbugs are being found so often that a few hospitals are swabbing and culturing microbes from the skin, fingernails, and nostrils of incoming patients to identify *Staphylococcus aureus* carriers so as to provide special care. Today's more sophisticated searches for resistant bacteria are finding a few superbugs almost everywhere. Apparently the evil genie is out and wandering about in the community at large. But for all we know it has been there all along.

While the use of antibiotics in humans is the main source of resistance problems, agricultural uses almost certainly contribute in the form of resistant, food-born pathogens and contribute to the overall antibiotic resistome. Because agricultural use is mostly far from urban areas, resistant bacteria must either gain access to significant human populations via the food chain, by transport on/in the bodies of farm workers, or by traveling great distances through the general environment where selection to return to background levels of resistance is slow but inexorable. Consequently, the use of antibiotics in agriculture should contribute little to hospital resistance problems when compared to use of the same amount directly in humans. Although that is true, modern "super" farming uses antibiotics, and using antibiotics selects for antibiotic resistance. Sooner or later it causes super infections because some contributions through the food chain, through personal travel, and through the global resistome are unavoidable with today's technology. We need to know how important the contribution really is. The question is not does it happen. The questions is how serious is the contribution of farming to hospital problems, and what would happen if antibiotic use in food animals was discontinued.

Use of large amounts of sanitizers and disinfectants in homes, hospitals, restaurants, industry, and just about everywhere else is a contributor to the resistome. Although these antibacterials seem to be of less concern in causing selection for antibiotic resistance, those instances when they do can move resistant bacteria directly into the human population because they are used around humans. The amount of sanitizers and disinfectants used is apparently much greater than the amount of antibiotics used in animals or humans, but how much they contribute overall to resistance problems is obviously unknown.

Antibacterials applied in sublethal amounts as hurdles for control of bacteria in the production, processing, and distribution of food may also contribute because they can, to at least some extent, select for resistance. The use of sublethal amounts seems on its face to set conditions where selective pressures are maximized. The use of antibiotics in humans at less than the full therapeutic dose for the full term of treatment is usually considered irresponsible except in a few cases, such as acne, where treatment may continue for months or years. Yet food production and processing are very different from treating hospitalized patients, and we just do not have enough data on the contribution to resistance problems to make informed decisions.

Most of the complex DNA recipes for resisting antibiotics probably originated in the natural world eons before humans discovered penicillin. A superbug can be defined as a bacterium with several DNA recipes for antibiotic resistance. Most chance mutations occurring today probably are little more than slight modifications that uncover or activate a muted sequence on a chromosome or that provoke an increase in the activity of a sequence, both actions simply coding for the biochemistry needed turn on a complex gene(s) to prevent the bacterium from being adversely affected by an antibiotic. Simply stated, use of antibacterials adversely affects bacteria that bear no resistant genes and thereby allows for overgrowth of bacteria that do bear resistance genes, including bacteria with the ability to transfer those genes to other bacteria.

The use of antibacterials anywhere on the planet can increase the incidence of antibiotic resistance encountered anywhere on the planet. Resistance may reside in the worldwide pool of microbial genes, delivered there by every conceivable mechanism, such as the migration of birds and other animals or the movement of people, wind, and water. Antimicrobial resistance was widespread before civilization existed, and distinguishing between resistance genes present because of human activity and those present because of purely non-human forces of nature is not possible. As the number of resistant bacteria worldwide increases, the global bacterial gene pool probably includes more and more genes ready for use by bacterial strains on their way to becoming superbugs. We know many probable sources of these resistant genes, but we do not know how much each source contributes or how fast the genes are removed from the environmental resistome by selective pressure to return to the natural background level. Maybe we just need to find out how those ants managed to successfully use antibacterials for the last 50 million years.

Dealing with antibacterial resistance in humans and animals requires a comprehensive documentation of the role played by commensal bacteria (harmless bacteria normally present in animals and humans) present in both. We must also recognize that use of a specific antibacterial can result in the overgrowth of bacteria with genes for resistance to that antibacterial as well as to many others. Commensal bacteria and pathogenic bacteria are present in animals and humans, although all animal pathogens do not affect humans, and all human pathogens do not affect animals. One key to dealing with resistance is to recognize commensals carry resistance genes just as do pathogens, and those commensals often have the same ability as pathogens to transfer genes to pathogens as well as to other commensals. Their genetics are intertwined.

The apparent presence of many superbugs in recent years but not in the early years of antibiotic use may also be due to the way we have dealt with patients and the pathogens affecting them. In the 1950s, patients who were treated with what seemed to be an appropriate antibiotic and failed to respond often died, but in such cases we lacked the technology to determine whether the bacteria were superbugs because methicillin was still years away. Those cases were just treatment failures. Today we have, and use, technologies that allow determination of the presence of antibiotic resistance and the DNA sequence(s) responsible.

Our knowledge of the nature and origins of superbugs is truly impressive although incomplete. We do know antibacterials have been in use for millions of years and that resistance genes are routinely culled from the resistome by competition and natural selection if the genes are present in an environment where they are of no value, that is, an environment where there is competition and no antibacterials in use. Such microenvironments are to be found almost everywhere; however, our knowledge of the rapidity of gene removal in non-antibacterial environments is limited. We only know they persist long enough to be of concern.

Minimizing pathogen populations in companion and food animals is generally agreed to be important to human health, and we know with great confidence the use of antibacterials in animals is critical to keeping pathogen populations low. Sadly, antibacterial use in treating both animals and humans is deeply intertwined with housing, population density, sanitation, and hygiene. Antibiotics have been used by all parties to compensate for shortcomings in these areas. Unfortunately, we do not know how much our various uses of antibacterials, both true antibiotics and non-antibiotics, in animals contributes to human health problems, and even if we knew, we would face many decisions involving difficult social, economic, and ethical issues. Allowing animals to suffer and die in vast numbers to avoid possible problems at the hospital is probably unethical; however, some activist groups have concluded that discontinuing the use of antibacterials for disease prevention, disease control, increased rate of weight gain, and improved efficiency of feed utilization in food animals are uses that should be banned immediately. These so-called "subtherapeutic" uses have become a major point of contention. Many scientists warn that banning such uses will adversely affect human health by increasing the frequency of animal and human disease while others warn that failure to ban them will lead to the end of the antibiotic era. Thus we know where superbugs come from but don't quite know what to do about it. This is where politics takes over.

REFERENCES

AHI (Animal Health Institute). 2007. News release: Trends in sales of lifesaving animal medicines continue. October 3, 2007. http://ahi.timberlakepublishing.com/files/Media%20Center/Antibiotic%20use%202006.pdf (accessed October 18, 2007). The AHI reported 26.4 million pounds of antibiotics were sold by member firms of the Institute in 2006 for use in companion and farm animals. The total presented here was adjusted to 30 million pounds to allow for the estimated amount of antibiotics sold for animal use by several small firms that were not members of the Institute.

Cano, Raul J. and Monica K. Borucki. 1997. *Ancient microorganisms*. U.S. Patent 5593883. January 14. http://www.freepatentsonline.com/5593883.html (accessed August 15, 2007).

CDC. 2000. *Hospital infections cost U.S. billions of dollars annually*. March 6. http://www.cdc.gov/od/oc/media/pressrel/r2k0306b.htm (accessed October 18, 2007).

———. 2005. *Center for Disease Control campaign to prevent antimicrobial resistance in healthcare settings*. http://www.cdc.gov/drugresistance/healthcare/ltc.htm (accessed June 29, 2005).

———. 2007. *CDC estimates 94,000 invasive drug resistant staph infections occurred in the U.S. in 2005*. http://www.cdc.gov/od/oc/media/pressrel/2007/r071016.htm (accessed October 18, 2007).

COAH (The Coalition on Animal Health). 2001. Antibiotics and safeguarding the Food Supply Statement by Coalition on Animal Health Regarding 'Keep antibiotics working'. *Press Conference U.S. Newswire.* October 30 (http://www.pmac.net/AM/safeguarding.html).

Collignon, Peter J., M. Lindsay Grayson, and Paul D.R. Johnson. 2007. Methicillin-resistant *Staphylococcus aureus* in hospitals: Time for a culture change. *The Medical Journal of Australia* 187(1):4–5.

Currie, Cameron R., Bess Wong, Alison E. Stuart, Ted R. Schultz, Stephen A. Rehner, Ulrich G. Mueller, Gi-Ho Sung, Joseph W. Spatafora, Neil A. Straus. 2003. Ancient tripartite coevolution in the attine ant-microbe symbiosis. *Science* 299:386–88.

D'Costa, Vanessa M., Katherine M. McGrann, Donald W. Hughes, and Gerard D. Wright. 2006. Sampling the antibiotic resistome. *Science* 311:374–77.

Dantas, Gautam, Morten O. A. Sommer, Rantimi D. Oluwasegun and George M. Church. 2008. Bacteria subsisting on antibiotics. *Science* 320:100–3.

De Vincent, Stephen J. and Christina Viola. 2006. Deliberations of an advisory committee regarding priorities, sources, and methods for collecting animal antimicrobial use data in the United States. *Preventive Veterinary Medicine* 73:133–151.

EPA. 2001. 2000–2001 Pesticide market estimates. http://www.epa.gov/oppbead1/pestsales/01pestsales/usage2001_4.htm (accessed August 31, 2007).

FDA. 1977. Diamond Shamrock Chemical Co., et al. Penicillin-containing premixes: Opportunity for a hearing. *Federal Register* 42:43775.

Grabow, W.O.K. and O.W. Prozesky. 1973. Drug resistance of coliform bacteria in hospital and city sewage. *Antimicrobial Agents and Chemotherapy* 3:175–80.

Halford, Bethany. 2008. What to do with your unused pharmaceuticals. *Chemical & Engineering News* 86: 13–17.

Hanselman, Beth A., Kruth Stephen, and Weese J. Scott. 2007. Methicillin-resistant staphylococcal colonization in dogs entering a veterinary teaching hospital. *Veterinary Microbiology* 126: 277–81.

Hecker, Michelle T., David C. Aron, Nilam P. Patel, Meghan K. Lehmann, and Curtis J. Donskey. 2003. Unnecessary use of antimicrobials in hospitalized patients: Current patterns of misuse with an emphasis on the antianaerobic spectrum of activity. *Archives of Internal Medicine* 163:972–78.

IFT (Institute of Food Technology). 2006. Antimicrobial resistance: Implications for the food system. http://www.blackwell-synergy.com/doi/full/10.1111/j.1541-4337.2006.00004.x (accessed December 1, 2007).

IOM (U.S. Institute of Medicine). 1989. Human health risks with the subtherapeutic use of penicillin or tetracyclines in animal feed. Washington D.C., *National Academy Press*.

Khanna, T., R. Friendship, C. Dewey, and J.S. Weese. 2007. Methicillin-resistant *Staphylococcus aureus* colonization in pigs and pig farmers. *Veterinary Microbiology* 128:298–303.

Klevens, R. Monina, Melissa A. Morrison, Joelle Nadle, Susan Petit, Ken Gershman, Susan Ray, Lee H. Harrison, Ruth Lynfield, Ghinwa Durnyati, Townes, Allen S. Craig, Elizaberth R. Zell, Gegory E. Fosheim, Lindia K. McDougal, Roberta B. Carey, and Scott K. Fridkin, 2007. Invasive methicillin-resistant *staphylococcus aureus* infections in the United States. *Journal of the American Medical Association* 298:1763–71. http://jama.ama-assm.org/cgi/reprint/298/15/1763.pdf (accessed December 17, 2007).

Landro, Laura 2008. Curbing antibiotic use in war on 'Superbugs'. *The Wallstreet Journal On Line*. September 3, page D1. http://online.wsj.com/article/SB122039916170892933.html

Loomis, Vader M. 2008. Personal communication.

McDonalds 2003. Global policy on antibiotic use in food animals. http://www.mcdonalds.com/corp/values/purchasing/antibiotics/global_policy.html (accessed October 8, 2007).

Price, Christopher T.D., Vignette K. Singh, Radheshyam K. Jayaswal, Brian J. Wilkinson, and John E. Gustafson. 2002. Pine oil cleaner-resistant *Staphylococcus aureus*: Reduced susceptibility to vancomycin and oxacillin and involvement of SigB. *Applied and Environmental Microbiology* 68:5417–21.

Rutala, William A. 2006. Disinfectants resistance: Is there a relationship between use and resistance. http://www.unc.edu/depts/spice/dis/DisinfectantsResistance.pdf (accessed October 7, 2007).

Salvage, Bryan. 2008. Pork products found containing "super bug." *Meat and Poultry*, March 20. http://www.meatpoultry.com/news/headline_stories_print.asp?ArticleID=92223 (accessed March 21, 2008).

Sjolund, Maria, Bonnedahl J, Hernandez J, Bengtsson S, Cederbrant G, Pinhassi J., et al. 2008. Dissemination of multidrug-resistant bacteria into the Arctic. *Emerging Infectious Diseases* 14(1):70–72. http://www.cdc.gov/EID/content/14/1/70.htm (accessed April 13, 2008).

Smith, Stephen. 2007. A tale of pigs, people, and a shared germ. *The Boston Globe: Home/News/Science.*November 12.http://www.boston.com/news/science/articles/2007/11/12/a_tale_of_pigs_and_a_shared_germ/

Steinman, Michael A., et al. 2003. Changing use of antibiotics in community-based outpatient practice 1991–1999. *Annals of Internal Medicine* 138:525–33.

Suller, M.T.E. and A.D. Russell. 2000. Triclosan and antibiotic resistance in *staphylococcus aureus*. *Journal of Antimicrobial Chemotherapy* 46:11–18.

CHAPTER IV

TRADING ANTIBIOTICS FOR MONEY

A Faustian Bargain?

In the book *Faust: A Tragedy*, Johann Wolfgang von Goethe presented Faust as a man thoroughly versed in all the subjects in which a Renaissance scholar could receive a degree and a man torn between knowledge and experience. Mephistopholes is a subordinate of the devil who tempts Faust into trading his soul for wealth and power. In this there are parallels for any discussion of the use of antibiotics. Are we trading something of enormous value for something of passing importance? The Union of Concerned Scientists, the Environmental Defense, the Sierra Club, and the Alliance for the Prudent Use of Antibiotics all apparently think the use of antibiotics to control or prevent diseases or improve productivity in food crops and food animals is just such a bargain, and although they know the available data do not really support them, they state their case in passionate terms, often because of their hidden agendas. A strong aversion to modern agriculture, ethical concerns about humane treatment of animals, and serious doubts about capitalism are examples of common hidden agendas. Nevertheless, we should be appreciative for the shrill concerns expressed about resistant, potentially lethal bacteria in patients being treated with antibiotics. Suffering and death in men, women, children, and babies due at least in part to the failure of

51

antibiotics to have their intended effect is shocking, heartbreaking, and tragic. The CDC and the Institute of Medicine have estimated the cost to be four to five billion dollars per year in human medicine. The cost in animal medicine and plant medicine seems not to have been estimated by reliable authorities but is probably considerably less than the cost in human medicine. And how much value do we receive for the effectiveness of antibiotics? Obviously, this is not something we can really estimate without an enormous and concerted effort by representatives of several disciplines. But the number is surely a big one, especially if the value in human medicine is added to the value in industry as well as animal and plant medicine.

The most vivid and passionate book on antibiotic resistance is the 2002 *The Killers Within* by Michael Shnayerson, contributing editor to *Vanity Fair, Condi Nast Traveler*, and *National Geographic*, and Mark J. Plotkin, research associate at the Smithsonian Institution and president of the Amazon Conservation Team. The authors take the reader on a depressing, patient-by-patient, exhausting search for something or somebody to blame. The book is a terrifying story of disease, suffering, and death. In the end they place that blame on corporate greed, corporate lobbying, an abysmal lack of knowledge, use of antibiotics in agriculture and industry, overuse and misuse of antibiotics in humans, and finally, weakly and lastly, on unsanitary practices of physicians, nurses, hospitals, clinics, and nursing homes.

The other book that must be mentioned is *The Antibiotic Paradox* by Stuart B. Levy, a physician and Tufts University professor, published in 1992 with a second edition by the same title published in 2002. Although poorly written, the first edition shocked the medical community with its gloom and doom message, and the second edition has been described as a clarion call for immediate action to prevent the total demise of the antibiotic era. As a physician at Tufts University, one would not expect Levy to have an in-depth knowledge of the agricultural sciences; however, his general lack of understanding about what is going on and his use of pejorative language are revealing (animal feeds are not described as "treated" with antibiotics, and antibiotics are not "added" to animal feeds—Levy says feeds are "*laced*" with antibiotics) (Levy 2002 163). The sad part of it all is that even textbook writers pick up on such language and bias the next generation (Goldsmith 2007, 66–67).

In any case, physicians have such a heavy financial stake in the use of antibiotics that a conflict of interest is manifest to most observers. Antibiotics really are the "crown jewels" of human and veterinary medicine because they improved medical practice so drastically. Loosing them due to improper use would be outrageous and financially disastrous. Before the discovery of sulfonamides and true antibiotics, physicians and veterinarians were poorly paid bedside companions who could do little more than comfort and reassure. Some vaccines were available and pain killers, principally morphine, could be used to relieve pain and, when appropriate, permit patients to die with dignity—as in the case of Sigmund Freud. Antibiotics largely changed that. At first, physicians and veterinarians administered sulfonamides and antibiotics with abandon, including for diseases that were known not to be affected in the least by the drugs, but as time went by they became diagnosticians who simply examined the patient, diagnosed the problem, prescribed an appropriate antibiotic within minutes, and promptly moved on to the next patient. Their concerns and hospital administrators' concerns about personal hygiene and sanitation were vastly reduced because infections were not so fearful anymore. Suddenly the practice of medicine became not only a respected profession but also a very profitable one indeed. If a patient contracted another infection, just prescribe another antibiotic. Largely as a consequence of the antibiotic era, physicians and veterinarians went from lower-middle-class incomes to upper-middle-class and upper-class incomes. Antibiotics changed the practice of medicine from one of public service to a highly profitable profession. Much of that could be lost if all antibiotics become useless, a horrible embarrassment and an economic crisis for the profession. Surgery without antibiotics is inherently dangerous. The authors of the above-mentioned books are to be commended for their untiring dedication to exposing what they envisioned as the sources of antibiotic failures. Their contributions to the general alarm are valid even though most of their fearful conjectures are not justified. As almost everyone in the pharmaceutical industry knows, when the economics of developing new antibiotics becomes favorable, the industry will bring them to market. Although resistance is troublesome, antibiotics developed many years ago are still marketed and still valuable in human medicine if the patient's diagnosis includes a profile of the resistance genes the infective organism is carrying. Such diagnoses are now available and becoming practical. A lot of antibacterials are sitting undeveloped on the laboratory shelf, and a lot more are out there to be discovered. It really is that simple, but the authors of these and several similar books seem not to be aware of this simple fact. Plus, for too many academicians and too many bureaucrats it is fun to abuse pharmaceutical companies and farmers and absolutely anathema to provide economic incentives to "big pharma." Sadly, many patients pay with their lives because of it.

As is often the case when an author's primary goal is to persuade and frighten rather than to inform, both books go to extremes and both books go around and beyond the existing scientific data to permit unsupported conclusions or conclusions that are correct but misleading in the context presented. One example of correct but misleading conclusions is that the use of antibiotics in agriculture results in increases in the incidence of resistant bacteria (correct) and therefore should be sharply and immediately curtailed or entirely eliminated (misleading and probably would have catastrophic results). Their arguments are similar to "The Precautionary Principle," an idea which states that if a serious adverse effect is seen to possibly occur due to a particular technology then that technology should be abolished although scientific data to support such a decision is not available. This principle has been a political weapon for a long time and was actually used in Europe to terminate usage of certain antibiotics in animals. That decision has been much praised and much criticized because it is not science based.

But physicians, veterinarians, livestock and poultry producers, horticulturalists, environmentalists, housewives, and everyone who uses antibacterials have some economic motives underlying their actions. The question before us is whether a given economic use of an antibacterial is tragic like Faust or a prudent use of modern technology. Unfortunately, there are no animal uses of antibacterials that do not also entail medical (health) issues. Even the use of antibacterials in kitchens and bathrooms and the lowest doses of antibacterials (2 to 20 grams per ton of feed) for enhanced growth and feed efficiency in food animals are almost certainly promoting antibiotic resistance and suppressing disease organisms. It is true that directions for use of 2 to 20 grams of antibiotics per ton of animal feed to suppress disease-causing bacteria cannot be found on the labels of marketed products because firms who sponsor research to support such label claims don't elect to spend their resources on such claims. Proving to FDA's satisfaction that a very low dose of an antibacterial will suppress a disease that is subclinical or that occurs only intermittently and somewhat randomly is expensive and difficult. After all, livestock and poultry producers are interested in seeing their animals grow fast on less feed and will worry about disease control only if they find the use of the antibiotic leads to more disease. In short, producers will use the antibiotics to increase profitability whether or not the disease-reduction claim is on the label. The value of a chicken, for example, is small enough that just having an employee catch a chicken for treatment costs more than the profit to be made on that bird. If using an antibiotic holds down morbidity and mortality in the herd or flock, then that is just a nice economic add-on.

Before antibiotics were discovered, man-made substances useful in the control of bacteria were named "antibacterials," but when antibiotics were discovered their chemical structure was far more complex than previously known antibacterials and too complicated for anyone to synthesize them. The only source of those complex first antibiotic molecules was living things such as fungi and bacteria. That is why large fermentation tanks were and still are used for producing most antibiotics. Thus a new name seemed to be needed. The scientific community settled on "antibiotics" as a new class of antibacterials. Today the distinction between antibiotics and other antibacterials is mostly lost because chemists can now synthesize complex antibiotics and modify those produced by fermentation. It is just a matter of cost. When considering the rise of "antibiotic" resistance, the distinction is also misleading. Bacterial gene pools react to various threats in the same way as they react to antibiotics: in time, they become resistant. That resistance is sometimes found to be a broadly effective mechanism that bacteria can use to resist the effects of many environmental insults, including some of the antibiotics.

The first date when antibiotics were administered to animals for profit is probably lost to history. In the case of true antibiotics, we do know animals have long been treated with investigational drugs in order to evaluate safety. Probably healthy mice, rabbits, rats, and dogs were the first animals to receive sulfanilamide and penicillin in toxicity studies. By 1943 four pharmaceutical firms were producing penicillin, something inconceivable without toxicity reports regarding safety to humans handling the drug, even for that early period in pharmaceutical development. As penicillin became widely available for human use in 1943 and 1944, one can be confident veterinarians promptly began treating domestic animals with that yellow magic. No FDA approval was needed for duly licensed practitioners to acquire and use penicillin. But antibiotic resistance has been linked not just to antibiotics but also to antibacterial substances widely used in human and animal healthcare long before Fleming published his initial findings in 1929. Many such antibacterials have been in use for a very long time. For example, in 1924 Haver-Glover Laboratories, Kansas City, Missouri, published a catalogue (Haver and Glover 1924) loaded with antibacterials for sale to veterinarians. Included were iodine, camphor, hypochlorites, acriflavine, proflavine, eucalyptus oil, bichloride of mercury, boric acid, phenol, methyl salicylate, methylene blue, benzoic acid, mercuric iodide, potassium iodide, potassium orthoxyquinoline sulphonate, chloramine-T, and potassium chlorate, among others. At first glance none of these antibacterials may appear threatening as regards resistance to antibiotics, but that is not the case. It is true that sulfonamides are missing, as are all the true antibiotics. The same antibacterials, and more, were being offered in the 1936 edition of the same firm's catalogue (Haver 1936) and we have plenty of reasons to believe anything used to control bacteria will, in time, lead to resistance either on the chromosome or in the DNA of those highly mobile plasmids, or both. Keeping in mind the bacterial genome is dynamic, it should be clear both chromosomal antibiotic resistance and the presence of resistance plasmids with DNA coding for antibiotic resistance were being promoted by the use of various antibacterials. Acriflavine, introduced by Paul Ehrlich in 1912 as an antiseptic, for example, was widely used to help control infections, but acriflavine is more than just an antibacterial. It is a bacterial mutagen, meaning it causes a higher than normal rate of mutations in bacteria. That alone would be expected to accelerate the development of resistance. More recent studies have shown selecting the bacteria *Streptococcus cremoris* for resistance to acriflavine also results in cross-resistance to neomycin, streptomycin, ethidium bromide, mitomycin C, and proflavine (Smith 1977a). Thus the mechanism whereby this species of bacteria resisted acriflavine was also effective in protecting it against several antibiotics. Similarly, researchers at St. Jude reported in 1999 that *E. coli* bacteria were able to become resistant to triclosan, an antibacterial widely used in sanitizers, bath soaps, and body washes, by a chromosomal mutation in a gene named fabI (Rock and Heath 1999). St. Jude researchers sounded the alarm that widespread use of triclosan could lead to a serious public health concern. That led to several studies and to the conclusion that cross-resistance mechanisms in several bacterial species and strains are known to confer a wide range of antibiotic resistance onto bacteria that have developed resistance to triclosan, benzalkonium chloride, pine oil, and chlorhexidine (Braoudaki and Hilton 2004) and pine oil (Price, Singh, Jayaswal, et al. 2002). A detailed review of the mechanisms of action and bacterial resistance to antiseptics and disinfectants helps one to understand the linkage (McDonnell and A. Denver Russell 1999). Any useful listing of antibacterial products that are likely to be the source of resistance must therefore include identification of all antibacterial animal drugs currently approved by the FDA, all antimicrobial pesticides approved by the EPA for use on inanimate surfaces, all antimicrobials approved by the United States Department of Agriculture (USDA) for use on raw agricultural commodities, all antibacterials approved by the FDA for food additive use, and all antibacterial substances approved by the FDA for use in humans. The sheer number of different approvals for various antibacterials to be used for so many purposes since the 1940s can be overwhelming. With the high level of concern over the spread of pathogens such as *Staphylococcus aureus*, *C. diff.* (*Clostridium difficile*), and *Salmonella*, the use of antimicrobials outside the U.S. is also of concern. International movement of humans, animals, and foods is so extensive that what happens anywhere can affect us all. But stopping the movement of humans, animals, and food internationally would have horrific economic consequences.

Numerous antibiotics have been widely used to treat countless numbers of food animals for four or five decades. That alone should serve as a warning to those who would assume resistance developed on the farm and ranch is a critically important phenomenon that threatens to soon render all antibiotics ineffective. A lot of years have passed with many tons of antibiotics used in animals each year. Much attention has been focused on transfer of resistant bacteria from the farm to the table, but it is rare for antibiotic resistance problems to be traced to agricultural use. The principal source of antibiotic resistance problems in human medicine is and has always been the transfer of resistant bacteria from patients repeatedly and/or inappropriately medicated with antibiotics to other patients as well as to caretakers and friends. A powerful way to select for multiple antibiotic resistances in a disease organism is to treat an immunocompromised patient with an antibiotic and then when the few resistant bacteria in that patient's body grow out to cause a relapse, treat the patient with another antibiotic and repeat the process several times. Because normal patients have enough natural defenses to wipe out the few resistant bacteria that seem to always remain after antibiotic treatment, the treatment is fully effective, but not so in the immunocompromised patient. That seems to be how we got MRSA and highly resistant TB, gonorrhea, and syphilis.

We are forced to recognize the use of antibacterials in humans promotes resistance, and that resistance may be specific to a single antibacterial or it may be effective in resisting a wide variety of related or unrelated antibacterials. Treatment of farm animals is no different. As noted earlier, the use of a high level of streptomycin in turkey feed shortly after it was first marketed resulted in immediate resistance. We must also keep in mind that physicians and veterinarians have full access to any drug legally sold. The veterinarians' need to make a profit sometimes leads them to use the cheapest available antibacterials that are likely to be effective. Most of this usage is in treating companion animals that are soon returned to the home environment, and distribution of resistance in homes is not harmless. It should be avoided whenever feasible.

In the 1960s, the FDA became concerned about the possibility that subtherapeutic use of antibiotics in animals was not a good deal (Van Houwelling 1977a). Subsequently, the agency funded research, held symposia, and consulted experts to determine the severity of the matter. In April 1970, the commissioner of the FDA established a task force of scientists to undertake a comprehensive review of the use of antibiotic drugs in animal feeds. That task force concluded that the use of antibiotic and sulfonamide drugs favored the selection and development of single and multiple antibiotic-resistant and R-factor (plasmid) bearing bacteria, treated animals served as a reservoir of resistant bacteria, the increase in the prevalence of resistant bacteria was related to the use of antibiotics, and that resistant bacteria had been found on meat and meat products (Edwards 1972). In 1970 the British Government Joint Committee (the "Swann Committee") issued a report on "The Use of Antibiotics in Animal Husbandry and Animal Medicine" expressing real concern about antibiotic use in feeds. On February 1, 1972, the FDA issued proposed rulemaking to require pharmaceutical firms to conduct additional research into the subtherapeutic use of antibiotics, nitrofurans, and sulfonamides. Nitrofuran use in animal feeds has since been terminated due to unresolved human food safety issues, thereby making the possible restriction of their use in animal feeds moot. The rules concerning the remaining antibacterials were made final on April 20, 1973 (Gardiner 1973). On October 21, 1977, the FDA proposed to withdraw all approvals of subtherapeutic use of tetracyclines with the exception of a few applications with disease claims where no alternative drugs were available (such as control of fowl cholera and infectious synovitis) (Van Houwelling 1977b). In that document the FDA stated its criteria for human and animal safety as follows:

1. Transfer of drug resistance: (a) an antibacterial drug fed at subtherapeutic levels to animals must be shown not to promote increased resistance to antibacterials used in human medicine. Specifically, increased multiple resistance capable of being transferred to other bacteria in animals or man should not occur. (b) If increased transferable multiple resistance is found in coliforms, studies may be done to show whether this resistance is transferable to man.

2. The *Salmonella* reservoir: The use of antibacterial drugs at subtherapeutic levels in animal feed must be shown not to result in (a) an increase in quantity, prevalence or duration of shedding of *Salmonella* in medicated animals as compared to nonmedicated controls; (b) an increase in the number of antibiotic-resistant *Salmonella* or in the spectrum of antibiotic resistance; (c) disease (caused by *Salmonella* or other organisms) that is more difficult to treat with either the same medicated (sic) or other drugs.

3. The use of subtherapeutic levels of an antibacterial drug should not enhance the pathogenicity of bacteria, e.g., by increasing enterotoxin production. The association of toxin production characteristics with transfer factors must be investigated in well-designed studies. (Final resolution of this question was not

expected within the 2-year period. Drug sponsors were expected to show evidence of work underway which would lead toward answers to this question).

4. An antibacterial drug used at subtherapeutic levels in the feed of animals shall not result in residues in food ingested which may cause either increased numbers of pathogenic bacteria or an increase in the resistance of pathogens to antibacterial agents used in human medicine. Hypersensitivity to residues was to be addressed by a literature survey.

Because of our expanded knowledge of bacterial genetics, we can now see that document set an impossible standard. Years ago Chief Justice Burger, who served on the Supreme Court from 1969 to 1986, observed, "Absolute safety is a chimera," but that is precisely the standard set when the criteria for a decision on safety requires the use of antibacterials in feed produce no increase in antibiotic resistance and no increase in the prevalence of plasmids. Thus antibiotics in feed were to be considered safe only if they were *absolutely* safe. But it was of little consequence because Congress elected to stay the FDA's hand in the matter.

Recently the FDA decided one therapeutic product, Baytril® (enrofloxacin), approved in 1996 for use in poultry drinking water was creating problems that made it a Faustian bargain. According to the FDA's "Final Decision of the Commissioner (Docket No. 2000N-1571)" to ban, effective September 12, 2005, the use of enrofloxacin to control mortality in chickens associated with *Escherichia coli* and mortality in turkeys associated with *Escherichia coli* and *Pasteurella multocidia* because its use promoted resistant *Campylobacter jejuni* and *Campylobacter coli*, common and apparently harmless residents of poultry intestines, a few of which can then move through poultry processing plants and along the food chain into restaurants and homes. According to the FDA, unsanitary handling of raw meat then occasionally passes those intestinal bacteria along to consumers who, unlike poultry, may become ill with fever, headache, abdominal pain, and diarrhea, an especially dangerous condition if the patient is very young, very old, or immunocompromised and thus requires antibacterial treatment. Unfortunately, the antibacterials of choice in such patients are fluoroquinolones, close relatives of enrofloxacin. Naturally, they don't work well in such patients when the *Campylobacter* are already highly resistant. In banning Baytril (enrofloxacin) the FDA acknowledged that offsetting benefits, such as fewer *Escherichia coli*, *Pasteurella multocidia*, and fewer *Campylobacter* (and reduced pathogenicity of *Campylobacter*) on or in food, may exist but were not taken into consideration in the decisions to ban use of the drug in chickens and turkeys because the Food, Drug, and Cosmetic Act did not require balancing of risks and benefits in this case. Thus there was no weighing of potential risks against potential benefits. The costs and the benefits were not identified. Maybe it was a Faustian bargain and maybe not. But the real lesson to be learned from the Baytril ban is that if the same criteria are applied to other antibacterials then *all must be banned from any animal use*. No one actually proposes that because it would obviously be disastrous.

The sulfonamides were discovered and in widespread use before the first antibiotics were employed, and resistance to sulfonamides developed but has not been a serious problem because newer sulfonamides and antibiotics have been developed and used whenever therapeutic failures were encountered. Sulfonamide resistance seems not to have been shown to confer cross-resistance to true antibiotics, at least in part because the mechanism of action (inhibition of folic acid synthesis) is different from the true antibiotics; however, sulfonamides do encourage the spread of plasmids. Any antibacterial capable of promoting the spread of plasmids that can carry such properties as virulence and antibiotic resistance genes should be of concern. The presence of antibiotic resistance within the plasmid is not necessary to cause concern. The mere presence of increased numbers of plasmids must be a concern.

Likewise, organic arsenicals (arsanilic acid, roxarsone, nitarsone, carbarsone) enjoy widespread use in poultry and swine because their antibacterial and antiprotozoal activity makes their use profitable. Originally introduced to combat human venereal disease, organic arsenicals are today used in animals to control dysentery, prevent histomoniasis, improve pigmentation in chickens, and to enhance growth and feed efficiency. At the high dosages currently approved by the FDA for feed use, arsanilic acid and roxarsone are clearly antibacterial, and their role(s) in developing antibiotic resistance, if any, has not been reported. At the reduced doses at which roxarsone is approved for pigmentation, growth promotion, and feed efficiency in chickens and the reduced dosages at which arsanilic acid is used to enhance growth and feed efficiency in swine, little or no antibacterial activity has been reported. The mechanism of action whereby arsanilic acid and roxarsone enhance rate of weight gain and improved efficiency of feed utilization remains unknown although efforts have been made to elucidate it. A reduction in intestinal peristalsis has been documented and suggests nutrients have more time to be digested and absorbed before excretion; however, one must not forget the level of true antibiotics used to enhance growth and feed efficiency is also below the minimum concentration needed to inhibit bacterial growth. A reduction in intestinal wall thickness has been reported for both the arsenicals and the antibiotics. Thus the worries over use of true antibiotics, such as the tetracyclines, for enhanced growth and feed efficiency at doses below the minimum inhibitory level should trigger similar worries that non-antibiotic antibacterials used below the minimum inhibitory levels may also contribute to the overall problem of antibiotic resistance.

Concern about use of antibiotics in animals tends to focus on feed additive use of true antibiotics for enhanced growth and efficiency of feed utilization because these are presumed to be purely economic uses, but that focus uniformly ignores any role of other high- and low-level non-antibiotic antibacterials in possible promotion of antibiotic resistance. Data to support that lack of concern is largely missing, and data to support an alarm is everywhere. Similarly, numerous feed additive and water additive anticoccidials have been developed for preventing (continuous low dosage use) or treating (intermittent high dosage use) intestinal diseases caused by protozoa of the *Eimeria* species in poultry, sheep, goats, and cattle, not primarily for antibacterial effects. Nevertheless, some anticoccidials do affect the balance of microorganisms involved in digestion, especially in ruminants, and some have been found to be profitable because of their antibacterial activity. Currently approved anticoccidials include aklomide, amprolium, clopidol, decoquinate, diclazuril, ethopabate, halofuginone, laidlomycin, lasalocid, maduramicin, monensin, narasin, nicarbazin, nitromide, ormetoprim, robenidine, salinomycin, semduramicin, sulfadimethoxine, sulfanitran, sulfaquinoxaline, and zoalene. Their contribution to antibiotic resistance in human and veterinary medicine has not been much considered; however, recent studies by scientists at the USDA's National Animal Disease Center have shown protozoa such as *Ophyroscolex* species that live in the gastrointestinal system of cattle are implicated in transferring antibiotic resistance to bacteria (including *Salmonella*) that are susceptible to the antibiotics. Some of the above coccidiostats are indeed administered to cattle to control coccidiosis as well as to increase rate of weight gain and improve the efficiency of feed utilization. They affect the rumen microflora although at least some have been shown not to have noticeable activity against *Salmonella* or *E. coli*. Whether they select for bacteria with transferable plasmids seems to be unexplored at this time. They probably do.

The FDA has not approved all currently marketed antibacterials for humans or animals. Unapproved products are relatively few and not discussed in detail here because there is no useful record of them. Some of these may be the subject of current legal action, some may be marketed without coming to the attention of regulatory officials, some may have come to the attention of regulatory officials but no action has been taken because of other agency priorities, and some may be unapproved and illegally sold but not removed from the market because their role in preventing suffering or death is overwhelmingly important. Those products should be identified insofar as possible and their potential for inducing antibiotic resistance evaluated.

The days when the managers of hospitals and clinics thought the display of aquarium fish in lobbies and sitting rooms was a nice touch seem to have finally passed. Managers now seem to recognize the practice of adding medicines, including antibiotics, to the water in bubbling aquariums to treat the fish for various diseases was an aerosolized source of antibiotic-resistant bacteria originating from their own actions and right under their noses. Medicated water in fish aquariums bubbling in hospital waiting rooms was clearly a Faustian bargain, and it was rightfully stopped. Yes, it was calming and rather pretty but not worth the cost.

But there is still much work to do in preventing patient-to-patient movement of resistant bacteria in nursing homes, clinics, hospitals, hospices, and in private care facilities. Dogs and other pets are often brought to human health care facilities, much to the delight of patients. The animals are petted, often kissed by adoring patients, and then moved along to the next patient where the process is repeated. One can only wonder how many bacteria are thus transported from room to room and whether the benefits could possibly outweigh the costs. Animal visits are probably best restricted to patients with non-infectious diseases.

Although the scientific and medical communities are generally aware of the dangers associated with antibacterial treatment of pets such as dogs, cats, aquarium fish, and pet birds, few homeowners recognize any risk there at all, and data to measure the real risk seem to be weak or unavailable. Likewise, families working with livestock and poultry on the farm, in poultry processing plants, or in restaurants and grocery stores, and families living near animal production facilities remain mostly oblivious to the risk of antibiotic resistance by direct contact as well as from resistant bacteria carried by insects, rodents, and birds or simply borne on the wind. Perhaps that is best until sufficient studies are completed to determine where and when the danger is real and, when real, how serious. The little data we have is far from comprehensive. Until we have good data from well-controlled studies, we are just guessing about costs and benefits.

CONCLUSIONS

If trading antibacterials for money is a Faustian bargain, it is a big one although no final overall judgment is now possible in most cases. Still, without that bargain civilization just might lose its war with bacteria. After all, antibacterials, especially antibiotics, made possible the medical profession as we know it. With that bargain we must select our uses of antibacterials carefully and, even when we do, we must endure the curse of rolling the stone up the mountain of antibacterial research and development only to watch it roll back down as the bacteria become resistant to our latest inventions.

REFERENCES

Braoudaki, M. and A.C. Hilton. 2004. Adaptive resistance to biocides in *Salmonella enterica* and *Escherichia coli* O157 and cross-resistance to antimicrobial agents. *Journal of Clinical Microbiology* 42:73–78.

Doyle, Michael P., Francis (Frank) Busta, Bruce R. Cords, et al. 2006. Antimicrobial resistance: Implications for the food system, an expert report, funded by the IFT Foundation. *Comprehensive Reviews of Food Science and Food Safety* 5:71–137.

Edwards, Charles C. 1972. Antibiotics and sulfonamide drugs in animal feeds. *Federal Register* 37:2444–45.

Gardiner, Sherwin 1973. Antibiotics and sulfonamide drugs in the feed of animals. *Federal Register* 38:9811–14.

Goldsmith, Connie. 2007. *Superbugs strike back: When antibiotics fail*. Minneapolis. Twenty-First Century Books. This book is intended for middle school and high school students.

Haver, C.V. and E.K. Glover. 1924. *Catalogue issued by Haver-Glover Laboratories, manufacturers of special veterinary preparations, biologicals, pharmaceuticals, instruments and appliances.* Catalogue No. 4310.

Levy, Stuart B. 2002. *The antibiotic paradox*. Cambridge: Persus Publishing.

McDonnell, Gerald and A. Denver Russell. 1999. Antiseptics and disinfectants: Activity, action, and resistance. *Clinical Microbiology Reviews* 1999:147–79.

Price, Christopher T.D., Vignette K. Singh, Radheshyam K. Jayaswal, Brian J. Wilkinson, and John E. Gustafson. 2002. Pine oil cleaner-resistant *Staphylococcus aureus*: Reduced susceptibility to vancomycin and oxacillin and involvement of SigB. *Applied and Environmental Microbiology* 68:5417–21.

Richard J. Heath, Richard J., J. Ronald Rubin, Debra R. Holland, et al. 1999. Mechanism of triclosan inhibition of bacterial fatty acid synthesis. *Journal of Biological Chemistry* 274:11110–14.

Sinha, B.P. 1977. Acriflavine-resistant mutant of *Streptococcus cremoris*. *Antimicrobial Agents and Chemotherapy* 12:383–89.

The Haver-Glover Laboratories. 1936. *Catalogue issued by the Haver-Glover Laboratories, Kansas City Missouri, manufacturers and distributors of special veterinary products—Biological, pharmaceutical and surgical*. Fifth Edition.

Van Houwelling, C.D. 1977a. Tetracycline (chlortetracycline and oxytetracycline)-containing premixes: Opportunity for hearing. *Federal Register* 42:56264–89.

Van Houwelling, C.D. 1977b. Penicillin-containing premixes: Opportunity for hearing. *Federal Register* 42:43772–93.

CHAPTER V

OUTSMARTING THE SUPER BACTERIA

What Scientists, Farmers, And Food Processors

Are Doing About Resistance

While legislation aimed at banning the use of important antibiotics for disease control, disease prevention, growth, and feed efficiency is bogged down in Congress, the agricultural community is very much aware of public concerns and concerns in the medical community as well as the urgent demands of activist organizations. And the agricultural community has been taking steps to voluntarily reduce use of antibiotics. Data to guide rational decision-making about reducing the use of antibiotics in agriculture is still missing, and that is a great concern to most agriculturalists; therefore, the process is slow.

Although absurd, consumer images of "antibiotic soaked" meat are important to farmers. Threats from activist organizations about picketing large poultry and swine producers as well as fast-food retail outlets are well known and widely discussed. Farmers have long had biosecurity programs to reduce diseases, but in recent years these have been refined and more rigorously enforced in an effort to reduce the need for antibiotics. Tyson Foods, Gold Kist, Perdue, and Foster Farms, firms that account for 38 percent of all U.S. poultry production, have drastically reduced antibiotic use. For example, Tyson Foods reportedly reduced its use of antibiotics from 853,000 pounds per year in 1997 to just 59,000 pounds per year in 2007 at least in part by eliminating subtherapeutic uses and treating only poultry diagnosed with or clearly threatened with clinical disease (Wise 2006).

Swine and cattle producers are also reducing antibiotic use but are finding that discontinuing subtherapeutic uses is more difficult than has been the case with poultry. Worries about a possible and potentially dangerous rise in pathogen counts on food products if subtherapeutic use should be discontinued or significantly reduced have been widespread, but until recently definitive data has not been available. Wondwossen A. Gebreyes, Associate Professor of Veterinary Preventive Medicine at Ohio State University, Peter B. Bahnson of the University of Wisconsin School of Veterinary Medicine, Julie A. Funk and James McKean of the College of Veterinary Medicine at Iowa State University, and Prapas Patchanee of Ohio State's Department of Veterinary Preventive Medicine conducted a large, controlled study to compare pathogen levels in antibiotic-treated versus non–antibiotic-treated swine in North Carolina, Ohio, and Wisconsin to determine whether discontinuing antibiotic use might result in increases in pathogen levels. The results published in the journal *Foodborne Pathogens and Disease*, show conclusively that both pathogenic bacteria levels and dangerous parasite levels increased in pigs raised without antibiotics in their feed. Reducing the population density by putting the pigs on pasture complicates interpretation of the results but is probably needed to hold down infections in the pigs (Gebreyes, Bahnson, Funk, et al. 2008). This study will need to be confirmed by more studies, and similar studies are needed in other species. Cattle producers have not been able to reduce antibiotic use greatly because they mostly use antibiotics for serious respiratory diseases, mastitis control in dairy cattle, and for growing calves for slaughter as veal.

Antibiotic use in plant production is relatively minor and involves the use of tetracycline, streptomycin, and sulfonamides. When there is good reason to suspect a given crop will be exposed to a known bacterial disease, antibiotics are used to prevent loss of the crop. Because the amount used annually is small, not particularly controversial, and because crop producers have no apparent options to control disease, the use of antibiotics has not been much reduced.

The use of antibiotics in aquaculture is somewhat unique in that antibiotics are added to animal feed and thus distributed in the water. Worldwide use in aquaculture and the worldwide distribution of fresh fish and seafood makes this use of antibiotics a serious concern. The addition to water via feed also causes more of an ecological concern than for uses in land animals because the water often moves directly into the environment. Only in poultry production and a bit in swine production has serious reduction of antibacterial use occurred. The concern over antibiotic use is well known, the efforts to reduce their use are very real, and agriculturalists are gradually moving ahead. Some of the dangers of moving too fast are being identified.

STAYING ONE ANTIBIOTIC AHEAD

Another obvious way to outsmart the super bacteria is to develop new antibacterials faster than the bacteria can develop resistance. That way, resistant strains of any bacterial species can be quickly dealt with anytime and anywhere they are troublesome. But in fact that is what we have been trying to do since 1947; that is, we have been switching to an alternate antibiotic whenever resistance was encountered. We have done that in humans, in animals, in crops, and in industry. We have even done that with sanitizers and disinfectants. It has helped, but the bacteria seem capable of carrying resistance to more and more substances—with no end in sight.

We have at least 203 antibacterial substances for human use, about 275 for use on inanimate surfaces and on crops, several dozen for use in food processing and preservation, and approximately 95 for use in animals.

The problem now is that the flood of new antibacterials from industry to the market in the 1950s and 1960s has slowed to a trickle due to difficulty in finding really new ones, the high cost of developing them into products, the shocking cost of performing the necessary safety and effectiveness studies, and the cost and time for obtaining federal and state approvals to market the products. For human drugs the cost is about 500 million dollars but often hits a billion dollars; for animal drugs the cost is variable but usually runs between 20 million and 400 million dollars for a single new antibiotic product.

For an antibiotic to be approved for use in humans for any purpose other than its current approved purpose(s), the cost is again variable but ranges from about 20 to 250 million dollars. Fortunately, antibacterials studied for one market can sometimes be sold in a different presentation into another market. For example, a substance developed as an ointment for treating humans may also be useful as an aerosol spray for disinfecting hard surfaces. Thus the cost for research and development can be shared in two markets, but differences in the final formulation and differences in registration requirements imposed by different federal agencies can easily make the savings small. For example, the FDA is almost entirely science-driven so that requirements are variable, depending on the type of drug whereas the EPA has gone to considerable lengths to standardize their requirements across products lines in a manner that is reminiscent of a "checklist" approach. Of course, the EPA supplements the checklist when they decide additional studies are needed.

In the last three or four years, a resurgence of interest has developed for bringing new antibiotics to market for treating humans infected with resistant bacteria; however, return on investment has been low in recent years and remains problematic. Patients are almost always treated with antibiotics for a couple of weeks, during which time the pharmaceutical company must recoup the appropriate share of its investment from that patient. A cured patient may never again need another dose of any antibiotic of any sort. Animals are usually treated the same way, but some differences do exist. For example, in growing pigs antibiotics are used over long periods of time to prevent or control diseases. In growing chickens antibiotics and coccidiostats are often used continuously, while in plant agriculture antibiotics are used sporadically, for example, only during bloom in fruit trees. Industrial uses are often continuous but are mostly limited to non-antibiotic antibacterials.

Pharmaceutical companies have to be careful about investing in antibacterials because current U.S. law permits *generic* copies of pioneer drugs to be approved by the FDA (the agency typically requires no safety or effectiveness data from the generic sponsor and instead relies on the pioneer sponsor's data) as soon as the pioneer company's patents expire. Some exceptions exist but are not important for the present discussion. Patents are granted for 17 years and are usually extended to allow for time spent in product development. Setting the price of a new antibiotic high enough to recover a 800-million-dollar investment within about seven to ten years on a drug that is likely to be held in reserve by physicians until all other antibiotics have failed—and then only be used for two weeks—is possible, but pricing the drug at $800 per day of dosing results in very bad publicity for the drug's sponsor. Efforts to explain the reasons for charging that much almost invariably fail to impress patients and consumer advocates. In most cases firms choose to develop other types of drugs unless some rationale other than profit can be developed. That only occasionally happens.

Making a desperately needed, lifesaving drug available at a reasonable price gets lots of praise and establishes good relationships with physicians, patients, and the general public. The firm's sales agents can usually more easily get their foot in the hospital's purchasing door to sell their unique new antibiotic and, perhaps, use the opportunity to take orders for some of the firm's other products as well. Firms viewed as serious contributors to saving lives are respected, but it is difficult to explain serious financial losses to the firm's stockholders. These really great public relations products can put a firm into bankruptcy. Thus continued introduction of new antibiotics is clearly possible, but under existing constraints probably not likely to allow us enough really new antibiotics to outsmart the several different types of super bacteria. We can and must do a lot better (Payne 2008).

In the 2009 fiscal year, the up-front fee to be paid to the FDA for review of a marketing application for a new antibiotic drug for animal use is $246,300, and any supplement to the application that includes data on safety or effectiveness costs an additional $123,150. Once approved, the sponsor also must pay an annual FDA fee of $4,925 to maintain the approval, $59,450 for the privilege of being a drug establishment, plus an additional annual fee of $52,700 for being the sponsor of an animal drug approval (Shuren 2008a).

Similar fees to be paid for prescription drugs for fiscal year 2009 for human use are: for review of a marketing application requiring clinical data $1,247,200; for applications not requiring clinical data $623,600; for a supplement to the application that includes clinical data an additional $623,600. Once approved, the sponsor of a human drug application also must pay an annual FDA fee of $71,520 to maintain the approval and $425,600 for the privilege of being a registered drug establishment (Shuren 2008b).

All such fees should be waived for new antibacterial drugs until we get far ahead of the resistant bacteria. Additional steps such as placing antibiotics in orphan drug status, grants to universities for antibacterial research, and funding of government agencies for the conduct of clinical studies are needed. Patent extensions and other similar steps to give pioneer research companies a lot more time to recover the cost of new antibacterial drug development could be great incentives for top managers to turn their research armamentariums back to focus on new antibacterial discovery and development. When real incentives are in place, the superbug problem will probably disappear and the plague of antibiotic resistance will go away. At least that is the case if medical professionals can become more diligent about their hygiene programs.

Naturally occurring antibacterial substances isolated from fruits, vegetables, and herbs (such as garlic, salsa, yogurt, etc.) are commodities that cannot be patented so as to provide the sponsor a period of exclusive time to recover costs and can only be adequately researched if special circumstances exist or a governmental agency serves as the sponsor and performs the needed research and development. Even then, persuading a drug company to dedicate the necessary funds to sponsor the FDA approval and market such a new antibacterial can be difficult if not impossible because the exclusivity provisions of the act allow copycat products to be marketed after three years and many consumers can be expected to acquire the active ingredient(s) from food and related sources at food or condiment prices, not by buying the FDA approved drug product.

SCREENING PATIENTS

Because MRSA has been found in the community generally, and especially on swine and poultry farms as well as on the people who work on farms, screening of patients upon entrance to the hospital is being tried by several hospitals. Swabbing skin and nostrils has apparently helped hospitals to get better control because patients carrying staph can be given special treatment to avoid contaminating other patients and the hospital generally. Using antibiotics produces resistance, so anything that reduces the need to use one extends its effective lifetime. But staph is not the only super bacteria, and many additional steps will be needed. Some of those steps have already been taken by a few hospitals, steps such as sealing off areas where a patient has been treated for resistant bacterial so that extreme steps can be taken to decontaminate the area and all equipment used there. Attacking the super bacteria problem in the larger community (outpatient clinics, nursing homes, and residences in general) is another way to extend the effective life of an antibiotic, but apparently the efforts currently underway are mostly limited to programs that are educational in nature, that is, the focus is on training homeowners, patients, caretakers, doctors, and nurses in hygiene and disinfection procedures to reduce spreading of pathogens to family, to visitors, and to other patients.

REDUCING EXPOSURE TO FOOD-BORNE RESISTANT BACTERIA

While Americans mostly assume the foods they purchase are safe to eat, they are gradually losing confidence due to the alarming outbreaks of illness traced to food and the dramatic, detailed media depictions of each occurrence. The CDC has estimated the annual cost of all food-borne illness due to *Salmonella*, *Listeria monocytogenes*, and *Escherichia coli* O157:H7, including medical costs, productivity losses, and premature deaths in the United States, to be $2.9, $2.3 and $0.7 billion, respectively; however, the specific the cost for treating patients having food-derived *antibiotic-resistant* pathogens is not well documented, in part because antibiotics are not appropriate for such patients unless the patient first gets into serious trouble because these gastrointestinal diseases are self-limiting. Normal patients who are treated usually suffer more than non-treated patients. Occasional transmission of antibiotic-resistant pathogenic bacteria "from the farm to the fork" is real.

Control measures for food-borne bacteria and other microorganisms have been mandated by the United States government; however, food additives intended to prevent bacterial growth in/on foods have themselves been suggested as another probable source of increasing antibiotic resistance. The Institute of Food Technologists sponsored a comprehensive report on risks from food additives (Doyle, Busta, et al. 2006). For many years the composition and all uses of food additives has been reviewed for safety and utility—and approved by the FDA's Center for Food Safety and Nutrition (CFSAN) through the food additive petition process or in the case of raw (unprocessed) agricultural commodities by the EPA. With respect to meat and poultry additives, additional regulatory review and regulatory approval from the USDA's Plant and Animal Health Inspection Service (APHIS) has been required.

To reduce product liability risks and meet government requirements, manufacturers have used various processing techniques, added antimicrobials, applied antimicrobial treatments to the surface of products, applied post-pasteurization treatments, and have irradiated foods. Comments on these interventions and additional general reference websites for further information are provided in the following discussion.

Drying

New drying technologies are intended to lower the unbound or free water in a food or perishable material. This method relies on the fact that most microorganisms cannot multiply if there is little or no available water for their metabolism and reproduction. Available water or free water is quantified as water activity (aw). Water activity is defined as "free," "bound," or "available water" in a package environment. Water activity—not water content—determines the lower limit of available water for microbial growth and is a critical factor in shelf life for many foods. While temperature, pH, and other factors can influence if and how fast organisms will grow in a product, water activity may be the most important factor in controlling spoilage. Most bacteria, for example, do not grow at water activities below 0.91, and most molds cease to grow at water activities below 0.80. By measuring water activity, it is possible to predict which microorganisms will and will not be potential sources of problems in a packaging system. In addition to influencing microbial spoilage, water activity can play a significant role in determining the activity of enzymes and vitamins in foods and can have a major impact on their color, taste, and aroma. It can also significantly impact the potency and consistency of pharmaceuticals. More information about water activity can be obtained from Decagon Devices, Inc., by visiting their web site at http://www.decagon.com.

Packaging

Packaging seeks to limit the exposure of products to environmental contamination. Dramatic advances in packaging materials and procedures have resulted in reduced contamination during processing and substantially increased shelf lives for perishable products and fresh foods, even at temperatures of 40 degrees C. New types of plastic film technologies have led to the development of "active packaging." These flexible packaging materials not only serve as a barrier to the entry of contaminants and gases but also can scavenge oxygen to reduce the rate of oxidation or ethylene to slow ripening in the intra-package environment. The structural barrier and oxygen management nature of the flexible packaging material can reduce the proliferation of pathogens and dramatically extend the fresh appearance and shelf life of the packaged food. More information about active packaging can be obtained from Sealed Air Corporation which may be contacted by visiting www.cryovac.com.

Refrigeration and Freezing

Cooling perishable material has been around for a long time. It changes the water activity and can create a temperature environment not conducive to microbial growth. Refrigeration combined with packaging has allowed the food distribution infrastructure to develop from a local to a regional to a global food-delivery enterprise. The major problem with temperature control is that it is an active preservation method requiring energy and operating equipment. Additionally, there are a few important spoilage and food-borne pathogens that can grow in refrigerated foods. Freezing can further delay the growth of these organisms; however, it is even more expensive and difficult to maintain. Information about refrigeration and freezing to control microorganisms on food is available from The Air-Conditioning, Heating, and Refrigeration Institute (AHRI).

Lyophilization (Freeze Drying)

Freeze drying perishables relies on the combination of packaging, then freezing, drying, and sealing the package as well as creating a controlled intra-package atmosphere. Freeze dried materials support little or no bacterial growth, have greatly extended shelf life under extreme conditions, and can provide a reliable source of nutrition for extended periods. The most famous diet transition from traditional methods to freeze drying was the evolution of military rations C and K to Meals Ready to Eat (MREs). MREs have greatly extended shelf life.

Irradiation

Many foods, such as poultry, spices, vegetables, and grain products, are irradiated to control insects and bacteria. The radiation not only destroys the insect eggs and bacterial and fungal spores but also inactivates spoilage enzymes that naturally occur in the food. Radiation must be combined with a packaging system to prevent recontamination. Some foods cannot be irradiated without causing negative organoleptic (taste and odor) effects. Also, the public fears radiation of any sort and continues to be uncomfortable with irradiated foods. Some bacteria are known to be able to flourish in the presence of extremely high levels of radiation and should therefore be considered "resistant;" however, no link or cross-resistance between antibiotic resistance and radiation resistance has been reported. Because public acceptance of irradiation is not complete the use of radiation is limited, but if really needed it can be a major addition to our tool kit for control of food-borne bacteria (Tauxe 2000).

Acidification

The addition of acids to foods is a proven method of preventing bacterial growth; however, some bacteria can survive at low pH. The development of super acids that literally protonate a food product is an important new method for food preservation and decontamination.

These super acids, such as acidic calcium sulfate, kill bacteria by over-whelming the proton pump. These acids only kill the vegetative state of microorganisms and not the spores. The combination of super acids and radiation in food preservation and packaging is a developing area of interest for shelf-stable products.

Processing Aids

The bacteriophage is a tiny, virus-like organism that parasitizes bacteria. Phages were discovered in 1917 and are present almost everywhere, including in the intestinal tract of animals. And, phages may help animals defend themselves against pathogenic bacteria (Core 2001). In 2006 the USDA approved the use of a phage-based product as an additive for treatment of *Listeria* in ready-to-eat meat and poultry products and in 2007 approved a similar phage product to be applied as a mist, spray, or wash to the skin and hair of animals prior to their entering the slaughter facility. The latter product targets *E. coli* 0157:H7 and helps prevent cross-contamination of animal products and the processing facility. Additional uses include treatment of holding areas, transportation vehicles, containers, and living quarters of animals. The goal is to reduce overall *E. coli* 0157:H7 contamination of the animals and the facilities where they are processed (ElAmin 2007). Studies are currently in progress to determine the safety and effectiveness of using phages directly in human medicine. That is feasible because phages are not known to attack animal cells, only specific bacteria.

Animal Feed Additives

We know one source of *Salmonella* and other pathogens carried by food animals is their feed and therefore non-antibiotic antimicrobials are being added to animal feed to reduce contamination in the feed during manufacture, storage, and distribution. Acidification of feed is also a method to not only preserve the feed but to influence the bacterial makeup of the animal's digestive tract. For example, buffered formic acid was recently approved as a feed additive for swine in some countries where growth-promoting antibiotics have been banned. These organic acids can cause disturbances in the animal's metabolism as well as increases in the incidence of gastrointestinal ulcers. Some members of taste panels can taste the organic acid in the food products produced from these animals. Various organic acid combinations have also been advocated; however, problems with uniform mixing in the feed and palatability problems continue to be negatives for their use. Recently a new technology combining a superacid with toxin-adsorbing clay seems to have overcome most of these delivery and palatability issues while providing the benefits of an acidified feed. This combination seems to offer the possibility of reducing animal-to-animal or litter-to-animal transmission of pathogens as well as reducing carcass contamination at slaughter and processing.

Food Additives

Common food additives have also been implicated in contributing to antibiotic resistance as a matter of principle, however specific data seem to be missing. The efficacy of these preservatives is easy to observe and validate, but the effects of their long-term use is a more difficult problem. Because of currently approved methods and product liability issues, most manufacturers are reluctant to try any new technologies. When research results on new food additive materials indicate compliance with approved methods and when minimization of product liability issues has been achieved, manufacturers will then become more receptive to using new food additives.

One of the most promising new food additives is "cationic antimicrobial peptides." Most organisms manufacture cationic peptides to avoid opportunistic infections. These cationic peptides are small, positively charged molecules that kill or inhibit the growth of bacteria, fungi, and protozoa. These peptides are responsible for a potent, non-specific immune response that protects the host against invading microorganisms. This important "host-defense" system has been highly conserved throughout evolution, and cationic antimicrobial peptides have been isolated from a diverse array of organisms that include bacteria, plants, insects, amphibians, and mammals (including humans). To date more than 300 natural antimicrobial peptides have been identified by researchers around the world. Because most species throughout the evolutionary scale continue to use peptides as antimicrobial agents, many experts believe it is likely that resistance to peptide antibacterial agents will be manageable. One of the most promising of the cationic antimicrobial peptides for direct food additive applications is epsilon-polylysine (ε-PL), a short-chain polypeptide. These peptide antibiotics hold significant promise as drugs and food preservatives of the future; however, should resistance become significant then such bacteria would not only be resistant to the drug but also one of the body's normal ways of defending itself. That is just plain frightening. In this area one must be careful.

The market for "organic foods" is growing in the United States and Europe. Since standards of identity for meat products must be maintained and synthetic chemical preservatives cannot be added without losing their "organic" status, the only known alternative is irradiation. A provider-consumer conflict results because many consumers will not buy irradiated food on the assumption that it might not be safe; however, that perception may change in the future. Nevertheless, the application of cationic proteins such as epsilon-polylysine (ε-PL) to Ready To Eat (RTE) meats and other refrigerated products promises to provide extended shelf life without increasing the risk of antibiotic resistance in food-borne pathogens and other organisms.

<u>Blocking Quorum Sensing and Biofilms</u>

Many disease-causing bacteria use chemical languages to alert other bacteria when a sufficient population is present to successfully produce disease or to trigger production of biofilms that cloak the bacteria so as to make them less sensitive to antibiotics. Researchers have recently identified a group of small molecules call N-acylated L-homoserine lactones that are involved in bacterial communications and are currently working on substances that interfere with these communications. This work is ongoing and specifically aimed at antibiotic-resistant bacteria (Peplow 2006).

Herbal and Other Feed Additives

Lactic acid, formic acid, probiotics, yeast, minerals, and more than 500 different herbs are being tested for their ability to provide the benefits of antibiotics in animal feed while avoiding the build up of antibiotic resistance. The addition of these ingredients to ruminant, swine, poultry, and fish feeds is being tested for a variety of effects on metabolism, weight gain, feed efficiency, and disease prevention; however, the presumption that such ingredients are safe because they are natural is obviously dangerous and potentially catastrophic. The European Union and some commercial firms are funding such projects in an effort to compensate for bans on antibiotic use in food-producing animals because European farmers are complaining that they are unable to compete with farmers in countries where antibiotics are still in use. Considerable research is underway in this area but nothing very promising has yet emerged.

Super Plants, Super Livestock, and Super Poultry

While environmental contamination of food during processing is a major target of food additives and preservatives used in processing plants, these products may not be effective against disease organisms actually contained within the tissues of food animals and plants. Antibiotics fed to animals are intended to control these subclinical cases of disease in production species; however, the most logical approach to combat the subclinical disease state may be to develop disease-resistant production animals. Natural selection and intentional breeding practices have produced highly productive plants and animals, but the emphasis on inherent disease resistance in breeding plants and animals has been relatively low. In almost every disease outbreak there are survivors. One of the reasons for their survival is genetic-based resistance. Now that we have nearly complete genetic maps of most of the food production species, it is possible to detect genes that are directly responsible for or associated with disease resistance. One method for discovering these genes is to look for differences in plants and animals that are susceptible to disease and those that are not. An interesting example is bovine spongiform encephalitis (BSE) which has never been found in a cow heterozygous at a certain BSE susceptibility locus. Every cow that has developed BSE and been tested for this trait has been found to be homozygous at this locus. Now it should be possible to test cows for this genetic marker, identify the susceptible calves, and not retain them for breeding purposes and/or to remove susceptible cows from the herd. BSE is not caused by bacteria, but the same principles can be applied to controlling bacterial diseases.

Expansion of a disease resistance gene in a population in the past has been hampered by the time required to expand the gene through customary breeding practices. With cloning and embryo transfer techniques, desirable and stable genes for disease resistance can be expanded into a population in as little as three generations. These identification and genetic expansion techniques will allow scientists and producers to introduce desirable traits and disease resistance into their crops, flocks, and herds more quickly—thereby reducing the risk of spontaneous or bioterrorism-induced diseases in production plant and animal populations (Whitelaw and Sang 2005).

SUMMARY

The technologies discussed are just a few of the innovations in food and feed production and safety. The technologies can reduce the number of antibiotic-resistant bacteria worldwide, and some of these technologies are currently available. Implementation relies on a number of factors, but most importantly, widespread adoption will require continued consumer demand and support as well as government-funded research to better understand how we can outsmart resistant bacteria in hospitals, clinics, homes, agriculture, and industry. Many microbiologists and chemists are actively searching for novel ways to control resistant bacteria, and many of these are promising. Super hospitals and super farms create circumstances where selection for resistant bacteria is inevitable. Our war with bacteria is on-going, not lost.

REFERENCES

Core, Jim 2001. Bacteriophages a possible alternative to antibiotics in animal production. *USDA Agriculture Research Service News &Events*. September 21. http//:www.ars. usda.gov/is/pr/2001/010921.htm

ElAmin, Ahmed, 2007. Bacteriophage approved for hide washing. *PPM Technologies: Breaking News On Food Processing & Packaging*. January 4. http://www.foodproduction-daily.com/news/ng.asp?id=73105-omnilytics-bacteriophage-e-coli.

Gebreyes, Wondwossen A., Peter B. Bahnson, Julie A. Funk, James McKean, Prapas Patchanee 2008. Seroprevalence of Trichinella, Toxoplasma, and Salmonella in antimicrobial-free and conventional swine production systems. *Foodborne Pathogens and Disease* 5:199-203.

Payne, David J. 2008. Desperately seeking new antibiotics. *Science* 321: 1644-45.

Shuren, Jeffrey 2008a. Animal drug user fee rates and payment procedures for fiscal year 2009. *Federal Register* 73: 53254-60.

Shuren, Jeffrey 2008b. Prescription drug user fee rates for fiscal year 2009. *Federal Register* 73: 45017-22.

Peplow, Mark 2006. Bacteria silenced by conversation stoppers. *Royal Society of Chemistry, Chemistry World*. September 12. http://www.rsc.org/chemistryworld/News/2006/September/12090601.asp.

Tauxe, Robert V. 2000. Food safety and irradiation: Protecting the public from foodborne infections. *Emerg Infect Dis*. 2001, 7(3Suppl) 516-21.

Whitelaw, C.B.A. and H.M. Sang 2005. Disease-resistant genetically modified animals. *Rev. Sci. Tech. Off. Int. Epiz*. 24 (2) 275-83. http://www.oie.int/eng/publicat/rt/2401/24-1%20pdfs/24-whitelaw275-284.pdf.

Wise, Elizabeth 2006. Natural chickens take flight. *USA Today*. http://www.usatoday.com/news/health/2006-01-23-natural-chickens_x.htm. Posted 1/23/2006 9:52PM. Updated 1/24/2006 12:06 PM.

APPENDIX A. TABLE OF ANTIBACTERIALS WITH USE DESIGNATIONS

Antibacterial	Human Use	Animal Use	Disinfect/ Sanitizer/ Plants
1-Decanaminium, N, N-dimethyl-N-octyl-, chloride			√
1-Decanaminium, N-decyl-N,N-dimethyl-, chloride			√
1-Octanaminium, N, N-dimethyl-N-octyl-, chloride			√
2-Benzyl-4-chlorophenol			√
4-Chloro-3,5-xylenol			√
4-Tert amylphenol			√
Acetic acid	√		
Acetylsalicylic acid			√
Acyclovir	√		
Aklomide		√	
Alatrofloxacin	√		
Alkyl amine acetate (5% C8, 7% C10, 54% C12, 19% C14, 8% C16, 7% C18)			√
Alkyl amino-3-aminopropane (42% C12, 26% C18, 15% C14, 8% C16, 5% C10, 4% C8)			√
Alkyl dimethyl 1-naphthymethyl ammonium chloride (98% C12, 2% C14)			√
Alkyl dimethyl benzyl ammonium chloride (58% C14, 28% C16, 14% C16)			√
Alkyl dimethyl benzyl ammonium chloride (61% C12, 23% C14, 11% C16, 5% C18)			√
Alkyl dimethyl benzyl ammonium chloride (67% C12, 25% C14, 7% C16, 1% C8, C10)			√
Alkyl dimethyl benzyl ammonium chloride (70% C12, 30% C14)			√
Alkyl dimethyl benzyl ammonium chloride (90% C14, 5% C12, 5%C16)			√
Alkyl dimethyl benzyl ammonium chloride (93% C14, 4% C12, 3% C16)			√
Alkyl dimethyl benzyl ammonium chloride (95% C14, 3% C12, 2% C16)			√
Alkyl dimethyl benzyl ammonium chloride (as in fatty acids of coconut oil)			√
Alkyl dimethyl benzyl ammonium chloride (50% C12, 30% C14, 17% C16, 3% C18)			√

Alkyl dimethyl benzyl ammonium chloride (50% C14, 40% C12, 10% C16)			√
Alkyl dimethyl benzyl ammonium chloride (60% C14, 30% C16, 5% C12)			√
Alkyl dimethyl benzyl ammonium chloride (60% C14, 30% C16, 5% C18, 5% C12)			√
Alkyl dimethyl benzyl ammonium chloride (60% C14, 30% C18, 5% C12)			√
Alkyl dimethyl benzyl ammonium chloride (60% C14, 40% C12, 10% C16)			√
Alkyl dimethyl benzyl ammonium chloride (68% C12, 32% C14)			√
Alkyl dimethyl benzyl ammonium saccharinate (50% C14, 40% C12, 10% C16)			√
Alkyl dimethyl dimethylbenzyl ammonium chloride (50% C12, 30% C14, 17% C16)			√
Alkyl dimethyl dimethylbenzyl ammonium chloride (68% C 12, 32% C14)			√
Alkyl dimethyl ethyl ammonium bromide (90% C14, 5% C16, 5% C12)			√
Alkyl dimethyl ethylbenzyl ammonium chloride (50% C12, 30% C14, 17% C16, 3% C18)			√
Alkyl dimethyl ethylbenzyl ammonium chloride (68% C12, 30% C14)			√
Alkyl dimethyl ethylbenzyl ammonium chloride (68% C12, 32% C14)			√
Alkyl-omega-hydroxypoly (oxyethylene) iodine complex (100% C12-C15)			√
Amikacin	√	√	
Amines, coco alkyl trimethylene diacetates			√
Amines, coco alkyl, hydrochlorides			√
Amines, N-coco alkyl trimethylene diacetates			√
Amines, N-coco alkyl trimethylene glycolates			√
Aminocrine	√		
Aminosalicylate	√		
Aminosalicylic acid	√		
Ammonia			√
Ammonium, N-alkyl (9-15) tolyl methyltrimethyl chloride			√
Amoxicillin	√	√	
Amphomycin		√	
Ampicillin	√	√	
Amprolium		√	

Amylphenol, potassium salt			√
Amylphenol, sodium salt			√
Anthracene oil			√
Apramycin		√	
Arsanilic Acid		√	
Arsenic acid anhydride			√
Atovaquone	√		
Aziocillin	√		
Azithromycin	√		
Aztreonam	√		
Bacampicillin	√		
Bacitracin	√	√	
Bambermycins		√	
Barium metaborate			√
Benzalkonium chloride	√	√	√
Benzene dicarboxaldehyde			√
Benzisothiazolin-3-one			√
Benzoyl peroxide	√		
Benzyl dimethyl tetradecyl ammonium chloride			√
Benzyl-4-chlorophenol			√
Bicyclohexylammonium Fumagillin		√	
Bis (bromoacetoxy)-2-butene dantoin			√
Bis (tributyltin) oxide			√
Bis (tributyltin) salicylate			√
Bis (trichloromethyl) sulfone			√
Bismuth tribromophenate	√		
Boron zinc oxide			√
Bromine			√
Bromine chloride			√
Bromo-1-(bromomethyl)-1,3-propanedicarbonitrile			√
Bromo-3-chloro-5,5-dimethyl hydantoin			√
Bromo-41-hydroxyacetophenone			√
Bromo-beta-nitrostyrene			√
Bronopol			√
Butoxy polypropoxy polyethoxy ethanol-iodine complex			√
Butylparaben	√		
Butylphenol	√		
Calcium hypochlorite			√
Calcium oxide			√
Calcium sulfate			√

SUPERBUGS

Capreomycin	√		
Caprylic acid			√
Carbamide peroxide	√		
Carbendazim			√
Carbenicillin	√		
Carbomycin		√	
Carbonic acid, monopotassium salt			√
Cefaclor	√		
Cefadroxil	√	√	
Cefalexin	√		
Cefamandole	√		
Cefazolin	√		
Cefdinir	√		
Cefditoren	√		
Cefepime	√		
Cefixime	√		
Cefixime	√		
Cefmetazole	√		
Cefonicid	√		
Cefoperazone	√		
Ceforanide	√		
Cefotaxime	√		
Cefotetan	√		
Cefovecin		√	
Cefoxitin	√		
Cefpodoxime	√		
Cefprozil	√		
Ceftazidime	√		
Ceftazidime	√		
Ceftibuten	√		
Ceftiofur		√	
Ceftizoxime	√		
Ceftriaxone	√		
Cefuroxime	√		
Cephadine	√		
Cephalexin	√		
Cephalothin	√		
Cephapirin	√	√	
Cephradine	√		
Cetyldimethylammonium bromide	√		

Cetylpyridinium chloride	√		
Chloramphenicol	√	√	
Chlorhexidine	√	√	
Chlorinated trisodium phosphate			√
Chlorine			√
Chlorine dioxide			√
Chloroallyl-3,5,7-triaza-1-azoniaadamantane chloride			√
Chloro-2-(2,4-dichlorophenoxy) phenol			√
Chloro-2-methyl-3 (2H)-isothiazolone			√
Chloro-2-propenyl-3,5,7-triaza-1-azoniatricyclo (3.3.1.1 superscript 3,7) decane			√
Chlorobutanol		√	
Chloropene			√
Chlorothymol	√		
Chloroxylenol			√
Chlortetracycline	√	√	
Chromic acid			√
Cilastatin	√		
Cinoxacin	√		
Ciprofloxacin	√		
Citric acid			√
Clarithromycin	√		
Clavulanate	√	√	
Clindamycin	√	√	
Clofazimine	√		
Cloflucarban	√		
Clopidol		√	
Cloroxine	√		
Cloxacillin	√	√	
Coal tar			√
Coal tar creosote			√
Copper as metallic chelates of copper citrate			√
Colistimethate (Colistin)	√		
Copper ethanolamine complex			√
Copper ethylene diamine tetraacetate			√
Copper naphthenate		√	√
Copper (I) oxide			√
Copper (II) oxide			√
Copper triethanolamine complex			√
Creosote oil			√

91

Cuprimyxin		√	
Cuprous thiocyanate			√
Cyclopropyl-N,-(1,1-dimethylethyl)-6-(methylthio)-1,3,5-tri-azine-2,4-diamine			√
Cycloserine	√		
Cyclosporine		√	
Dalbavacin	√		
Dalfopristin	√		
Danofloxacin		√	
Dapsone	√		
Daptomycin	√		
Dazomet, sodium salt			√
Decoquinate		√	
Decyl isononyl dimethyl ammonium chloride			√
Decylthio ethanamine hydrochloride			√
Demeclocycline	√		
Dialkyl methyl benzyl ammonium chloride (60% C14, 30% C16, 5% C18, 5% C12)			√
Dibromo-3-nitrilopropionamide			√
Dibromo-5, 5-dimethylhydantoin			√
Dicecyl-N-methyl-3-(trimethoxysilyl) propanaminium (trimethoxysilyl) propanaminium chloride			√
Dichloro-2-n-octyl-3 (2H)-isothiazolone			√
Dichloro-5,5-dimethylhydantoin			√
Dichloro-5-ethyl-5-methylhydantoin			√
Dichloro-s-triazinetrione			√
Dichromic acid			√
Diclazuril		√	
Dicloxacillin	√	√	
Didecyl dimethyl ammonium chloride			√
Difloxacin		√	
Dihydrostreptomycin	√	√	
Diisobutylcresoxyethoxyethyl dimethy benzyl ammonium chloride			√
Diisobutylphenoxyethyl dimethyl benzyl ammonium chloride			√
Dimethyl-m-dioxan-4-ol acetate			√
Dimethyloxazolidine			√
Dioctyl decyl dimethyl ammonium chloride			√
Dioctyl dimethyl ammonium chloride			√
Dioctyl sodium sulfosuccinate			√

Dipropylene glycol			√
Dirithromycin	√		
Disodium cyanodithioimidocarbonate			√
Dithiol-3-one, 4,5-dichloro			√
Diuron			√
DMDM hydantoin			√
Dodecyl alcohol			√
Dodecyl bis (2-hydroxyethyl) octyl hydrogen ammonium phosphate			√
Dodecyl bis (hydroxyethyl) dioctyl ammonium phosphate			√
Dodecylbenzenesulfonic acid			√
Dodecylbenzyl trimethyl ammonium chloride			√
Dodecylguanidine hydrochloride			√
Doxycycline	√	√	
EDTA tetrasodium salt			√
Enrofloxacin		√	
Ertapenem	√		
Erythromycin	√	√	
Ethambutol	√		
Ethanol	√	√	√
Ethionamide	√		
Ethopabate		√	
Ethyl-2-nitrotrimethylene dimorpholine			√
Ethylene oxide			√
Ethylparaben	√		
Eucalyptol	√		
Famciclovir	√		
Florfenicol		√	
Folpet			√
Formaldehyde	√	√	√
Fosfomycin	√		
Furazolidone	√	√	
Fusidate	√		
Gatifloxacin	√		
Gemifloxacin	√		
Gentamicin	√	√	
Gentian violet	√		
Glutaraldehyde			√
Gramicidin	√		
Halazone			√

SUPERBUGS

Halofuginone		√	
Hetacillin	√	√	
Hexachlorophene	√		√
Hexylresorcinol	√		
Hydrochloric acid			√
Hydrogen peroxide	√	√	√
Hydroxy-2-(1H)-pyridinethione, sodium salt			√
Hydroxyethyl-2-alkyl-2-imidazoline			√
Hydroxymethly-1-aza-3,7-dioxabicyclo (3.3.0) octane			√
Hydroxymethoxymethyl-1-1-aza-3,7-dioxabicyclo (3.3.0) octane			√
Hydroxymethyl (amino) ethanol			√
Hydroxymethyl (amino)-2-methyl-1-propanol			√
Hydroxymethyl-2-nitro-1,3-propanediol			√
Hydroxypoly (methyleneoxy) methyl-1-1-aza-3,7-dioxabicyclo (3.3.0) octane			√
Hydroxypropyl thiomethane sulfonate			√
Hydroxyquinoline	√		
Imipenim	√		
Iodine	√	√	√
Iodine-potassium iodine complex			√
Iodo-2-propynyl butylcarbamate			√
Iodochlorhydroxyquin		√	
Isoniazid	√		
Isopropanol	√	√	√
Kanamycin	√	√	
Laidlomycin		√	
Lasalocid		√	
Levofloxacin	√		
Lime, chlorinated			√
Lincomycin	√	√	
Linezolid	√		
Lithium hypochlorite			√
Lomefloxacin	√		
Loracarbef	√		
Maduramicin		√	
Mafenide	√		
Marbofloxacin		√	
MDM Hydantoin			√
Meclocycline	√		

94

Menthol	√		
Mercaptobenzothiazole		√	
Meropenem	√		
Methacycline	√		
Methanol			√
Methenamine hippurate	√		√
Methicillin	√		
Methyl alcohol			√
Methyl salicylate	√		√
Methyl-3 (2H) –isothiazolone			√
Methyl-4-5–trimethylene-4-isothiazolin-3-one			√
Methylbenzethonium chloride	√	√	√
Methylene bis (thiocyanate)			√
Methylparaben			√
Methyltrimethylenedioxy bis (4-methyl-1,3,2-dioxaborinate)			√
Metronidazole	√		
Meziocillin	√		
Minocycline	√		
Monensin		√	
Moxalactam	√		
Moxifloxacin	√		
Muphocin	√	√	
Myristyl-Gamma-Picolinium Chloride		√	
Nabam			√
Nafcillin	√		
Nalidixic acid	√		
Narasin		√	
Neomycin	√	√	
Netilmicin	√	√	
Nicarbazin		√	
Nitarsone		√	
Nitazoxanide		√	
Nitrobutyl morpholine			√
Nitrofurantoin	√		
Nitrofurazone	√	√	
Nitromide		√	
Nitrophenol			√
Nonylphenoxypolyethanol – iodine complex			√
Nonylphenoxypolyethoxyethanol - iodine complex			√
Norfloxacin	√		

Novobiocin	√	√	
Octanoic acid			√
Octhilinone			√
Octyl decyl dimethyl ammonium chloride			√
Ofloxacin	√		
Oleandomycin	√	√	
o-Phenylphenol			√
Orbifloxacin		√	
Ormetoprim		√	
Oxacillin	√		
Oxazolidine E			√
Oxine-copper			√
Oxybis (4,4,6-trimethyl-1,3,2-dioxaborinane)			√
Oxybisphenoxarsine			√
Oxychlorosene sodium	√		√
Oxydiethylenebis (alkyl dimethyl ammonium chloride)			√
Oxytetracycline	√	√	√
Parachloromethaxylenol	√		
Parachlorophenol	√		
Paraformaldehyde			√
Pefloxacin	√		
Penicillin G	√	√	
Penicillin V	√	√	
Pentachlorophenol			√
Pentylphenol	√		
Peroxyacetic acid			√
Phenazopyridine	√		
Phenol			√
Phenyl mercuric borate			√
Phenylmercuric acetate	√		
Phenylmercuric nitrate	√		
Phenylphenol			√
Phosphoric acid			√
Phosphoric acid, bis (2-ethylhexyl) ester			√
Phosphoric acid, mono (2-ethylhexyl) ester			√
Pine oil			√
Piperacillin	√		
Pirlimycin		√	
Poly (iminoimidocarbonyliminoimidocarbonylmino hexa-methylene) hydrochloride			√

Poly (methylmethacrylate-co-tributyltin methacrylate)			√
Poly (oxyethylene (dimethyliminio) ethylene (dimethyliminio) ethylene dichloride			√
Poly-ethoxypoly-propoxyethanol iodine complex			√
Polymyxin B	√	√	
Potassium 2-benzyl-4-chlorophenate			√
Potassium bromide			√
Potassium cresylate			√
Potassium dichloro-s-triazinetrione			√
Potassium dichromate			√
Potassium dimethyldithiocarbamate			√
Potassium iodide			√
Potassium N-hydroxymethyl-N-methyldithiocarbamate			√
Potassium N-methyldithiocarbamate			√
Potassium permanganate	√		√
Potassium peroxymonosulfate			√
Povidone iodine	√	√	√
Propen-1-aminium, N, N-dimethyl-N-2-propenyl chloride, homopolymer			√
Propylene glycol			√
Propylene oxide	√		
Pryazole-1-methanol, 3,5-dimethyl			√
PVP iodine			√
Pyrazinamide	√		
Pyrithione zinc	√		
Quinupristin	√		
Retapamulin	√		
Rifabutiin	√		
Rifampin	√		
Rifapentine	√		
Rifaximin	√		
Robenidine		√	
Roxarsone		√	
Salinomycin		√	
Selenium sulfide	√	√	
Semduramicin		√	
Silver			√
Silver oxide			√
Soaps, stocks, vegetable oil, acidulated			√
Sodium 2-benzyl-4-chlorophenate			√

Sodium 2-mercaptobenzothiolate			√
Sodium arsenate			√
Sodium bisulfate			√
Sodium bromide			√
Sodium chlorate			√
Sodium chloride			√
Sodium dichloroisocyanurate dihydrate			√
Sodium dichloro-s-triazinetrione			√
Sodium dichromate			√
Sodium dimethyldithiocarbamate			√
Sodium dodecylbenzenesulfonate			√
Sodium hypochlorite	√		√
Sodium metasilicate			√
Sodium o-phenyphenate			√
Sodium perforate monohydrate			√
Sodium phenate			√
Sparfloxin	√		
Spectinomycin	√	√	
Spiramycin	√		
Streptomycin	√	√	
Sulbactam	√		
Sulfabenzamide	√		
Sulfabromomethazine		√	
Sulfacetamide	√		
Sulfachloropyrazine	√	√	
Sulfachlorpryidazine	√	√	
Sulfacytine	√		
Sulfadiazine	√	√	
Sulfadimethoxine		√	
Sulfadoxine	√		
Sulfaethoxypyridazine		√	
Sulfamerazine	√	√	
Sulfameter	√		
Sulfamethazine	√	√	
Sulfamethizole		√	
Sulfamethizole	√		
Sulfamethoxazole	√		
Sulfanilamide	√		
Sulfanitran		√	
Sulfapyridine	√		

Sulfaquinoxaline		√	√
Sulfasalazine	√		
Sulfathiazole	√	√	
Sulfisoxazole	√	√	
Sulfomyxin		√	
Sulfonated oleic acid, sodium salt			√
Sulfoxone	√		
Tazobactam	√		
Telavancin	√		
Telithromycin	√		
Tetrachlorophenyl			√
Tetracycline	√	√	
Tetradecyl alcohol			√
Tetraglycine hydroperiodide			√
Tetrakis (hydroxymethyl) phosphonium sulphate			√
Thimersal	√		
Thiocyanomethylthio benzothiazole			√
Thymol	√	√	√
Tiamulin		√	
Ticarcillin	√	√	
Tilmicosin		√	
Tobramycin	√		
Tolyl diiodomethyl sulfone			√
Triaza-1-azoniatricyclo (3.3.1.1 superscript 3,7) decane, 1-methyl-chloride			√
Tributyltin benzoate			√
Tributyltin fluoride			√
Tributyltin maleate			√
Tributyltin methacrylate			√
Trichloromelamine			√
Trichloro-s-triazinetrione			√
Triclocarban	√		
Triclosan (Irgasan)	√	√	√
Triethanolamine			√
Triethylene glycol			√
Triethylhexahydro-s-triazine			√
Trimethoprim	√	√	
Trimethoxys ilyl propyl dimethyl octadecyl ammonium chloride			√
Tripropyltin oxide			√

Trisodium (2-hydroxyethyl) ethylenediaminetriacetate			√
Trisodium phosphate			√
Trisulfapyrimidine	√		
Troleandomycin	√		
Trovafloxacin	√		
Tulathromycin		√	
Tylosin		√	
Undecylenic acid			√
Valacyclovir	√		
Vancomycin	√		
Virginiamycin		√	
Xylenol			√
Zinc			√
Zinc 2-pyridinethiol-1-oxide			√
Zinc chloride			√
Zinc naphthenate			√
Zinc oxide			√
Zinc sulfate	√		√
Zinc sulfate monohydrate			√
Ziram			√
Zoalene		√	

APPENDIX B. FEDERAL
LEGISLATION PENDING

Two important bills have recently been introduced in the U.S. Congress for the purpose of addressing the problem of growing resistance to antimicrobials used in human medicine.

On November 6, 2007, Senators Hatch and Brown introduced S. 2313, a bill to amend the Public Health Service Act to establish an "Office of Antimicrobial Resistance, Task Force, and Advisory Board" to gather and publish information about the amount of antimicrobials used, trends in the development of resistance, and to recommend procedures to mitigate resistance. The law would authorize expenditures of $45,000,000 the first year, $65,000,000 the second years, $120,000,000 the third year, and "such sums as may be necessary for each subsequent fiscal year"; however, at least one-third of the funds are to go to the Center for Disease Control and Prevention.

On February 12, 2007 Senators Kennedy, Snowe, Reed, and Brown introduced S. 549, a bill intended to preserve the effectiveness of medically important antibiotics by phasing out use of certain antibiotics for nontherapeutic purposes in food animals. It also proposes to defray the expense of such action to farmers.

These two bills are reproduced in the following pages.

LEGISLATION TO FUND RESEARCH AND INFORMATION COLLECTION ON ANTIMICROBIAL RESISTANCE

110TH CONGRESS

1ST SESSION

S. 2313

To amend the Public Health Service Act to enhance efforts to address antimicrobial resistance.

IN THE SENATE OF THE UNITED STATES
NOVEMBER 6, 2007
A BILL

To amend the Public Health Service Act to enhance efforts to address antimicrobial resistance.

Be it enacted by the Senate and House of Representatives of the United States of America in Congress assembled,

SECTION 1. SHORT TITLE.

This Act may be cited as the "Strategies to Address Antimicrobial Resistance Act".

SEC. 2. FINDINGS.

The Congress finds as follows:

(1) The advent of the antibiotic era has saved millions of lives and allowed for incredible medical progress; however, the increased use and overuse of anti-microbial drugs have correlated with increased rates of antimicrobial resistance.

(2) Through mutation as well as other mechanisms, bacteria and other infectious disease-causing organisms—viruses, fungi, and parasites—develop resistance to antimicrobial drugs over time. The more antimicrobial drugs are used, whether appropriately or inappropriately, the more this contributes to the development of antimicrobial resistance.

(3) Scientific evidence suggests that the source of antimicrobial resistance in humans is not just limited to use of antimicrobial drugs in humans, but may in fact also be from food-producing animals which are exposed to antimicrobial drugs.

(4) A study estimates that in 2005 more than 94,000 invasive methicillin-resistant Staphylococcus aureus (MRSA) infections occurred in the United States and more than 18,500 of these infections resulted in death.

(5) Each year, nearly 2,000,000 people contract bacterial infections in hospitals and approximately 22 90,000 of these people die from these infections.

(6) The costs of antimicrobial-resistant bacterial diseases are hard to quantify, but a 1995 report by the Office of Technology Assessment of and agency of Congress, which looked at 6 different antimicrobial-resistant strains of bacteria, calculated that the minimum nationwide hospital costs of just these strains of bacteria accounted for $1,300,000,000 annually in 1992 dollars ($1,870,000,000 in 2006 dollars).

(7) The cost to society of antimicrobial-resistant infections will only rise as antimicrobial resistance continues to spread.

SEC. 3. ANTIMICROBIAL RESISTANCE TASK FORCE.

(a) IN GENERAL.—Section 319E of the Public Health Service Act (42 U.S.C. 247d–5) is amended—

(1) in subsection (a)—

(A) in the subsection heading, by striking "TASK FORCE" and inserting the following: "OFFICE OF ANTIMICROBIAL RESISTANCE, TASK FORCE, AND ADVISORY BOARD";

(B) in paragraph (1)—

(i) by striking "as of the date of the enactment of this section" and inserting "September 30, 2006"; and

(ii) by adding at the end the following: "The Secretary shall, not later than 1 year after the date of enactment of the Strategies to Address Antimicrobial

Resistance Act, establish an Office of Antimicrobial Resistance in the Office of the Secretary and appoint a director to that Office. The Secretary shall, not later than 1 year after the date of enactment of such Act, establish the Public Health Antimicrobial Advisory Board as an advisory board to the Director of the Office of Antimicrobial Resistance. The Director of the Office of Antimicrobial Resistance shall serve as the Director of the task force and supervise the activities of the Office, task force, and advisory board.";

(C) by amending paragraph (2) to read as follows:

"(2) MEMBERS.—

"(A) MEMBERS OF THE ANTIMICROBIAL RESISTANCE TASK FORCE.—The task force described in paragraph (1) shall be composed of representatives of such Federal agencies as the Secretary determines necessary, including representation of the following:

"(i) The Office of Antimicrobial Resistance.

"(ii) The Assistant Secretary of Preparedness and Response.

"(iii) The Centers for Disease Control and Prevention.

"(iv) The Food and Drug Administration.

"(v) The National Institutes of Health.

"(vi) The Agency for Healthcare Research and Quality.

"(vii) The Centers for Medicare & Medicaid Services.

"(viii) The Health Resources and Services Administration.

"(ix) The Department of Agriculture.

"(x) The Department of Education.

"(xi) The Department of Defense.

"(xii) The Department of Veterans Affairs.

"(xiii) The Environmental Protection Agency.

"(xiv) The Department of Homeland Security.

"(B) MEMBERS OF THE PUBLIC HEALTH ANTIMICROBIAL ADVISORY BOARD.—

"(i) IN GENERAL.—The Public Health Antimicrobial Advisory Board shall be composed of 13 voting members, appointed by the Secretary. Such members shall include experts from the medical professions (including hospital and community-based physicians), public health, veterinary, research, and international health communities.

"(ii) TERMS.—Each member appointed under clause (i) shall be appointed for a term of 3 years, except that of the 13 members first appointed—

"(I) 4 shall be appointed for a l5 term of 12 months; and

"(II) 4 shall be appointed for a term of 2 years.

"(iii) CHAIR.—The Secretary shall appoint a Chair of the Public Health Antimicrobial Advisory Board from among its members to lead and supervise the activities of the advisory board.";

(D) in paragraph (3)(B), by striking "in consultation with the task force described in paragraph (1) and" and inserting "acting through the Director of the Office of Antimicrobial Resistance and the Director of the Centers for Disease Control and Prevention, and in consultation with"; and

(E) by amending paragraph (4) to read as follows:

"(4) MEETINGS AND DUTIES.—

"(A) OFFICE OF ANTIMICROBIAL RESISTANCE DUTIES.—The Director of the Office of Antimicrobial Resistance, working in conjunction with the Federal agencies that are represented on the task force described in paragraph (1), shall issue an update to the Public Health Action Plan to Combat Antimicrobial Resistance within months of the establishment of the Office and biennial updates thereafter. The updates shall include enhanced plans for addressing antimicrobial resistance in the United States and internationally. The

Director of the Office shall post on a website these updates as well as summaries of all non-proprietary data the Task Force makes available. The Director of the Office of Antimicrobial Resistance shall, as appropriate—

"'(i) establish benchmarks for achieving the goals set forth in the action plan;

"(ii) assess the ongoing, observed patterns of emergence of antimicrobial resistance, and their impact on clinical outcomes in terms of how patients feel, function, or survive;

"(iii) assess how antimicrobial products are being used in humans, animals, and plants, and the impact of such use in furthering the development of resistance and the implications thereof for patient safety and public health;

"(iv) establish a priority list of human infectious diseases with the greatest need for development of new point-of-care and other diagnostics, antimicrobial drugs, and vaccines, and in particular serious and life threatening bacterial diseases, for which there are few or no diagnostic or treatment options;

"(v) recommend basic, clinical, epidemiological, prevention, and translational research where additional federally supported studies may be beneficial;

"(vi) recommend how to support antimicrobial development through the Food and Drug Administration's Critical Path Initiative;

"(vii) recommend how best to strengthen and link antimicrobial resistance-related surveillance and prevention and control activities; and

"(viii) collaborate with the Assistant Secretary for Preparedness and Response to ensure that strategies to address antimicrobial-resistance are coordinated with initiatives aimed at Severe Acute Respiratory Syndrome, bioterrorism, and other emerging health threats.

"(B) ANTIMICROBIAL RESISTANCE TASK FORCE MEETINGS AND DU-
TIES.—

"(i) MEETINGS.—The Antimicrobial Resistance Task Force shall convene pe-
riodically as the Director of the Antimicrobial Resistance Task Force determines
to be appropriate, but not fewer than twice a year, to consider issues relating to
antimicrobial resistance.

"(ii) PUBLIC HEALTH ACTION PLAN.—At least twice a year, the task3 force
shall have a meeting to review, discuss, and further develop the Public Health
Action Plan to Combat Antimicrobial Resistance issued by the interagency task
force on antimicrobial resistance in 2001. Among other issues, the task force may
discuss and review, based on current need or concern—

"(I) antimicrobial clinical susceptibility concentrations proposed, established, or
updated by the Food and Drug Administration;

"(II) data obtained by government agencies and, as possible, by private sources
on emerging antimicrobial resistance related to clinical outcomes in terms of how
patients function, feel, or survive as well as data related to how antimicrobial drugs
may have been used inappropriately;

"(III) surveillance data and prevention and control activities regarding emerging
antimicrobial resistance from reliable sources including the Centers for Disease
Control and Prevention, the Food and Drug Administration, the Department of
Defense, the Department of Veterans Affairs, the Department of Agriculture, the
Environmental Protection Agency, and as feasible from private sources and inter-
national bodies;

"(IV) data on the amount of antimicrobial products used in humans, animals, and
plants from reliable sources including data from the Centers for Disease Control
and Prevention, the Food and Drug Administration, the Environmental Protection
Agency, the Department of Veterans Affairs, the Centers for Medicare & Medicaid Services, the Department of Homeland Security, and the Department of
Agriculture, and as feasible from private sources and international bodies;

"(V) reports of federally supported antimicrobial resistance research and antimicrobial drug development research activities (including clinical, epidemiological,
prevention, and translational research) obtained from Federal agencies, as well as

reports of research sponsored by other countries, industry, and non-governmental organizations;

"(VI) reports on efforts by the Food and Drug Administration to develop policies and guidances which encourage antimicrobial drug development and appropriate use while maintaining high standards for safety and effectiveness;

"(VII) health plan employer data and information set (HEDIS) measures pertaining to appropriate use of antimicrobial drugs; and

"(VIII) other data and issues the task force identifies as relevant to the issue of antimicrobial resistance.

"(iii) PENDING APPLICATIONS.—The Food and Drug Administration may consult with the Director of the Office of Antimicrobial Resistance concerning the pending application of any antimicrobial drug application submitted to the Secretary under section 505 or 512 of the Federal Food, Drug, and Cosmetic Act or the Public Health Service Act.

"(C) PUBLIC HEALTH ANTIMICROBIAL ADVISORY BOARD MEETINGS AND DUTIES.—

"(i) MEETINGS.—The Public Health Antimicrobial Advisory Board shall meet as the Chair of the Public Health Antimicrobial Advisory Board determines to be appropriate, but not fewer than 2 times each year.

"(ii) RECOMMENDATIONS.—The Public Health Antimicrobial Advisory Board shall make recommendations to the Secretary, and the Office of Antimicrobial Resistance, regarding—

"(I) ways to encourage the availability of an adequate supply of safe and effective antimicrobial products;

"(II) research priorities and other measures (such as antimicrobial drug resistance management plans) to enhance the safety and efficacy of antimicrobial products;

"(III) how best to implement and update the goals of the Public Health Action Plan to Combat Antimicrobial Resistance;

"(IV) incentives necessary to establish uniform mechanisms and data sets for State reporting of resistance data;

"(V) the adequacy of existing surveillance systems to collect antimicrobial resistance data and how best to improve the collection, reporting, and analysis of such data;

"(VI) the development of a national plan for the collection and analysis of isolates of resistant pathogens, including establishing priorities as to which isolates should be collected;

"(VII) the implementation and evaluation of interventions to promote appropriate antimicrobial drug use in both inpatient and outpatient settings; and

"(VIII) areas for government, nongovernment, and international cooperation to strengthen implementation of the Public Health Action Plan to Combat Antimicrobial Resistance.

"(D) AVAILABILITY OF INFORMATION.—

The Office of Antimicrobial Resistance shall ensure that all information shall be made available to the public on the website described in subparagraph (A) consistent with section 7 of the Strategies to Address Antimicrobial Resistance Act.";

(2) by amending subsection (b) to read as follows:

"(b) ANTIMICROBIAL RESISTANCE RESEARCH AND PRODUCT DEVELOPMENT.—The Secretary, acting through the Director of the Office of Antimicrobial Resistance, the Director of the Centers for Disease Control and Prevention, and the Director of the National Institutes of Health, and in consultation with other Federal agencies, shall develop an antimicrobial resistance strategic research plan that strengthens existing epidemiological, interventional, clinical, behavioral, translational, and basic research efforts to advance the understanding of—

"(1) the development, implementation, and efficacy of interventions to prevent and control the emergence and transmission of antimicrobial resistance;

"(2) how best to optimize antimicrobial effectiveness while limiting the emergence of resistance, including addressing issues related to duration of therapy, effectiveness of therapy in self-resolving diseases, and determining populations most likely to benefit from antimicrobial drugs;

"(3) the extent to which the use of antimicrobial products in humans, animals, plants, and other uses accelerates development and transmission of antimicrobial resistance;

"(4) the natural histories of infectious diseases (including defining the disease, diagnosis, severity, and the time course of illness)

"(5) the development of new therapeutics, including antimicrobial drugs, biologics, and devices against resistant pathogens, and in particular diseases for which few or no therapeutics are in development;

"(6) the development and testing of medical diagnostics to identify patients with infectious disease and identify the exact cause of infectious diseases syndromes, particularly with respect to the detection of pathogens resistant to antimicrobial drugs;

"(7) the epidemiology, pathogenesis, mechanisms, and genetics of antimicrobial resistance; and

"(8) the sequencing of the genomes, or other DNA analysis, or other comparative analysis of priority pathogens (as determined by the advisory board), in collaboration with the Department of Defense and the Joint Genome Institute of the Department of Energy."; and

(3) in subsection (c)—

    (A) by inserting "acting through the Director of the Office of Antimicrobial Resistance," after "The Secretary,"; and

    (B) by striking "members of the task force described in subsection (a),";

(4) in subsection (d)(1), by inserting ", through the Office of Antimicrobial Resistance," after "The Secretary"; and

(5) in subsection (e)—1 (A) in paragraph (1), by inserting ", acting through the Director of the Office of Antimicrobial Resistance," after "The Secretary";

(B) in paragraph (3), by inserting ", acting through the Office of Antimicrobial Resistance," after "The Secretary"; and

(C) by adding at the end the following:

"(4) PREFERENCE IN MAKING AWARDS.—In making awards under paragraph (1), the Secretary shall give preference to eligible entities that will use grant funds to establish demonstration projects to assess the scope of the antimicrobial resistance problem and the level of appropriate and inappropriate use of antimicrobial drugs especially related to acute bacterial otitis media and upper respiratory infections, and in particular acute exacerbation of chronic bronchitis, including the validation of models that may lead to the development of quality measures for health care providers prescribing antimicrobial drugs.".

(b) ENSURE ACCESS TO ANTIMICROBIAL DATA AND RESEARCH.—The Director of the Office of Antimicrobial Resistance shall work with the agencies represented on the Antimicrobial Resistance Task Force to identify relevant data and formats, and mechanisms for communicating such data to the Office of Antimicrobial Resistance and the Antimicrobial Resistance Task Force, including relevant data obtained by the agencies through contracts with other organizations, including—

(1) use and clinical outcomes data on patients receiving antimicrobial drugs for the treatment, prevention, or diagnosis of infection or infectious diseases;

(2) surveillance data regarding emerging antimicrobial drug resistance;

(3) susceptibility data related to antimicrobial drug use;

(4) data related to the amount of antimicrobial products used in humans, animals, and plants;

(5) data from federally funded research intended to support antimicrobial drug development;

111

(6) data demonstrating the impact of research, surveillance, and pre-vention and control initiatives in understanding and controlling antimicrobial resistance; and

(7) data regarding implementation and evaluation of interventions to improve antimicrobial drug prescribing practices.

SEC. 4. COLLECTION OF ANTIMICROBIAL DRUG DATA.

(a) SUBMISSION OF HUMAN AND ANIMAL DRUG DISTRIBUTION DATA.—Chapter V of the Federal Food, Drug, and Cosmetic Act (21 U.S.C. 351 et seq.) is amended by inserting after section 512 the following:

"SEC. 512A. SUBMISSION OF HUMAN AND ANIMAL DRUG DISTRI-BUTION DATA.

"(a) IN GENERAL.—Notwithstanding any other provision of law, the Secretary shall require that human drug distribution data required to be submitted for each calendar year under section 314.81(b)(ii) of title 21, Code of Federal Regulations (or any successor regulation) and the animal drug distribution data required to be submitted for each such calendar year under section 514.80(b)(4)(i) of title 21, Code of Federal Regulations (or any successor regulation) be—

"(1) submitted not later than 60 days after the beginning of the subsequent calendar year; and

"(2) made available to the Office of Antimicrobial Resistance, the Antimicrobial Resistance Task Force, and the Public Health Antimicrobial Advisory Board.

"(b) CONFIDENTIALITY.—The Office of Antimicrobial Resistance, the Antimicrobial Resistance Task Force, and the Public Health Antimicrobial Advisory Board shall sign a confidentiality agreement to protect proprietary information made available under subsection (a)(2).".

(b) COMPARABLE DATA.—

(1) IN GENERAL.—The Secretary, acting through the Director of the Office of Antimicrobial Resistance, shall explore opportunities to secure from private ven-

dors reliable and comparable animal and human antimicrobial drug consumption data (volume antimicrobial distribution data and antimicrobial use, including prescription data) by State or metropolitan area, as necessary, to supplement the antimicrobial drug consumption data to be collected under this section for the purpose of demonstrating how the consumption of antimicrobial drugs for human and animal uses may affect the development of resistance over time and within geographic locations and to institute preventive interventions.

(2) NEGOTIATIONS.—The Director of the Office of Antimicrobial Resistance may enter into negotiations with private vendors to determine acceptable formats for making summaries of antimicrobial drug consumption data that is collected under this section publicly available for research purposes while maintaining the confidentiality of any proprietary commercial data.

(3) OTHER MEANS TO SECURE DATA.—If the Director of the Office of Antimicrobial Resistance is not able to secure sufficient supplemental antimicrobial drug consumption data for human and animal uses through private vendors as provided for in this section, the Secretary shall consider other means to secure such consumption data, including through the conduct of surveys about how antimicrobial drugs are used in various settings and make such data available to the public consistent with section 7.

(c) COLLECTION OF ANTIMICROBIAL PRESCRIPTION

DATA.—

(1) CLINICAL OUTCOMES DATA.—The Director of the Office of Antimicrobial Resistance shall work with the Under Secretary for Health of the Department of Veterans Affairs and the Administrator of the Centers for Medicare & Medicaid Services to collect relevant drug utilization data and clinical outcomes data, as determined relevant by the Director of the Office of Antimicrobial Resistance, on patients who receive services funded by such agencies and who are receiving prescription antimicrobial agents for the treatment, prevention, or diagnosis of infection or infectious diseases.

113

(2) ORGANIZATION.—Any data collected under paragraph (1) shall be organized by—

(A) indication (including results of diagnostic studies when available);

(B) dosage;

(C) route of administration;

(D) duration;

(E) age of the patient; and

(F) geographic region.

(d) PUBLIC AVAILABILITY OF SUMMARIES.—The Director of the Office of Antimicrobial Resistance shall make summaries of the data received under this section publicly available by antimicrobial drug class and ensure that such summaries are updated and published, in a manner consistent with section 7, at least once annually on the website described in section 319E(a)(4)(A) of the Public Health Service Act (42 U.S.C. 247d–5(a)(4)(A)) in orde to support epidemiologic and microbiologic research. In the case of an antimicrobial drug class where only one antimicrobial drug has been approved, such summary data shall not be made public.

SEC. 5. ANTIMICROBIAL RESISTANCE CLINICAL RESEARCH AND PUBLIC HEALTH NETWORK.

(a) IN GENERAL.—The Secretary, through the Director of the Centers for Disease Control and Prevention and the Director of the National Institutes of Health, shall establish at least 10 Antimicrobial Resistance Clinical Research and Public Health Network sites to strengthen the national capacity to—

(1) describe and confirm regional outbreaks through surveillance of locally available clinical specimens;

(2) assess, integrate, and address local and national antimicrobial resistance patterns;

(3) facilitate research on prevention, control, and treatment of resistant organisms; and

(4) serve as a clinical trials network for optimizing antimicrobial drug effectiveness.

(b) GEOGRAPHIC DISTRIBUTION.—The sites established under subsection (a) shall be geographically distributed across the United States, based in academic centers, health departments, and existing surveillance sites.

(c) RESPONSIBILITIES.—The sites established under subsection (a) shall—

(1) monitor the emergence and changes in the patterns of antimicrobial resistant pathogens in individuals;

(2) study the molecular epidemiology of such pathogens;

(3) evaluate the efficacy of new and existing interventions to prevent or limit the emergence of antimicrobial resistance throughout the geographic region of the site;

(1) provide to the Centers for Disease Control and Prevention isolates of resistant pathogens, and in particular, pathogens that show new or atypical patterns of resistance adversely affecting public health;

(5) conduct clinical research to develop natural histories of infectious disease and to study duration of antimicrobial use related to resistance development, among other things;

(6) assess the feasibility, cost-effectiveness, and appropriateness of surveillance and screening programs in differing health care and institutional settings, such as schools; and

(7) evaluate current treatment protocols and make appropriate recommendations on best practices for treating drug resistant infections.

(d) COORDINATION.—The sites established under subsection (a) may share data and cooperate with the Centers for Disease Control and Prevention and the National Institutes of Health.

(e) DATA ACCESS.—The Director of the Centers for Disease Control and Prevention and the Director of the National Institutes of Health shall ensure that summary reports of data obtained by the Antimicrobial Resistance Clinical Research and Public Health Network sites are made accessible to the Antimicrobial Task Force for review on an ongoing basis.

SEC. 6. AUTHORIZATION OF APPROPRIATIONS.

Section 319E(g) of the Public Health Service Act (42 U.S.C. 247d–5(g)) is amended to read as follows:

"(g) AUTHORIZATION OF APPROPRIATIONS.—

"(1) AUTHORIZATION.—There are authorized to be appropriated to carry out this section (other than subsection (b)) $45,000,000 for fiscal year 2008, $65,000,000 for fiscal year 2009, $120,000,000 for fiscal year 2010, and such sums as may be necessary for each subsequent fiscal year.

"(2) ALLOCATION.—Of the amount appropriated to carry out this section for a fiscal year, not less than one-third of such amount shall be made available for activities of the Centers for Disease Control and Prevention under subsections (a)(3)(B) and (c), of which at least one-third of such amount shall be made available for the Centers for Disease Control and Prevention educational programs dedicated to the reduction of inappropriate antimicrobial use.".

SEC. 7. PROTECTION OF CONFIDENTIAL AND NATIONAL SECURITY INFORMATION.

Except as otherwise required by law, this Act (and the amendments made by this Act) shall not permit public disclosure of trade secrets, confidential commercial information, or material inconsistent with national security that is obtained by any person under this Act.

Thomas K. Shotwell

LEGISLATION PROHIBITING SUBTHERAPEUTIC USE OF ANTIBIOTICS IN FOOD PRODUCING ANIMALS

110th CONGRESS

1st Session

S. 549

To amend the Federal Food, Drug, and Cosmetic Act to preserve the effectiveness of medically important antibiotics used in the treatment of human and animal diseases.

IN THE SENATE OF THE UNITED STATES
February 12, 2007

A BILL

To amend the Federal Food, Drug, and Cosmetic Act to preserve the effectiveness of medically important antibiotics used in the treatment of human and animal diseases.

Be it enacted by the Senate and House of Representatives of the United States of America in Congress assembled,

SECTION 1. SHORT TITLE; TABLE OF CONTENTS.

(a)　Short Title- This Act may be cited as the 'Preservation of Antibiotics for Medical Treatment Act of 2007'.

(b)　Table of Contents- The table of contents of this Act is as follows:

117

SUPERBUGS

TITLE I – SAFETY OF CRITICAL ANTIMICROBIAL ANIMAL DRUGS

Sec. 101. Proof of safety of critical antimicrobial animal drugs.

TITLE II – USE OF CRITICAL ANTIMICROBIAL ANIMAL DRUGS IN AGRICULTURE

Sec. 201. Assistance to defray expenses of livestock or poultry producers in phasing out nontherapeutic use of critical antimicrobial animal drugs.

Sec. 202. Research and demonstration programs.

Sec. 203. Collection of data on critical antimicrobial animal drugs.

SEC. 2. FINDINGS.

Congress Finds that –

(1)(A) in January 2001, a Federal interagency task force released an action plan to address the continuing decline in effectiveness of antibiotics against common bacterial infections, referred to as antibiotic resistance;

(B) the task force determined that antibiotic resistance is a growing menace to all people and poses a serious threat to public health; and

(C) the task force cautioned that if current trends continue, treatments for common infections will become increasingly limited and expensive, and, in some cases, nonexistent;

(2) antibiotic resistance, resulting in a reduced number of effective antibiotics, may significantly impair the ability of the United States to respond to terrorist attacks involving bacterial infections or a large influx of hospitalized patients;

(3)(A) any overuse or misuse of antibiotics contributes to the spread of antibiotic resistance, whether in human medicine or in agriculture; and

(B) recognizing the public health threat caused by antibiotic resistance, Congress took several steps to curb antibiotic overuse in human medicine through amendments to the Public Health Service Act (42 U.S.C. 201 et seq.) made by section 102 of the Public Health Threats and Emergencies Act (114 Stat. 2315), but has not yet addressed antibiotic overuse in agriculture;

(4) in a March 2003 report, the National Academy of Sciences stated that –

(A) a decrease in antimicrobial use in human medicine alone will have little effect on the current situation; and

(B) substantial efforts must be made to decrease inappropriate overuse in animals and agriculture;

(5)(A) an estimated 70 percent of the antibiotics and other antimicrobial (sic) used in the United States are fed to farm animals for nontherapeutic purposes, including—

(i) growth promotion; and

(ii) compensation for crowded, unsanitary, and stressful farming and transportation conditions; and

(B) unlike human use of antibiotics, these nontherapeutic uses in animals typically do not require a prescription;

(6)(A) many scientific studies confirm that the nontherapeutic use of antibiotics in agricultural animals contributes to the development of antibiotic-resistant bacterial infections in people;

(B) the periodical entitled 'Clinical Infectious Diseases' published a report in June 2002, based on a 2-year review by experts in human and veterinary medicine, public health, microbiology, biostatistics, and risk analysis, of more than 500 scientific studies on the human health impacts of antimicrobial use in agriculture; and

(C) the report recommended that antimicrobial agents should no longer be used in agriculture in the absence of disease, but should be limited to therapy for diseased individual animals and prophylaxis when disease is documented in a herd or flock;

(7)(A) the United States Geological Survey reported in March 2002 that antibiotics were present in 48 percent of the streams tested nationwide; and

(B) almost half of the tested streams were downstream from agricultural operations;

(8) an April 1999 study by the General Accounting Office concluded that resistant strains of 3 microorganisms that cause food-borne illness or disease in humans--Salmonella, Campylobacter, and E. coli--are linked to the use of antibiotics in animals;

(9)(A) in January 2003, Consumer Reports published test results on poultry products bought in grocery stores nationwide showing disturbingly high levels of Campylobacter and Salmonella bacteria that were resistant to antibiotics used to treat food-borne illnesses; and

(B) further studies showed similar results in other meat products;

(10) in October 2001, the New England Journal of Medicine published an editorial urging a ban on nontherapeutic use of medically important antibiotics in animals;

(11)(A) in 1999, the European Union banned the practice of feeding medically important antibiotics to animals other than for disease treatment or control, and prior to that, individual European countries had banned the use of specific antibiotics in animal feed; and

(B) those countries have experienced no significant impact on animal health or productivity, food safety, or meat prices, and more importantly, levels of resistant bacteria have declined sharply;

(12) in 1998, the National Academy of Sciences noted that antibiotic-resistant bacteria generate a minimum of $4,000,000,000 to $5,000,000,000 in costs to United States society and individuals yearly;

(13) a year later, the National Academy of Sciences estimated that eliminating the use of all antibiotics as feed additives would cost each American consumer less than $5 to $10 per year;

(14) the American Medical Association, the American Public Health Association, the National Association of County and City Health Officials, and the National Campaign for Sustainable Agriculture, are among the more than 300 organizations representing health, consumer, agricultural, environmental, humane, and other interests that support enactment of legislation to phase out nontherapeutic use in farm animals of medically important antibiotics;

120

(15) the Federal Food, Drug, and Cosmetic Act (21 U.S.C. 301 et seq.)—

    (A)   requires that all drugs be shown to be safe before the drugs are approved; and

    (B)   places the burden on manufacturers to account for health consequences and prove safety;

(16)(A) the Food and Drug Administration recently modified the drug approval process for antibiotics to recognize the development of resistant bacteria as an important aspect of safety;

(B) however, most antibiotics currently used in animal production systems for nontherapeutic purposes were approved before the Food and Drug Administration began giving in-depth consideration to resistance during the drug-approval process; and

(C) the Food and Drug Administration has not established a schedule for reviewing those existing approvals;

(17)(A) the Food and Drug Administration has begun a process of evaluating the safety of antibiotics used in animal agriculture; and

(B) that process —

    (i) is a valuable contribution to public health; and

    (ii) may determine that there is a reasonable certainty of no harm from the use of certain antibiotics in animal agriculture;

(18)(A) an April 2004 study by the General Accounting Office concluded that Federal agencies do not collect the critical data on antibiotic use in animals that they need to support research on human health risks; and

(B) the report recommends that the Department of Agriculture and the Department of Health and Human Services develop and implement a plan to collect data on antibiotic use in animals; and

(19) certain nonroutine uses of antibiotics in animal agriculture to prevent animal disease are legitimate.

SUPERBUGS

SEC. 3. PURPOSE.

The purpose of this Act is to preserve the effectiveness of medically important antibiotics used in the treatment of human and animal diseases by phasing out use of certain antibiotics for nontherapeutic purposes in food-producing animals.

TITLE I – SAFETY OF CRITICAL ANTIMICROBIAL ANIMAL DRUGS

SEC. 101. PROOF OF SAFETY OF CRITICAL ANTIMICROBIAL ANIMAL DRUGS.

(a) Definitions- Section 201 of the Federal Food, Drug, and Cosmetic Act (21 U.S.C. 321) is amended by adding at the end the following:

'(rr) Critical Antimicrobial Animal Drug- The term 'critical antimicrobial animal drug' means a drug that–

'(1) is intended for use in food-producing animals; and

'(2) is composed wholly or partly of–

'(A) any kind of penicillin, tetracycline, macrolide, lincosamide, streptogramin, aminoglycoside, sulfonamide; or

'(B) any other drug or derivative of a drug that is used in humans or intended for use in humans to treat or prevent disease or infection caused by microorganisms.

'(ss) Nontherapeutic Use- The term 'nontherapeutic use', with respect to a critical antimicrobial animal drug, means any use of the drug as a feed or water additive for an animal in the absence of any clinical sign of disease in the animal for growth promotion, feed efficiency, weight gain, routine disease prevention, or other routine purpose.'

(b) Nontherapeutic Use- Section 512(d)(1) of the Federal Food, Drug, and Cosmetic Act (21 U.S.C. 360b(d)(1)) is amended–

(1) in the first sentence–

(A) in subparagraph (H), by striking 'or' at the end;

122

(B) by redesignating subparagraph (I) as subparagraph (J); and

(C) by inserting after subparagraph (H) the following:

'(I) with respect to a critical antimicrobial animal drug or a drug of the same chemical class as a critical antimicrobial animal drug, the applicant has failed to demonstrate that there is a reasonable certainty of no harm to human health due to the development of antimicrobial resistance that is attributable, in whole or in part, to the nontherapeutic use of the drug; or'; and

(2) in the second sentence, by striking '(A) through (I)' and inserting '(A) through (J)'.

APPENDIX C. ANTIBACTERIALS USED IN OR ON ANIMALS

General

The classification of animal drugs as "antibacterials" is complex because a great many products with label claims for something other than therapeutic use against bacteria contain active ingredients that have antibacterial activity. Antifungals, antiprotozoals, and drugs intended for control of parasites often have some ability to affect an animal's microflora, either internally or externally or both. Unfortunately, hard data are not always available on such drugs to determine how much antibacterial activity they may have, plus, decisions are difficult due to the well established fact that antibacterials added to medicated feeds at doses well below the amount needed to inhibit bacterial growth in the laboratory produce drastic changes in intestinal flora as well as improving growth and feed efficiency. Anticoccidials such as nitromide, aklomide, zoalene and amprolium are not likely to have enough antibacterial activity to be of concern; however, in an abundance of caution all anticoccidials are included in the following listing even though only coccidiostats classified as ionophores are widely recognized as antibiotics. While some will object to their inclusion, the need for understanding that almost everything we use has some antibacterial activity at some dose and if we are to understand how bacterial gene pools evolve we need the broadest picture possible. For example, we know bacteria, protozoa and fungi exchange genes, to some uncertain extent, for resistance to substances we use to keep animals healthy and to improve their performance. Antifungals and products for the control of internal and external parasites are not included although there is a risk that some of these may have antibacterial activity or the ability to select for resistance through plasmids or specific genes. In due time these should be evaluated also.

125

SUPERBUGS

Underlining of Antibiotics to be Banned Under Proposed Legislation

Many efforts have been made to use legislation to restrict antibacterial uses but most have failed in the end. However, at the urging of consumer activists Senators Edward Kennedy and Olympia Snowe and Representative Louise Slaughter recently proposed legislation to ban all non-therapeutic uses of antibiotics in food-producing animals if those antibiotics are considered essential for protecting human health. Their proposed legislation defines non-therapeutic use as "use in the absence of any clinical sign of disease in the animal for growth promotion, feed efficiency, weight gain, routine disease prevention, or other routine purpose." It also defines "essential for protecting human health" to include penicillins, tetracyclines, macrolides, lincosamides, streptogramins, aminoglycosides, and sulfonamides, as well as some drugs related to them. In the following pages the non-therapeutic uses of those specific antibiotics have been underlined to illustrate exactly how many and which antibiotic uses the activists and legislators propose to ban. Non-therapeutic uses of other antibacterials have been listed but not underlined because the proposed legislation is restricted to antibiotics described in the legislation as essential to human health. All antibacterials are listed because they are all of concern in the control of antibiotic resistance. Although ionophore coccidiostats are classified as antibiotics by the scientific community and although resistance to at least one of them results in cross resistance to an antibiotic used in human medicine, the legislation seems unclear as to whether these are to be banned. Therefore these have not been underlined. Of course, non-therapeutic uses in non-food animals have not been underlined because the legislation does not address such uses.

Notices & Disclaimers

1. Sources

This itemization of FDA approved uses of antibiotics and other antibacterials was developed through personal contact with the manufacturers and FDA employees, by reviewing *Federal Register* notices regarding new animal drug application approvals and withdrawals, by reviewing *The Green Book* (FDA's semi-official listing of approved animal drugs published in cooperation with the University of Virginia), by reviewing *The Complete Handbook of Approved New Animal Drug Applications in the United States* published by Shotwell & Carr, Inc., by use of the *Freedom of Information Act*, and other sources such as company catalogues and advertisements that brought the existence of products to attention. Assembly and editing of this listing was a difficult task and sustained efforts have been made to avoid errors; however, with more than 1,300 entries some errors probably remain. The final authority on approved animal drugs is the FDA itself.

2. Multiple Approvals

Each FDA approval is product specific, that is, penicillin does not get approved for general use but rather for use in specific products at specific dosages for specific purposes in specific species. Likewise, many of the approvals issued by FDA are for products consisting of a fixed combination of antibacterials and, frequently, other active ingredients, sometimes as many as a total of four in a single product, two or three of which may be antibacterial to some extent. For example, many products contain an anticoccidial, an organic arsenical, and an antibiotic, all of which have some known or probable antibacterial activity when used as directed. Thus one product approval may appear separately under the generic names of each of the ingredients. The result is more than 1,300 entries for about 99 antibacterials in the following listing, even though the total number of formal FDA approvals actions for antibacterial products is considerably less than 1,300. One FDA action can approve the concurrent use of more than one antibacterial.

3. Format

Each approved antibacterial ingredient is listed in alphabetical order. Many ingredients are enhanced in some specific way when combined with another suitable molecule. In cases were an antibacterial may be combined with something else, that additional substance is identified in parentheses immediately following the generic name of the active ingredient. For example, bacitracin is marketed as bacitracin zinc or as bacitracin methylene disalicylate.

The following format is used throughout the listing:

FDA File (FDA issues this number upon receipt of an application for marketing of a product and it is a permanent reference for the drug product and the sponsor.)

Firm: (The name of the sponsor firm to whom the approval was issued.)

Use: (Lists the species to be treated and the dosage form. Antibacterial products restricted to prescription use only are indicated by "Rx only" or "VFD only". "VFD only" means the product can only be used in feed when such use is prescribed by a licensed veterinarian. All other feed additives are sold OTC.)

Dosage: (Provides the amount of antibacterial to be used and the duration of treatment - when available.)

Purpose: (Indicates whether the antibacterial is to be used to control, prevent, treat, etc., and the medical condition for which the drug is indicated.)

In reviewing the use of antibacterials in animals the terminology used to describe the intended purpose(s) of use is important. Additionally, the dosage and directions for use have been condensed or paraphrased to conserve space and to remove wording not relevant to the issues surrounding antibacterial resistance problems. When more than one antibacterial is present in a fixed combination product, "best efforts" have been employed to state the intended effect (claim) for the ingredient under which the listing occurs.

4. Intended Use(s)

The Center for Veterinary Medicine at the FDA controls labeling of approved drugs and makes various distinctions that are not always obvious. For example, the stated purpose may be "reduction in the severity of", "reduction in the incidence of", "prevention", "control", or "treatment", all of which have different implications for antibiotic use. For example, "prevention" indicates the antibacterial is to be used in healthy animals to prevent the occurrence of a specified disease. The dosage is usually lower than the full therapeutic dose and is usually at or higher than the minimum inhibitory level. This use may be limited to those cases where medical history of the premises, the herd, or the flock indicates there is a reasonable expectation the animals will contract the disease if they are not treated. "Control" is the term used to indicate the product is to be used in a flock or herd when a few animals have been diagnosed with a given disease that is likely to spread to the rest of the group if no action is taken. The dosage is usually at or above the minimum inhibitory level and near or at therapeutic levels. "Treatment" is used to indicate the product is to be used with one animal or a group of animals diagnosed with a specific disease and the full therapeutic dose and the treatment regimen are specified.

Of course, "increased rate of weight gain" (sometimes referred to as "growth promotion") is reserved for drugs that can be expected to result in more rapid weight gain and thereby cause the animals to complete the growing period at an earlier date. The dosage ranges from about one to 50 grams per ton of feed and is usually below the minimum inhibitory concentration. The terms "improved feed efficiency" and "increased feed efficiency" refer to the ability of an antibacterial to cause animals to gain more weight per unit of feed consumed. Again, the dosage ranges from about one to 50 grams per ton of feed. One cannot overemphasize that the weight of an antibiotic is a convenient but poor guide to the amount of antibacterial activity used.

Some FDA approvals are simply for use in the treatment or control of unnamed diseases caused by bacteria susceptible to that antibacterial. In some cases no specific bacteria are named. Thus the use is mostly left to the veterinarian's discretion based on information about the antibiotic's activity. Veterinarians are not permitted to write prescriptions for antibiotics or any other drug to be added to feed unless FDA has approved over-the-counter feed additive use of that product or, if not, has specified that veterinarians may write prescriptions in its approval of the drug product. Only a few such approvals have been issued and these are identified herein as "Rx (VFD) only".

Licensed veterinarians routinely use antibacterial drugs in ways that are not specifically included in the FDA approved labeling for the product and such uses are obviously not included here; however, FDA has prohibited extra-label use of chloramphenicol, dimetridazole, ipronidazole, furazolidone, nitrofurazone, sulfonamides in lactating dairy cattle (except approved use of sulfadimethoxine, sulfabromomethazine, and sulfaethoxypyridazine), fluoroquinolones, and glycopeptides.

The following product listing is organized alphabetically by antibacterial. It reveals a wide variety of antibacterials are approved, including the sulfonamides and many other products, such as chlorhexidine, a drug often considered to be an antiseptics or disinfectant, and a few (especially organic arsenicals and anticoccidials) with antibacterial activity even though the stated purpose for using the products seldom includes their antibacterial activity. Some of the listed anticoccidials reportedly have no antibacterial activity at the levels used in feed (nicarbazin, for example); however, antibiotics used at very low levels seem to have some antibacterial activity even though the minimum inhibitory concentration (MIC) is not reached in the feed. The question is not whether the anticoccidial is used at or above the MIC when added to feed or water but whether the drug has effects on the intestinal microflora at the level used. Until the full spectrum of antibacterial activity is reported for such substances one must assume there is a good chance such coccidostats may promote selection for some sort of antibiotic resistance or at least encourage selection for plasmids that can carry resistance and therefore must be of concern.

5. Duplications

Apparent duplications of entries attributed to the same firm should be understood as various combinations of antibacterials with other drugs that are not identified in that particular entry. For example, coccidiostats are universally used in chicken feed and any firm wishing to market an antibacterial growth promotant to also be mixed into the same feed must obtain FDA approval. Also, some products already contain more than one antibacterial. If so, the additional antibacterial ingredients can be found listed separately under the appropriate generic name. The repetition of the same drug used at the same dosage for the same condition in the same species occurs because sponsor firms develop a drug, an anticoccidial for example, and obtain FDA approval to market the product. The firm can then increase their share of the total market if the original drug can be approved for use in combination with one or two other drugs that expand the benefits, such as promoting growth and improving feed efficiency. FDA treats each of these applications for marketing as a different file. For this reason the same drug may appear repeatedly and a given FDA File number may appear under more than one antibacterial heading. Information on fixed combinations of all animal drugs may be found in the *Code of Federal Regulations* at Part 21; however, a user-friendly and often more current source of such information is the handbook of approved animal drugs maintained by the author *(The Complete Handbook of Approved New Animal Drug Applications in the United States*, ix + 913 pgs. Published and updated quarterly since 1980 by Shotwell & Carr, Inc., 1415 Halsey Way, Suite 304, Carrollton, Texas 75007-4455. www.shotcarr.com.).

6. General

The descriptions of intended use(s) and dosage(s) are condensed and often paraphrased to provide species to be treated, dosage, dosage form, duration of treatment, and purpose of use in as few words as possible, but includes information needed by anyone interested in antibiotic usage and antibiotic resistance. It does not reflect all the wording or the exact wording of the officially approved labeling.

This listing reveals bacitracin, roxarsone, and bambermycins are widely approved for growth promotion and feed efficiency in poultry while other antibacterials are approved for prevention, control, and therapy. In swine, tylosin is commonly used for disease prevention and control as well as growth promotion and feed efficiency, and, in combination with certain sulfonamides, for other disease treatments. In cattle, gentamicin and the tetracyclines remain popular for control or treatment of respiratory disease because of their low cost but newer antibiotics, such as tulathromycin, enrofloxacin and danofloxacin, are increasingly important. While identification of drug products approved by FDA under the generic drug act has relatively little bearing on antibiotic resistance they are easily identified because only generic drugs are assigned FDA File numbers of 200-000 and higher.

The presence of an FDA approval of an antibacterial for animal use does not necessarily indicate the product is being marketed, only that it is FDA approved for marketing. However, firms currently pay FDA $4,125 for an annual product fee and $52,700 for an annual drug establishment fee. Thus firms are unlikely to maintain FDA approvals very long if the product which is the subject of the approval is not marketed and is unlikely to be needed in the future.

This large file undergoes constant revisions as FDA acts to add new antibacterials, revise dosages, modify use directions, and withdraw or transfer approvals. Visit the website http://www.biontogeny.com to download and print (in PDF format) the most recent version of this appendix. Word searching is easy after downloading the file. Updated versions of this appendix will be available every six months.

ANTIBACTERIAL DRUG PRODUCTS APPROVED BY THE U.S. FOOD AND DRUG ADMINISTRATION FOR USE IN/ON ANIMALS

AKLOMIDE

FDA File **014-250**
Firm: **Fort Dodge Animal Health Division of Wyeth**
Use: **Chickens: Feed additive premix.**
Dosage: **227 Grams per ton of complete feed.**
Purpose: **Aid in the prevention of coccidiosis.**

FDA File **034-536**
Firm: **Fort Dodge Animal Health Division of Wyeth**
Use: **Chickens: Feed additive premix.**
Dosage: **227 Grams per ton of complete feed.**
Purpose: **Aid in the prevention of coccidiosis.**

FDA File **034-537**
Firm: **Fort Dodge Animal Health Division of Wyeth**
Use: **Chickens: Feed additive premix.**
Dosage: **227 Grams per ton of complete feed.**
Purpose: **Aid in the prevention of coccidiosis.**

FDA File **035-388**
Firm: **Fort Dodge Animal Health Division of Wyeth**

Use: **Chickens: Soluble Powder**
Dosage: **954 milligrams per gallon of water for 2 days followed by 5 days at 477 milligrams per gallon.**
Purpose: **Aid in the prevention and treatment of coccidiosis.**

AMIKACIN (SULFATE)

FDA File **127-892**
Firm: **Fort Dodge Animal Health Division of Wyeth**
Use: **Horses and Dogs:** Rx only **- Intrauterine, Intramuscular, Subcutaneous**
Dosage: **Horses: Infuse 400 milligrams per day for 3 days. Dogs: 5 milligrams twice daily for 7 to 21 days.**
Purpose: **Treatment of genital tract infections in mares and genitourinary tract infections and skin and soft tissue infections in dogs.**

FDA File **200-178**
Firm: **Phoenix Scientific, Inc.**
Use: **Horses and Dogs:** Rx only **- Intrauterine, Intramuscular, Subcutaneous**
Dosage: **Horses: Infuse 400 milligrams per day for 3 days. Dogs: 5 milligrams twice daily for 7 to 21 days.**

Purpose: **Treatment of genital tract infections in mares and treatment of genitourinary tract infections and skin and soft tissue infections in dogs.**

FDA File **200-181**
Firm: **Phoenix Scientific, Inc.**
Use: **Horses:** Rx only **- Intrauterine**
Dosage: **Infuse 400 milligrams per day for 3 days.**
Purpose: **Treatment of genital tract infections.**

AMOXICILLIN (TRIHYDRATE)

FDA File **055-078**
Firm: **Pfizer, Inc.**
Use: **Dogs:** Rx only **- Oral Tablet**
Dosage: **5 milligrams per pound of body weight daily for 5 to 7 days or 48 hours after all symptoms have subsided.**
Purpose: **For treatment of respiratory tract, genitourinary tract, gastrointestinal tract, soft tissue infections, and dermatitis.**

FDA File **055-080**
Firm: **Pfizer, Inc.**
Use: **Swine:** Rx only **- Oral Liquid**
Dosage: **40 milligrams twice daily until animal becomes asymptomatic but not to exceed 5 days.**
Purpose: **Treatment of colibacillosis in baby pigs weighing more than 10 pounds.**

FDA File **055-081**
Firm: **Pfizer, Inc.**
Use: **Cats:** Rx only **- Oral Tablet**
Dosage: **5 to 10 milligrams per pound of body weight per day for 5 to 7 days or until animal is asymptomatic.**

Purpose: **Treatment of upper respiratory, genitourinary, gastrointestinal tract, and skin and soft tissue infections.**

FDA File **055-085**
Firm: **Pfizer, Inc.**
Use: **Dogs and Cats:** Rx only **- Oral Suspension**
Dosage: **Dogs: 5 milligrams, cats 5 to 10 milligrams per pound of body weight. Administer twice per day for 5 to 7 days or until animal is asymptomatic.**
Purpose: **Treatment of upper respiratory, genitourinary, gastrointestinal tract, and skin and soft tissue infections.**

FDA File **055-087**
Firm: **Pfizer, Inc.**
Use: **Calves:** Rx only **- Oral Bolus**
Dosage: **400 milligrams per 100 pounds body weight twice daily. Continue for 48 hours after animal is asymptomatic but not to exceed 5 days.**
Purpose: **Treatment of bacterial enteritis in preruminating calves, including veal calves.**

FDA File **055-089**
Firm: **Pfizer, Inc.**
Use: **Cattle:** Rx only **- Sterile Suspension**
Dosage: **Inject intramuscularly or subcutaneously 3 to 5 milligrams per pound of body weight for up to 5 days. Continue for 48 to 72 hours after animal is asymptomatic but not to exceed 5 days.**
Purpose: **Treatment of respiratory tract infections and acute necrotic pododermatitis.**

FDA File **055-091**
Firm: **Pfizer, Inc.**
Use: **Dogs and Cats:** Rx only **- Sterile Suspension**
Dosage: **Intramuscularly or subcutaneously 5 milligrams per pound of body weight twice per day for up to 5 days or until animal is asymptomatic.**
Purpose: **Treatment of certain bacterial infections.**

FDA File **055-099**
Firm: **Pfizer, Inc.**
Use: **Dogs:** Rx only **- Oral Tablets**
Dosage: **5 milligrams per pound of body weight twice per day for 5 to 7 days or until 48 hours after animal is asymptomatic. Deep pyoderma may require treatment for 21 days. Do not treat for more than 30 days**
Purpose: **Treatment of skin and soft tissue infections such as wounds, abscesses, cellulitis, superficial juvenile and deep pyoderma, and for periodontal infections.**

FDA File **055-100**
Firm: **Schering-Plough Animal Health**
Use: **Cattle: Intramammary Infusion**
Dosage: **62.5 milligrams infused into each infected quarter every 12 hours for a maximum of 3 doses.**
Purpose: **Treatment subclinical infections of bovine mastitis.**

FDA File **055-101**
Firm: **Pfizer, Inc.**
Use: **Dogs:** Rx only **- Powder for Suspension**
Dosage: **5 milligrams per pound of body weight twice per day for 5 to 7 days or until 48 hours after animal is asymptomatic. Deep pyoderma may require treatment for 21 days. Do not treat for more than 30 days. Do not treat for more than 30 days.**
Purpose: **Treatment of skin and soft tissue infections such as wounds, abscesses, cellulitis, superficial juvenile and deep pyoderma, and for periodontal infections.**

FDA File **055-102**
Firm: **Pfizer, Inc.**
Use: **Dogs:** Rx only **- Oral Tablet**
Dosage: **5 milligrams per pound of body weight twice per day for 5 to 7 days or until 48 hours after animal is asymptomatic. Urinary tract infections may require treatment for 10 to 14 days or longer. Deep pyoderma may require treatment for 21 days. Do not treat for more than 30 days**
Purpose: **Treatment of skin and soft tissue infections such as wounds, abscesses, cellulitis, superficial juvenile and deep pyoderma, and for urinary tract infections (cystitis).**

FDA File **055-103**
Firm: **Pfizer, Inc.**
Use: **Cats:** Rx only **- Powder for Suspension**
Dosage: **50 milligrams per pound of body weight twice per day until 48 hours after animal is asymptomatic. Do not exceed 30 days.**
Purpose: **For treatment of skin and soft tissue infections such as wounds, abscesses and cellulitis/dermatitis.**

FDA File **065-492**
Firm: **Virbac Animal Health, Inc.**
Use: **Dogs:** Rx only **- Oral Tablet**

Dosage: **Dogs: 5 milligrams per pound of body weight twice per day for 5 to 7 days or until 48 hours after animal is asymptomatic.**

Purpose: **Treatment of bacterial dermatitis and soft tissue infections (abscesses, wounds, lacerations).**

FDA File **065-495**
Firm: **Virbac Animal health, Inc.**
Use: **Dogs:** Rx only **- Oral Suspension**
Dosage: **Dogs: 5 milligrams per pound of body weight twice per day for 5 to 7 days or until 48 hours after animal is asymptomatic.**

Purpose: **Treatment of dermatitis and soft tissue infections (abscesses, wounds, lacerations).**

FDA File **141-004**
Firm: **Fort Dodge Animal Health, Div. Wyeth**
Use: **Dogs:** Rx only **- Oral Suspension**
Dosage: **Dogs: 5 milligrams per pound of body weight twice per day for 5 to 7 days or until 48 hours after animal is asymptomatic.**

Purpose: **Treatment of bacterial dermatitis and soft tissue infections (abscesses, wounds, lacerations).**

FDA File **141-005**
Firm: **For Dodge Animal Health, Div. Wyeth**
Use: **Dogs:** Rx only **- Oral Tablet**
Dosage: **Dogs: 5 milligrams per pound of body weight twice per**
day for 5 to 7 days or until 48 hours after animal is asymptomatic.

Purpose: **Treatment of bacterial dermatitis and soft tissue infections (abscesses, wounds, lacerations).**

AMPHOMYCIN (CALCIUM)

FDA File **043-784**
Firm: **For Dodge Animal Health, Div. Wyeth**
Use: **Dogs:** Rx only **- Topical Ointment**
Dosage: **Each gram of ointment contains 5.0 milligrams amphomycin activity as the calcium salt. Apply to affected area at least twice daily initially, reducing frequency as conditions improve.**

Purpose: **Treatment of acute otitis externa, furunculosis, folliculitis, pruritis, anal gland infections, erythema, decubital ulcer, superficial wounds, and superficial abscesses.**

FDA File **047-997**
Firm: **For Dodge Animal Health, Div. Wyeth**
Use: **Dogs:** Rx only **- Topical Ointment**
Dosage: **Each gram of ointment contains 5.0 milligrams amphomycin activity as the calcium salt. Apply to affected area at least twice daily**
initially, reducing frequency as conditions improve.

Purpose: **Treatment of acute otitis externa and topical infections such as folliculitis, anal gland infections, superficial wounds, etc.**

AMPICILLIN (ANHYDROUS, TRI-HYDRATE, OR SODIUM)

FDA File **055-013**
Firm: **Wyeth Laboratories**
Use: **Dogs, Cats:** Rx only **- Oral Capsules**
Dosage: **Dogs: 5 to 10 milligrams per pound of body weight 2 to 4 times daily. Cats: 125 milligrams 2 times per day, in more acute conditions 3 times per day.**
Purpose: **Dogs: Treatment of respiratory and urinary tract infections, abscesses, tonsillitis and wounds. Cats: Treatment of respiratory tract infections abscesses and wounds.**

FDA File **055-030**
Firm: **Fort Dodge Animal Health Div. Of Wyeth**
Use: **Dogs, Cats, Cattle:** Rx only **- Sterile Injection**
Dosage: **Dogs and Cats: Inject intramuscularly or subcutaneously 3 milligrams per pound of body weight per day until 48 to 72 hours after animal is asymptomatic. Cattle: Inject intramuscularly 2 to 5 milligrams per pound of body weight per day, not to exceed 7 days. Continue treatment 48 to 72 hours after animal is asymptomatic.**
Purpose: **Dogs and Cats: Treatment of respiratory, urinary and gastrointestinal tract infections and skin and soft tissue infections. Cattle: Treatment of infections of the respiratory tract.**

FDA File **055-036**
Firm: **Norbrook Laboratories**

Use: **Dogs, Cats:** Rx only **- Oral Capsules**
Dosage: **Dogs: 5 to 10 milligrams per pound of body weight 2 to 3 times daily. Cats: 10-30 milligrams per pound of body weight 2 to 3 times per day. Continue treatment 48 hours after animal is asymptomatic.**
Purpose: **Dogs and Cats: Treatment of respiratory and urinary tract infections and generalized infections, and in dogs for the treatment of bacterial gastroenteritis and dermatitis.**

FDA File **055-042**
Firm: **Pfizer, Inc.**
Use: **Dogs:** Rx only **- Oral Tablets**
Dosage: **5 milligrams per pound of body weight 3 times daily. Continue for 36 to 48 hours after animal is asymptomatic.**
Purpose: **Treatment of respiratory and urinary tract infections, abscesses, lacerations and wounds.**

FDA File **055-050**
Firm: **Norbrook Laboratories**
Use: **Swine:** Rx only **- Soluble Powder**
Dosage: **5 milligrams per pound of body weight twice per day for up to 5 days.**
Purpose: **Treatment of colibacillosis and salmonellosis and bacterial pneumonia in swine up to 75 pounds body weight.**

FDA File **055-056**
Firm: **Norbrook Laboratories**
Use: **Cattle:** Rx only **- Oral Bolus**
Dosage: **5 milligrams per pound of body weight twice per day for up to 4 days.**

Purpose: **Treatment of bacterial enteritis in non-ruminating calves.**

FDA File **055-061**
Firm: **Norbrook Laboratories**
Use: **Dogs, Cats:** Rx only **- Oral Suspension**
Dosage: **Dogs: 5 to 10 milligrams per pound of body weight 2 to 3 times daily 1 to 2 hours prior to feeding. In severe infections increase dosage to 10 milligrams per pound of body weight 3 times per day. Cats: 10-30 milligrams per pound of body weight 2 to 3 times per day, 1 to 2 hours prior to feeding. Continue treatment 48 hours after animal is asymptomatic.**
Purpose: **Dogs and Cats: Treatment of respiratory and urinary tract infections and generalized infections, and in dogs for the treatment of bacterial gastroenteritis and dermatitis.**

FDA File **055-064**
Firm: **Fort Dodge Animal Health, Div. Of Wyeth**
Use: **Cattle, Swine:** Rx only **- Injection**
Dosage: **Inject calves and swine intramuscularly with 3 milligrams per pound of body weight per day until 48 hours after animal is asymptomatic.**
Purpose: **Treatment of colibacillosis and bacterial pneumonia.**

FDA File **055-066**
Firm: **Fort Dodge Animal Health, Div. Of Wyeth**
Use: **Dogs, Cats:** Rx only **- Injection**
Dosage: **Inject intramuscularly or subcutaneously 3 to 6 milligrams per pound of body weight 1 to 2 times per day until 48 hours after animal is asymptomatic.**
Purpose: **Treatment of generalized infections associated with abscesses, lacerations and wounds. In dogs for treatment of respiratory tract infections and tonsillitis.**

FDA File **055-071**
Firm: **Fort Dodge Animal Health, Div. Of Wyeth**
Use: **Swine:** Rx only **- Injection**
Dosage: **Inject intramuscularly 3 milligrams per pound of body weight per day until 48 hours after animal is asymptomatic or up to 3 days.**
Purpose: **Treatment of bacterial enteritis and bacterial pneumonia.**

FDA File **055-074**
Firm: **Pfizer, Inc.**
Use: **Calves:** Rx only **- Oral Bolus**
Dosage: **5 milligrams per pound of body weight twice per day until 48 hours after animal is asymptomatic, but not more than 4 days.**
Purpose: **Treatment of bacterial enteritis in non-ruminating calves.**

FDA File **055-079**
Firm: **Pfizer, Inc.**
Use: **Dogs:** Rx only **- Injection**
Dosage: **Inject intramuscularly 3 to 5 milligrams per pound of body weight per day for up to 5 days or until 48 hours after animal is asymptomatic.**
Purpose: **Treatment of bacterial upper respiratory tract and soft tissue infections.**

FDA File **055-084**
Firm: **Pfizer, Inc.**
Use: **Horses:** Rx only **- Injection**

Dosage: **Inject intramuscularly or intravenously 3 milligrams per pound of body weight per day until 48 hours after animal is asymptomatic.**
Purpose: **Treatment of respiratory tract, and skin and soft tissue infections.**

FDA File **200-180**
Firm: **G.C. Handford Mfg. Co.**
Use: **Dogs, Cats, Cattle:** Rx(dogs, cats)/OTC in cattle **- Injection**
Dosage: **Inject intramuscularly or subcutaneously 3 milligrams per pound of body weight per day in dogs and cats. For cattle inject 2-5 milligrams per pound of body weight per day intramuscularly, not to exceed 7 days. Continue treatment until 48 to 72 hours after animal is asymptomatic.**
Purpose: **Treatment of respiratory, urinary and gastrointestinal tract infections and skin and soft tissue infections in dogs and cats, and infections of the respiratory tract in cattle.**

AMPROLIUM

FDA File **012-350**
Firm: **Huvepharma AD**
Use: **Cattle, Chickens, Turkeys, Pheasants: Feed Additive Premix**
Dosage: **Calves: 5 or 10 milligrams per kilogram of body weight per day; Chickens and Turkeys: 36.3 to 113.5 grams per ton of feed; pheasants: 159 grams per ton of feed.**
Purpose: **Prevention and treatment of coccidiosis. For development of active immunity to coccidiosis.**

FDA File **013-149**
Firm: **Huvepharma AD**
Use: **Cattle, Chickens, Turkeys: Water Additive**
Dosage: **Calves: 5 or 10 milligrams per kilogram of body weight per day; Chickens and Turkeys: 0.12 to 0.24 percent in water.**
Purpose: **Prevention and treatment of coccidiosis.**

FDA File **013-663**
Firm: **Virbac AH, Inc.**
Use: **Chickens, Turkeys: Water Additive**
Dosage: **Chickens and Turkeys: Add to drinking water at the rate of 0.12 to 0.24 percent.**
Purpose: **Prevention and treatment of coccidiosis.**

FDA File **033-165**
Firm: **Huvepharma AD**
Use: **Cattle, Chickens, Turkeys: Water Additive**
Dosage: **Calves: 5 or 10 milligrams per kilogram of body weight per day; Chickens and Turkeys: 0.012 percent in water.**
Purpose: **Prevention and treatment of coccidiosis.**

FDA File **036-304**
Firm: **Merial Ltd.**
Use: **Chickens: Feed Additive Premix**
Dosage: **113.5 grams per ton of feed.**
Purpose: **Prevention of coccidiosis.**

FDA File **036-361**
Firm: **Merial Ltd.**
Use: **Chickens: Feed Additive Premix**

Dosage: **113.5 grams per ton of feed.**
Purpose: **Prevention of coccidiosis.**

FDA File **038-242**
Firm: **Cross Vetpharm Group Ltd.**
Use: **Chickens: Feed Additive Premix**
Dosage: **113.5 grams per ton of feed.**
Purpose: **Prevention of coccidiosis.**

FDA File **039-284**
Firm: **Swisher Feed Division**
Use: **Chickens: Feed Additive Premix**
Dosage: **113.5 grams per ton of feed.**
Purpose: **Prevention of coccidiosis.**

FDA File **040-920**
Firm: **Honeggers & Co., Inc.**
Use: **Chickens: Feed Additive Premix**
Dosage: **36.3 to 113.5 grams per ton of feed.**
Purpose: **Prevention of coccidiosis.**

FDA File **041-178**
Firm: **Pharmacia & Upjohn Co.**
Use: **Chickens: Feed Additive Premix**
Dosage: **113.5 grams per ton of feed.**
Purpose: **Prevention of coccidiosis.**

FDA File **044-820**
Firm: **Pharmacia & Upjohn Co.**
Use: **Chickens: Feed Additive Premix**
Dosage: **113.5 grams per ton of feed.**
Purpose: **Prevention of coccidiosis.**

FDA File **049-179**

Firm: **Merial Ltd.**
Use: **Chickens: Feed Additive Premix**
Dosage: **113.5 to 227 grams per ton of feed.**
Purpose: **Prevention of coccidiosis.**

FDA File **049-180**
Firm: **Merial Ltd.**
Use: **Chickens: Feed Additive Premix**
Dosage: **113.5 grams per ton of feed.**
Purpose: **Prevention of coccidiosis.**

FDA File **095-543**
Firm: **Huvepharma AD.**
Use: **Chickens: Feed Additive Premix**
Dosage: **113.5 grams per ton of feed.**
Purpose: **Prevention of coccidiosis.**

FDA File **095-547**
Firm: **Huvepharma AD.**
Use: **Chickens: Feed Additive Premix**
Dosage: **113.5 grams per ton of feed.**
Purpose: **Prevention of coccidiosis.**

FDA File **095-548**
Firm: **Huvepharma AD.**
Use: **Chickens: Feed Additive Premix**
Dosage: **113.5 grams per ton of feed.**
Purpose: **Prevention of coccidiosis.**

FDA File **095-549**
Firm: **Huvepharma AD.**
Use: **Chickens: Feed Additive Premix**
Dosage: **113.5 grams per ton of feed.**

Purpose: **Prevention of coccidiosis.**

FDA File **105-758**
Firm: **Alpharma Inc.**
Use: **Chickens: Feed Additive Premix**
Dosage: **113.5 grams per ton of feed.**
Purpose: **Prevention of coccidiosis.**

FDA File **114-794**
Firm: **Alpharma Inc.**
Use: **Chickens: Feed Additive Premix**
Dosage: **113.5 grams per ton of feed.**
Purpose: **Prevention of coccidiosis.**

FDA File **118-507**
Firm: **Merial Ltd.**
Use: **Turkeys: Feed Additive Premix**
Dosage: **113.5 grams per ton of feed.**
Purpose: **Prevention of coccidiosis.**

FDA File **122-822**
Firm: **Phibro Animal Health, Inc.**
Use: **Chickens: Feed Additive Premix**
Dosage: **113.5 grams per ton of feed.**
Purpose: **Prevention of coccidiosis.**

FDA File **130-185**
Firm: **Huvepharma AD**
Use: **Turkeys: Feed Additive Premix**
Dosage: **113.5 grams per ton of feed.**
Purpose: **Prevention of coccidiosis.**

FDA File **141-142**
Firm: **Alpharma Inc.**
Use: **Chickens: Feed Additive Premix**

Dosage: **36.3 to 113.5 grams per ton of feed.**
Purpose: **Prevention of coccidiosis.**

FDA File **141-156**
Firm: **Alpharma Inc.**
Use: **Chickens: Feed Additive Premix**
Dosage: **36.3 to 113.5 grams per ton of feed.**
Purpose: **Development of active immunity to coccidiosis.**

FDA File **200-205**
Firm: **Alpharma Inc.**
Use: **Chickens: Feed Additive Premix**
Dosage: **113.4 grams per ton of feed.**
Purpose: **Prevention of coccidiosis.**

FDA File **200-214**
Firm: **Alpharma Inc.**
Use: **Chickens: Feed Additive Premix**
Dosage: **113.5 grams per ton of feed.**
Purpose: **Prevention of coccidiosis.**

FDA File **200-217**
Firm: **Alpharma Inc.**
Use: **Chickens: Feed Additive Premix**
Dosage: **113.5 grams per ton of feed.**
Purpose: **Prevention of coccidiosis.**

FDA File **200-389**
Firm: **IVX Animal Health**
Use: **Cattle: Water Additive**
Dosage: **Calves: 5 or 10 milligrams per kilogram of body weight per day.**
Purpose: **Prevention and treatment of coccidiosis.**

APRAMYCIN (SULFATE)

FDA File **106-964**
Firm: **Elanco Animal Health, Div. Eli Lilly & Co.**
Use: **Swine: Soluble Powder**
Dosage: **11.4 milligrams per pound of body weight per day for 7 days in drinking water.**
Purpose: **Treatment of porcine colibacillosis.**

FDA File **126-050**
Firm: **Elanco Animal Health, Div. Eli Lilly & Co.**
Use: **Swine: Feed Additive premix**
Dosage: **150 grams per ton of feed for 14 days.**
Purpose: **Control of porcine colibacillosis in weanling pigs.**

ARSANILIC ACID

FDA File **008-966**
Firm: **Fleming Laboratories, Inc.**
Use: **Swine, Chickens, Turkeys: Feed Additive and Water Additive**
Dosage: **Water Additive: Administer 0.005 percent in water. In feed, 90 grams per ton.**
Purpose: **Increased rate of weight gain and improved feed efficiency in growing pigs. In chickens and turkeys for growth promotion and feed efficiency and improving pigmentation in chickens. For control of dysentery in swine.**

FDA File **038-241**
Firm: **Cross Vetpharm Group Ltd.**
Use: **Chickens: Feed Additive**
Dosage: **Feed Additive: 90 grams per ton of feed.**

Purpose: **Growth, feed efficiency and improved pigmentation.**

FDA File **038-242**
Firm: **Cross Vetpharm Group Ltd.**
Use: **Chickens: Feed Additive**
Dosage: **Feed Additive: 90 grams per ton of feed.**
Purpose: **Growth, feed efficiency and improved pigmentation.**

BACITRACIN (METHYLENE DISALICYLATE, OR ZINC)

FDA File **065-114**
Firm: **Pharmacia & Upjohn Co.**
Use: **Dogs, Cats:** Rx only **- Ophthalmic Ointment**
Dosage: **Apply a thin film 3 to 4 times per day over cornea.**
Purpose: **Treatment of superficial bacterial infections of the eyelid and conjunctiva.**

FDA File **036-304**
Firm: **Merial Ltd.**
Use: **Chickens: Feed Additive**
Dosage: **4 to 50 grams per ton of feed.**
Purpose: **Increased rate of weight gain.**

FDA File **038-647**
Firm: **Merial Ltd.**
Use: **Chickens: Feed Additive**
Dosage: **4 to 50 grams per ton of feed.**
Purpose: **Growth promotion and feed efficiency.**

FDA File **039-646**
Firm: **Merial Ltd.**
Use: **Turkeys: Feed Additive**
Dosage: **10 grams per ton of feed.**

Purpose: **Increased rate of weight gain.**

FDA File **041-541**
Firm: **Merial Ltd.**
Use: **Chickens: Feed Additive**
Dosage: **4 to 25 grams per ton of feed.**
Purpose: **Increased rate of weight gain.**

FDA File **046-592**
Firm: **Alpharma, Inc.**
Use: **Beef Cattle, Swine, Chickens, Turkeys, Pheasant, Quail: Feed Additive**
Dosage: **Beef Cattle: 70 grams per head per day. Swine: 10 to 30 grams per ton for increased feed efficiency, 250 grams per ton for control of swine dysentery and clostridial enteritis in suckling pigs when fed 14 days before and 21 days after farrowing; 50 grams per ton for prevention of necrotic enteritis and for control of necrotic enteritis use 100 to 200 grams per ton for 5 to 7 days. Chickens, Turkeys and Pheasants 4 to 50 grams per ton. Quail 5 to 20 grams per ton for improved feed efficiency and rate of weight gain and prevention of ulcerative enteritis.**
Purpose: **Increased rate of weight gain, improved feed efficiency, control of swine dysentery and clostridial enteritis. Control of necrotic enteritis and ulcerative enteritis. Reduction of liver condemnations due to abscesses in beef cattle.**

FDA File **049-180**
Firm: **Merial Ltd.**

Use: **Chickens: Feed Additive**
Dosage: **3 to 35 grams per ton of feed.**
Purpose: **Growth promotion and feed efficiency.**

FDA File **049-463**
Firm: **Elanco Animal Health, Div. Eli Lilly & Co.**
Use: **Chickens: Feed Additive**
Dosage: **5 to 25 grams per ton of feed.**
Purpose: **Increased rate of weight gain and improved feed efficiency.**

FDA File **049-464**
Firm: **Elanco Animal Health, Div. Eli Lilly & Co.**
Use: **Chickens: Feed Additive**
Dosage: **10 to 25 grams per ton of feed.**
Purpose: **Increased rate of weight gain and improved feed efficiency.**

FDA File **065-107**
Firm: **Veterinary Specialties, Inc.**
Use: **Dogs:** Rx only **- Oral**
Dosage: **One level teaspoon per 10 pounds body weight 3 times per day in a small quantity of liquid or feed.**
Purpose: **Treatment of bacterial enteritis and relief of associated diarrhea.**

FDA File **065-470**
Firm: **Alpharma, Inc.**
Use: **Swine, Chickens, Turkeys, Quail: Soluble Powder**
Dosage: Dosage: **Swine: 1 gram per gallon drinking water for up to 14 days. Chickens: To control transmissible gastroenteritis 200 to 400 milligrams per gallon of drinking water; for necrotic enteritis 100**

143

milligrams per gallon drinking water. Turkey and quail: 400 milligrams per gallon.

Purpose: **Increased rate of weight gain, improved feed efficiency, control of swine dysentery and clostridial enteritis. Control of necrotic enteritis and ulcerative enteritis.**

FDA File **097-085**
Firm: **Alpharma, Inc.**
Use: **Chickens: Feed Additive**
Dosage: **4 to 50 grams per ton of feed.**
Purpose: **Increased rate of weight gain and improved feed efficiency.**

FDA File **098-378**
Firm: **Phibro Animal Health, Inc.**
Use: **Chickens: Feed Additive**
Dosage: **30 grams per ton of feed.**
Purpose: **Increased rate of weight gain and improved feed efficiency.**

FDA File **099-150**
Firm: **Merial Ltd.**
Use: **Chickens: Feed Additive**
Dosage: **4 to 50 grams per ton of feed.**
Purpose: **Increased rate of weight gain.**

FDA File **100-853**
Firm: **Phibro Animal Health, Inc.**
Use: **Chickens: Feed Additive**
Dosage: **4 to 50 grams per ton of feed.**
Purpose: **Increased rate of weight gain and improved feed efficiency.**

FDA File **107-996**
Firm: **Phibro Animal health, Inc.**
Use: **Chickens: Feed Additive**

Dosage: **4 to 50 grams per ton of feed.**
Purpose: **Increased rate of weight gain and improved feed efficiency.**

FDA File **116-082**
Firm: **Alpharma, Inc.**
Use: **Chickens: Feed Additive**
Dosage: **4 to 50 grams per ton of feed.**
Purpose: **Prevention of necrotic enteritis.**

FDA File **116-088**
Firm: **Alpharma, Inc.**
Use: **Chickens: Feed Additive**
Dosage: **100 to 200 grams per ton of feed.**
Purpose: **Control of necrotic enteritis and increased rate of weight gain and improved feed efficiency.**

FDA File **131-894**
Firm: **Alpharma, Inc.**
Use: **Chickens: Feed Additive**
Dosage: **10 to 25 grams per ton of feed.**
Purpose: **Increased rate of weight gain and improved feed efficiency.**
FDA File **135-321**
Firm: **Alpharma, Inc.**
Use: **Chickens: Feed Additive**
Dosage: **4 to 50 grams per ton of feed.**
Purpose: **Increased rate of weight gain.**

FDA File **135-746**
Firm: **Alpharma, Inc.**
Use: **Chickens: Feed Additive**
Dosage: **4 to 50 grams per ton of feed.**

Purpose: **Increased rate of weight gain and improved feed efficiency.**

FDA File **138-456**
Firm: **Alpharma, Inc.**
Use: **Chickens: Feed Additive**
Dosage: **5 to 25 grams per ton of feed.**
Purpose: **Increased rate of weight gain and improved feed efficiency.**

FDA File **140-533**
Firm: **Intervet Inc.**
Use: **Chickens: Feed Additive**
Dosage: **10 to 50 grams per ton of feed.**
Purpose: **Increased rate of weight gain and improved feed efficiency.**

FDA File **140-584**
Firm: **Intervet, Inc.**
Use: **Chickens: Feed Additive**
Dosage: **10 to 50 grams per ton of feed.**
Purpose: **Improved feed efficiency.**

FDA File **140-823**
Firm: **American Cyanamid, Div. AHP Corp.**
Use: **Chickens: Feed Additive**
Dosage: **4 to 50 grams per ton of feed.**
Purpose: **Increased rate of weight gain and improved feed efficiency.**

FDA File **140-852**
Firm: **Alpharma, Inc.**
Use: **Chickens: Feed Additive**
Dosage: **50 to 200 grams per ton of feed.**
Purpose: **Prevention of necrotic enteritis and for increased rate of weight gain and improved feed efficiency.**

FDA File **140-853**
Firm: **Alpharma, Inc.**
Use: **Chickens: Feed Additive**
Dosage: **10 to 50 grams per ton of feed.**
Purpose: **Increased rate of weight gain and improved feed efficiency.**

FDA File **140-919**
Firm: **Intervet Inc.**
Use: **Turkeys: Feed Additive**
Dosage: **10 to 50 grams per ton of feed.**
Purpose: **Increased rate of weight gain.**

FDA File **140-926**
Firm: **Elanco Animal Health, Div. Eli Lilly & Co.**
Use: **Chickens: Feed Additive**
Dosage: **4 to 50 grams per ton of feed.**
Purpose: **Increased rate of weight gain and improved feed efficiency.**

FDA File **140-937**
Firm: **Elanco Animal Health, Div. Eli Lilly & Co.**
Use: **Turkeys: Feed Additive**
Dosage: **200 grams per ton of feed.**
Purpose: **Control of transmissible enteritis.**

FDA File **141-058**
Firm: **Phibro Animal Health, Inc.**
Use: **Chickens: Feed Additive**
Dosage: **10 to 50 grams per ton of feed.**
Purpose: **Improved feed efficiency.**

FDA File **141-059**
Firm: **Alpharma, Inc.**
Use: **Swine: Feed Additive**
Dosage: **10 to 30 grams per ton of feed.**

Purpose: **Increased rate of weight gain and improved feed efficiency; for treatment of bacterial enteritis and bacterial pneumonia.**

FDA File **141-065**
Firm: **Phibro Animal Health, Inc.**
Use: **Chickens: Feed Additive**
Dosage: **10 to 50 grams per ton of feed.**
Purpose: **Improved feed efficiency.**

FDA File **141-085**
Firm: **Alpharma Inc.**
Use: **Chickens and Turkeys: Feed Additive**
Dosage: **Chickens: 50 grams per ton of feed; Turkeys: 4 to 50 grams per ton of feed.**
Purpose: **Prevention of necrotic enteritis and increased rate of weight gain and improved feed efficiency.**

FDA File **141-088**
Firm: **Intervet Inc.**
Use: **Turkeys: Feed Additive**
Dosage: **4 to 50 grams per ton of feed.**
Purpose: **Increased rate of weight gain and improved feed efficiency.**

FDA File **141-097**
Firm: **Merial, Ltd.**
Use: **Swine: Feed Additive**
Dosage: **10 to 30 or 250 grams per ton of feed.**
Purpose: **Control of colostridial enteritis in suckling pgs; control of swine dysentery on premises with a history of the disease. Treat pregnant sows from 14 days before to 21 days after farrowing.**

FDA File **141-100**
Firm: **Alpharma, Inc.**
Use: **Chickens: Feed Additive**
Dosage: **50 grams per ton of feed.**
Purpose: **Prevention of necrotic enteritis and increased rate of weight gain and improved feed efficiency.**

FDA File **141-102**
Firm: **Alpharma Inc.**
Use: **Chickens: Feed Additive**
Dosage: **4 to 50 grams per ton of feed.**
Purpose: **Increased rate of weight gain and improved feed efficiency.**

FDA File **141-112**
Firm: **Alpharma Inc.**
Use: **Chickens: Feed Additive**
Dosage: **50 grams per ton of feed.**
Purpose: **Prevention of necrotic enteritis and increased rate of weight gain and improved feed efficiency.**

FDA File **141-121**
Firm: **Alpharma Inc.**
Use: **Chickens: Feed Additive**
Dosage: **50 grams per ton of feed.**
Purpose: **Prevention of necrotic enteritis and increased rate of weight gain and improved feed efficiency.**

FDA File **141-124**
Firm: **Alpharma Inc.**
Use: **Chickens: Feed Additive**
Dosage: **50 grams per ton of feed.**
Purpose: **Prevention or control of necrotic enteritis.**

FDA File **141-130**
Firm: **Alpharma Inc.**
Use: **Chickens: Feed Additive**

Dosage: **4 to 50 grams per ton of feed.**
Purpose: **Increased rate of weight gain and improved feed efficiency.**

FDA File **141-131**
Firm: **Alpharma Inc.**
Use: **Chickens: Feed Additive**
Dosage: **4 to 50 grams per ton of feed.**
Purpose: **Increased rate of weight gain and improved feed efficiency.**

FDA File **141-132**
Firm: **Alpharma Inc.**
Use: **Turkeys: Feed Additive**
Dosage: **4 to 50 grams per ton of feed.**
Purpose: **Increased rate of weight gain and improved feed efficiency.**

FDA File **141-136**
Firm: **Alpharma Inc.**
Use: **Chickens: Feed Additive**
Dosage: **4 to 200 grams per ton of feed.**
Purpose: **Increased rate of weight gain and improved feed efficiency; prevention and control of necrotic enteritis.**

FDA File **141-137**
Firm: **Pennfield Oil Co.**
Use: **Chickens, Turkeys, Quail: Feed Additive**
Dosage: **4 to 50 grams per ton of feed.**
Purpose: **Increased rate of weight gain and improved feed efficiency.**

FDA File **141-138**
Firm: **Alpharma Inc.**
Use: **Chickens: Feed Additive**
Dosage: **4 to 50 grams per ton of feed.**

Purpose: **Control of necrotic enteritis and increased rate of weight gain and improved feed efficiency.**

FDA File **141-140**
Firm: **Alpharma Inc.**
Use: **Chickens: Feed Additive**
Dosage: **100 to 200 grams per ton of feed.**
Purpose: **Increased rate of weight gain and improved feed efficiency and an aid in the prevention of necrotic enteritis.**

FDA File **141-142**
Firm: **Alpharma Inc.**
Use: **Chickens: Feed Additive**
Dosage: **50 grams per ton of feed.**
Purpose: **Increased rate of weight gain and improved feed efficiency and aid in the prevention of necrotic enteritis.**

FDA File **141-144**
Firm: **Alpharma Inc.**
Use: **Swine: Feed Additive**
Dosage: **10 to 30 or 250 grams per ton of feed.**
Purpose: **Increased rate of weight gain and improved feed efficiency, control of swine dysentery, and control of colostridial enteritis in suckling pigs.**

FDA File **141-153**
Firm: **Huvepharma AD**
Use: **Chickens: Feed Additive**
Dosage: **4 to 50 grams per ton of feed.**
Purpose: **Increased rate of weight gain and improved feed efficiency.**

FDA File **141-154**
Firm: **Alpharma Inc.**

Use: **Chickens: Feed Additive**
Dosage: **50 or 100 to 200 grams per ton of feed.**
Purpose: **Prevention of necrotic enteritis.**

FDA File **141-155**
Firm: **Alpharma Inc.**
Use: **Chickens: Feed Additive**
Dosage: **4 to 50 grams per ton of feed.**
Purpose: **Increased rate of weight gain and improved feed efficiency and control of necrotic enteritis.**

FDA File **141-156**
Firm: **Alpharma Inc.**
Use: **Chickens: Feed Additive**
Dosage: **4 to 50 grams per ton of feed.**
Purpose: **Increased rate of weight gain and improved feed efficiency.**

FDA File **141-179**
Firm: **Alpharma Inc.**
Use: **Turkeys: Feed Additive**
Dosage: **4 to 50 grams per ton of feed.**
Purpose: **Increased rate of weight gain and improved feed efficiency.**

FDA File **141-190**
Firm: **Schering-Plough Animal Health**
Use: **Chickens: Feed Additive**
Dosage: **Chickens: 4 to 50 grams per ton of feed.**
Purpose: **Prevention and control of necrotic enteritis and increased rate of weight gain and improved feed efficiency.**

FDA File **141-194**
Firm: **Schering-Plough Animal Health**

Use: **Turkeys: Feed Additive**
Dosage: **4 to 50 grams per ton of feed.**
Purpose: **Increased rate of weight gain and improved feed efficiency.**

FDA File **141-279**
Firm: **Alpharma, Inc.**
Use: **Chickens: Feed Additive**
Dosage: **4 to 50 grams per ton of feed.**
Purpose: **Increased rate of weight gain, improved feed efficiency, and prevention of necrotic enteritis.**

FDA File **200-081**
Firm: **Intervet, Inc.**
Use: **Chickens: Feed Additive**
Dosage: **4 to 50 grams per ton of feed.**
Purpose: **Increased rate of weight gain.**

FDA File **200-082**
Firm: **Intervet, Inc.**
Use: **Chickens: Feed Additive**
Dosage: **4 to 50 grams per ton of feed.**
Purpose: **Increased rate of weight gain and improved feed efficiency.**

FDA File **200-164**
Firm: **Planalquimica Industrial Ltd.**
Use: **Chickens: Feed Additive**
Dosage: **30 grams per ton of feed.**
Purpose: **Increased rate of weight gain and improved feed efficiency.**

FDA File **200-242**
Firm: **Alpharma Inc.**
Use: **Swine: Feed Additive**
Dosage: **10 to 30 grams per ton of feed.**

Purpose: **Increased rate of weight gain and improved feed efficiency, treatment of bacterial enteritis and bacterial pneumonia.**

FDA File **039-284**
Firm: **Swisher Feed Division**
Use: **Chickens: Feed Additive**
Dosage: **5 to 35 grams per ton of feed.**
Purpose: **Increased rate of weight gain.**

FDA File **044-016**
Firm: **Merial Ltd.**
Use: **Chickens: Feed Additive**
Dosage: **4 to 25 grams per ton of feed.**
Purpose: **Increased rate of weight gain and improved feed efficiency.**

FDA File **045-348**
Firm: **Alpharma, Inc.**
Use: **Chickens: Feed Additive**
Dosage: **10 to 50 grams per ton of feed.**
Purpose: **Increased rate of weight gain and improved feed efficiency.**

FDA File **046-920**
Firm: **Alpharma, Inc.**
Use: **Cattle, Swine, Sheep, Turkeys, Chickens, Pheasants and Quail: Feed Additive**
Dosage: **4 to 50 grams per ton of feed for chickens, turkeys and pheasants; 5-20 grams per ton for quail; 10 to 50 grams per ton for swine and 35 to 70 milligrams per head per day for cattle.**
Purpose: **Increased rate of weight gain and improved feed efficiency.**

FDA File **047-933**
Firm: **Elanco Animal Health, Div. Eli Lilly & Co.**
Use: **Chickens: Feed Additive**
Dosage: **10 to 30 grams per ton of feed.**
Purpose: **Increased rate of weight gain and improved feed efficiency.**

FDA File **049-034**
Firm: **Merial Ltd.**
Use: **Chickens: Feed Additive**
Dosage: **5 to 25 grams per ton of feed.**
Purpose: **Increased rate of weight gain and improved feed efficiency.**

FDA File **065-015**
Firm: **Altana, Inc.**
Use: **Dogs, Cats:** Rx only **- Ophthalmic Ointment.**
Dosage: **Apply a thin film over the cornea 3-4 times per day.**
Purpose: **Treatment of acute or chronic conjunctivitis.**

FDA File **065-016**
Firm: **Altana, Inc.**
Use: **Dogs, Cats:** Rx only **- Ophthalmic Ointment**
Dosage: **Apply a thin film over the cornea 3-4 times per day.**
Purpose: **Treatment of acute or chronic conjunctivitis.**

FDA File **065-313**
Firm: **Fort Dodge Animal Health, Div. Of Wyeth**
Use: **Chickens, Quail. Soluble Powder**
Dosage: **Chickens: 100 milligrams per gallon of drinking water for prevention and 200 to 400 milligrams per gallon for control. Quail: 500 milligrams per gallon**

of drinking water for 5 days followed by 165 milligrams per gallon for 10 days.
Purpose: **Chickens: Prevention and control of necrotic enteritis. Quail: Control of ulcerative enteritis.**

FDA File **065-476**
Firm: **Schering-Plough Animal Health**
Use: **Dogs, Cats:** Rx only **- Ophthalmic Ointment**
Dosage: **Apply a thin film over the cornea 3-4 times per day.**
Purpose: **Treatment of certain forms of conjunctivitis.**

FDA File **065-485**
Firm: **Schering-Plough Animal Health**
Use: **Dogs, Cats:** Rx only **- Ophthalmic Ointment**
Dosage: **Apply a thin film over the cornea 3-4 times per day.**
Purpose: **Treatment of superficial bacterial infections of the eyelid and conjunctiva.**

FDA File **091-326**
Firm: **Alpharma, Inc.**
Use: **Chickens: Feed Additive**
Dosage: **12 to 50 grams per ton of feed.**
Purpose: **Increased rate of weight gain and improved feed efficiency.**

FDA File **096-933**
Firm: **Alpharma, Inc.**
Use: **Chickens: Feed Additive**
Dosage: **4 to 50 grams per ton of feed.**
Purpose: **Increased rate of weight gain and improved feed efficiency.**

FDA File **098-452**

Firm: **Alpharma, Inc.**
Use: **Swine, Chickens, Turkeys, Pheasants, Quail: Feed Additive**
Dosage: **4 to 50 grams per ton of complete feed.**
Purpose: **Increased egg production, increased rate of weight gain and improved feed efficiency.**

FDA File **105-758**
Firm: **Alpharma, Inc.**
Use: **Chickens: Feed Additive**
Dosage: **50 grams per ton of feed.**
Purpose: **Increased rate of weight gain and improved feed efficiency.**

FDA File **114-794**
Firm: **Alpharma, Inc.**
Use: **Chickens: Feed Additive**
Dosage: **4 to 50 grams per ton of feed.**
Purpose: **Increased rate of weight gain and improved feed efficiency.**

FDA File **123-154**
Firm: **Alpharma, Inc.**
Use: **Chickens: Feed Additive**
Dosage: **4 to 50 grams per ton of feed.**
Purpose: **Increased rate of weight gain.**

FDA File **126-052**
Firm: **Alpharma, Inc.**
Use: **Chickens: Feed Additive**
Dosage: **4 to 50 grams per ton of feed.**
Purpose: **Increased rate of weight gain and improved feed efficiency.**

FDA File **128-550**
Firm: **Pennfield Oil Co.**
Use: **Chickens: Feed Additive**
Dosage: **4 to 50 grams per ton of feed.**

Purpose: **Increased rate of weight gain and improved feed efficiency.**

FDA File **134-830**
Firm: **Alpharma, Inc.**
Use: **Chickens: Feed Additive**
Dosage: **4 to 50 grams per ton of feed.**
Purpose: **Increased rate of weight gain and improved feed efficiency.**

FDA File **136-484**
Firm: **Alpharma, Inc.**
Use: **Turkeys: Feed Additive**
Dosage: **4 to 45 grams per ton of feed.**
Purpose: **Increased rate of weight gain and improved feed efficiency.**

FDA File **137-536**
Firm: **Alpharma, Inc.**
Use: **Chickens: Feed Additive**
Dosage: **4 to 50 grams per ton of feed.**
Purpose: **Increased rate of weight gain and improved feed efficiency.**

FDA File **138-703**
Firm: **Alpharma, Inc.**
Use: **Chickens: Feed Additive**
Dosage: **4 to 50 grams per ton of feed.**
Purpose: **Improved feed efficiency.**

FDA File **139-190**
Firm: **Alpharma, Inc.**
Use: **Chickens: Feed Additive**
Dosage: **10 to 50 grams per ton of feed.**
Purpose: **Increased rate of weight gain and improved feed efficiency.**

FDA File **139-235**
Firm: **Alpharma, Inc.**
Use: **Chickens: Feed Additive**

Dosage: **10 to 50 grams per ton of feed.**
Purpose: **Increased rate of weight gain.**

FDA File **140-865**
Firm: **Alpharma, Inc.**
Use: **Chickens: Feed Additive**
Dosage: **4 to 50 grams per ton of feed.**
Purpose: **Increased rate of weight gain and improved feed efficiency.**

FDA File **141-083**
Firm: **Alpharma, Inc.**
Use: **Chickens: Feed Additive**
Dosage: **4 to 50 grams per ton of feed.**
Purpose: **Increased rate of weight gain and improved feed efficiency.**

FDA File **141-109**
Firm: **Alpharma, Inc.**
Use: **Turkeys: Feed Additive**
Dosage: **4 to 50 grams per ton of feed.**
Purpose: **Increased rate of weight gain and improved feed efficiency.**

FDA File **141-132**
Firm: **Alpharma, Inc.**
Use: **Turkeys: Feed Additive**
Dosage: **4 to 50 grams per ton of feed.**
Purpose: **Increased rate of weight gain and improved feed efficiency.**

FDA File **141-146**
Firm: **Phibro Animal Health, Inc.**
Use: **Chickens: Feed Additive**
Dosage: **4 to 50 grams per ton of feed.**
Purpose: **Increased rate of weight gain and improved feed efficiency.**

FDA File **141-181**
Firm: **Alpharma, Inc.**
Use: **Turkeys: Feed Additive**
Dosage: **4 to 50 grams per ton of feed.**
Purpose: **Increased rate of weight gain and improved feed efficiency.**

FDA File **200-086**
Firm: **Intervet, Inc.**
Use: **Chickens: Feed Additive**
Dosage: **4 to 50 grams per ton of feed.**
Purpose: **Increased rate of weight gain and improved feed efficiency.**

FDA File **200-089**
Firm: **Intervet, Inc.**
Use: **Chickens: Feed Additive**
Dosage: **10 to 50 grams per ton of feed.**
Purpose: **Increased rate of weight gain.**

FDA File **200-143**
Firm: **Intervet, Inc.**
Use: **Chickens: Feed Additive**
Dosage: **10 to 50 grams per ton of feed.**
Purpose: **Increased rate of weight gain and improved feed efficiency.**

FDA File **200-203**
Firm: **Alpharma, Inc.**
Use: **Turkeys: Feed Additive**
Dosage: **4 to 45 grams per ton of feed.**
Purpose: **Increased rate of weight gain and improved feed efficiency.**

FDA File **200-204**
Firm: **Alpharma, Inc.**
Use: **Chickens: Feed Additive**
Dosage: **10 to 50 grams per ton of feed.**
Purpose: **Increased rate of weight gain.**

FDA File **200-205**
Firm: **Alpharma, Inc.**
Use: **Chickens: Feed Additive**
Dosage: **4 to 50 grams per ton of feed.**
Purpose: **Increased rate of weight gain and improved feed efficiency.**

FDA File **200-206**
Firm: **Alpharma, Inc.**
Use: **Chickens: Feed Additive**
Dosage: **12 to 50 grams per ton of feed.**
Purpose: **Increased rate of weight gain and improved feed efficiency.**

FDA File **200-207**
Firm: **Alpharma, Inc.**
Use: **Chickens: Feed Additive**
Dosage: **4 to 25 grams per ton of feed.**
Purpose: **Increased rate of weight gain and improved feed efficiency.**

FDA File **200-208**
Firm: **Alpharma, Inc.**
Use: **Chickens: Feed Additive**
Dosage: **30 grams per ton of feed.**
Purpose: **Increased rate of weight gain and improved feed efficiency.**

FDA File **200-209**
Firm: **Alpharma, Inc.**
Use: **Chickens: Feed Additive**
Dosage: **10 to 50 grams per ton of feed.**
Purpose: **Increased rate of weight gain and improved feed efficiency.**

FDA File **200-210**

Firm: **Alpharma, Inc.**
Use: **Chickens: Feed Additive**
Dosage: **10 to 50 grams per ton of feed.**
Purpose: **Increased rate of weight gain.**

FDA File **200-211**
Firm: **Alpharma, Inc.**
Use: **Chickens: Feed Additive**
Dosage: **4 to 50 grams per ton of feed.**
Purpose: **Increased rate of weight gain.**

FDA File **200-212**
Firm: **Alpharma, Inc.**
Use: **Chickens: Feed Additive**
Dosage: **4 to 50 grams per ton of feed.**
Purpose: **Increased rate of weight gain and improved feed efficiency.**

FDA File **200-213**
Firm: **Alpharma, Inc.**
Use: **Chickens: Feed Additive**
Dosage: **10 to 50 grams per ton of feed.**
Purpose: **Increased rate of weight gain and improved feed efficiency.**

FDA File **200-214**
Firm: **Alpharma, Inc.**
Use: **Chickens: Feed Additive**
Dosage: **50 grams per ton of feed.**
Purpose: **Increased rate of weight gain and improved feed efficiency.**

FDA File **200-215**
Firm: **Alpharma, Inc.**
Use: **Chickens: Feed Additive**
Dosage: **10 to 50 grams per ton of feed.**
Purpose: **Increased rate of weight gain and improved feed efficiency.**

FDA File **200-217**
Firm: **Alpharma, Inc.**
Use: **Chickens: Feed Additive**
Dosage: **5 to 35 grams per ton of feed.**
Purpose: **Increased rate of weight gain.**

FDA File **200-218**
Firm: **Alpharma, Inc.**
Use: **Chickens: Feed Additive**
Dosage: **5 to 25 grams per ton of feed.**
Purpose: **Increased rate of weight gain and improved feed efficiency.**

FDA File **200-223**
Firm: **Alpharma, Inc.**
Use: **Cattle, Chickens, Turkeys, Pheasants, Swine: Feed Additive**
Dosage: **Cattle: 35 to 70 milligrams per head per day; Chickens, Turkeys and Pheasants: 4 to 50 grams per ton; Laying hens: 10 to 25 grams per ton of feed.**
Purpose: **Increased rate of weight gain and improved feed efficiency and increased egg production in laying chickens.**

BAMBERMYCINS

FDA File **044-759**
Firm: **Intervet, Inc.**
Use: **Cattle, Chickens, Turkeys, Swine: Feed Additive**
Dosage: **1 to 4 grams per ton of feed.**
Purpose: **Increased rate of weight gain and improved feed efficiency.**

FDA File **095-543**
Firm: **Intervet, Inc.**
Use: **Chickens: Feed Additive**
Dosage: **1 to 3 grams per ton of feed.**
Purpose: **Increased rate of weight gain and improved feed efficiency.**

FDA File **095-547**
Firm: **Intervet, Inc.**
Use: **Chickens: Feed Additive**
Dosage: **1 to 3 grams per ton of feed.**
Purpose: **Increased rate of weight gain and improved feed efficiency.**

FDA File **095-548**
Firm: **Intervet, Inc.**
Use: **Chickens: Feed Additive**
Dosage: **1 to 3 grams per ton of feed.**
Purpose: **Increased rate of weight gain and improved feed efficiency.**

FDA File **095-549**
Firm: **Intervet, Inc.**
Use: **Chickens: Feed Additive**
Dosage: **1 to 3 grams per ton of feed.**
Purpose: **Increased rate of weight gain and improved feed efficiency.**

FDA File **098-340**
Firm: **Intervet, Inc.**
Use: **Chickens: Feed Additive**
Dosage: **1 to 2 grams per ton of feed.**
Purpose: **Increased rate of weight gain and improved feed efficiency.**

FDA File **098-341**
Firm: **Intervet, Inc.**
Use: **Chickens: Feed Additive**
Dosage: **2 grams per ton of feed.**
Purpose: **Increased rate of weight gain and improved feed efficiency.**

FDA File **101-628**
Firm: **Intervet, Inc.**
Use: **Chickens: Feed Additive**
Dosage: **1 gram per ton of feed.**
Purpose: **Increased rate of weight gain and improved feed efficiency.**

FDA File **101-629**
Firm: **Intervet, Inc.**
Use: **Chickens: Feed Additive**
Dosage: **1 gram per ton of feed.**
Purpose: **Increased rate of weight gain and improved feed efficiency.**

FDA File **112-687**
Firm: **Intervet, Inc.**
Use: **Chickens: Feed Additive**
Dosage: **1 gram per ton of feed.**
Purpose: **Increased rate of weight gain and improved feed efficiency.**

FDA File **130-185**
Firm: **Intervet, Inc.**
Use: **Turkeys: Feed Additive**
Dosage: **4 grams per ton of feed.**
Purpose: **Increased rate of weight gain and improved feed efficiency.**

FDA File **130-661**
Firm: **Intervet, Inc.**
Use: **Turkeys: Feed Additive**
Dosage: **1 or 4 grams per ton of feed.**
Purpose: **Increased rate of weight gain and improved feed efficiency.**

FDA File **131-413**
Firm: **North American Nutrition Companies, Inc.**
Use: **Swine, Turkeys: Feed Additive**
Dosage: **2 to 4 grams per ton of feed.**

Purpose: **Increased rate of weight gain and improved feed efficiency.**

FDA File **132-448**
Firm: **ADM Animal Health & Nutrition Div.**
Use: **Swine, Turkeys: Feed Additive**
Dosage: **2 or 4 grams per ton of feed.**
Purpose: **Increased rate of weight gain and improved feed efficiency.**

FDA File **132-705**
Firm: **Quali-Tech Products, Inc.**
Use: **Swine, Turkeys: Feed Additive**
Dosage: **2 to 4 grams per ton of feed.**
Purpose: **Increased rate of weight gain and improved feed efficiency.**

FDA File **134-185**
Firm: **Alpharma, Inc.**
Use: **Chickens: Feed Additive**
Dosage: **1 to 2 grams per ton of feed.**
Purpose: **Improved feed efficiency.**

FDA File **134-284**
Firm: **Roche Vitamins, Inc.**
Use: **Chickens: Feed Additive**
Dosage: **1 to 3 grams per ton of feed.**
Purpose: **Improved feed efficiency.**

FDA File **137-483**
Firm: **Intervet, Inc.**
Use: **Chickens: Feed Additive**
Dosage: **1 to 2 grams per ton of feed.**
Purpose: **Increased rate of weight gain and improved feed efficiency.**

FDA File **140-339**
Firm: **Intervet, Inc.**
Use: **Chickens: Feed Additive**

Dosage: **1 to 2 grams per ton of feed.**
Purpose: **Increased rate of weight gain and improved feed efficiency.**

FDA File **140-843**
Firm: **Intervet, Inc.**
Use: **Chickens: Feed Additive**
Dosage: **1 to 2 grams per ton of feed.**
Purpose: **Increased rate of weight gain and improved feed efficiency.**

FDA File **140-845**
Firm: **Intervet, Inc.**
Use: **Chickens: Feed Additive**
Dosage: **1 to 2 grams per ton of feed.**
Purpose: **Increased rate of weight gain and improved feed efficiency.**

FDA File **140-918**
Firm: **Intervet, Inc.**
Use: **Turkeys: Feed Additive**
Dosage: **2 grams per ton of feed.**
Purpose: **Increased rate of weight gain.**

FDA File **140-942**
Firm: **Elanco Animal Health Div. Eli Lilly & Co.**
Use: **Chickens: Feed Additive**
Dosage: **1 to 2 grams per ton of feed.**
Purpose: **Increased rate of weight gain and improved feed efficiency.**

FDA File **140-955**
Firm: **Elanco Animal Health Div. Eli Lilly & Co.**
Use: **Turkeys: Feed Additive**
Dosage: **2 grams per ton of feed.**
Purpose: **Improved feed efficiency.**

FDA File **141-034**

Firm: **Intervet, Inc.**
Use: **Cattle: Feed Additive**
Dosage: **10 to 40 milligrams per head per day. For cattle in confinement 1 to 4 grams per ton of feed, including liquid feeds.**
Purpose: **Increased rate of weight gain and improved feed efficiency in slaughter, stocker, and feeder cattle, and dairy and beef replacement heifers.**

FDA File **141-129**
Firm: **Huvepharma AD**
Use: **Chickens: Feed Additive**
Dosage: **1 to 2 grams per ton of feed.**
Purpose: **Increased rate of weight gain and improved feed efficiency.**

FDA File **141-158**
Firm: **Huvepharma AD**
Use: **Chickens: Feed Additive**
Dosage: **1 to 2 grams per ton of feed.**
Purpose: **Increased rate of weight gain and improved feed efficiency.**

FDA File **141-195**
Firm: **Huvepharma AD**
Use: **Turkeys: Feed Additive**
Dosage: **2 grams per ton of feed.**
Purpose: **Increased rate of weight gain and improved feed efficiency.**

FDA File **200-080**
Firm: **Intervet, Inc.**
Use: **Chickens: Feed Additive**
Dosage: **1 to 2 grams per ton of feed.**
Purpose: **Improved feed efficiency.**

FDA File **200-083**
Firm: **Intervet, Inc.**
Use: **Chickens: Feed Additive**

Dosage: **1 to 2 grams per ton of feed.**
Purpose: **Improved feed efficiency.**

BICYCLOHEXYLAMMONIUM FUMAGILLIN

FDA File **009-252**
Firm: **Mid-Continent Agrimarketing, Inc.**
Use: **Honey Bees: Soluble Powder**
Dosage: **0.5 grams in 5 to 6 gallons of 2:1 syrup for 5 to 6 colonies.**
Purpose: **Prevention of nosema.**

CARBOMYCIN

FDA File **032-946**
Firm: **Pfizer, Inc.**
Use: **Chickens: Soluble Powder**
Dosage: **1 gram per gallon of drinking water for up to 5 days.**
Purpose: **Prevention and** treatment **of complicated chronic respiratory disease, and to prevent and treat secondary infections due to** *E. coli.*

CEFADROXIL

FDA File **119-688**
Firm: **Fort Dodge Animal Health, Div. Wyeth**
Use: **Dogs, Cats:** Rx only **- Oral Tablets**
Dosage: **Dogs: 10 milligrams per pound of body weight twice daily for 3 to 7 days. Treat at least 48 hours after animal has become asymptomatic. Cats: 10 milligrams per pound of body weight once per day. Treat at least 48 hours after animal has become afebrile or asymptomatic. Do not treat for more than 21 days.**

Purpose: **Treatment of skin and soft tissue infections including wound infections and cellulitis. Dogs: Pyoderma, abscesses, and genitourinary tract infections. Cats: Abscesses and dermatitis.**

FDA File **140-684**
Firm: **Fort Dodge Animal Health, Div. Wyeth**
Use: **Dogs, Cats:** Rx only **- Sterile Oral Powder**
Dosage: **Reconstitute powder to form 50 milligram per milliliter aqueous suspension. Discard unused suspension after 14 days. Dogs: 10 milligrams per pound of body weight twice daily for 3 to 7 days. Cats: 10 milligrams per pound of body weight once per day. Treat at least 48 hours after animal has become afebrile or asymptomatic.**
Purpose: **Treatment of genitourinary tract infections, skin and soft tissue infections including wound infections and cellulitis. Dogs: Treatment of genitourinary tract infections (cystitis) and skin and soft tissue infections including cellulitis, pyoderma, dermatitis, wound infections, and abscesses. Cats: Treatment of abscesses, wound infections, cellulitis, and dermatitis.**

CEFOVECIN (SODIUM)

FDA File **141-285**
Firm: **Pfizer, Inc.**
Use: **Dogs, Cats:** Rx only **- Injection-Subcutaneous**
Dosage: **8 milligrams per kilogram of body weight as a single injection.**
A second injection may be given if response to therapy is not complete.
Purpose: **Treatment of skin infections caused by** *Staphlococcus intermedius* **and** *Streptococcus canis* **(Group G) in dogs and** *Pasteurella multocida* **in cats.**

CEFTIOFUR (CRYSTALLINE, HYDROCHLORIDE, OR SODIUM)

FDA File **141-209**
Firm: **Pharmacia & Upjohn Co.**
Use: **Cattle:** Rx only **- Subcutaneous Injection**
Dosage: **6.6 milligrams ceftiofur equivalents by a single, subcutaneous injection in the middle third of the posterior aspect of the ear.**
Purpose: **Treatment of bovine respiratory disease and shipping fever.** <u>Control of respiratory disease in cattle at high risk of developing respiratory disease</u> **and for treatment of bovine foot rot (interdigital necrobacillosis) in beef, non-lactating dairy, and lactating dairy cattle.**

FDA File **141-239**
Firm: **Pharmacia & Upjohn Co.**
Use: **Cattle:** Rx only **- Intramammary Infusion**
Dosage: **500 ceftiofur equivalents per affected quarter.**
Purpose: **Treatment of subclinical mastitis in dairy cattle at the time of drying off associated with** *Staphlococcus aureus, Streptococcus dysgalactiae,* **and** *Streptococcus uberis*.

FDA File **141-288**
Firm: **Pharmacia & Upjohn Co.**
Use: **Cattle, Swine:** Rx only **-Injectable Suspension**
Dosage: **1.1 to 2.2 milligrams per kilogram of body weight at 24-48**

hour intervals for 3 to 5 consecutive days for bovine respiratory disease and acute bovine interdigital necrobacillosis.

Purpose: **Cattle:Treatment of bovine respiratory disease associated with *Manneheimia haemolytica*, *Pasturella multocida*, and *Histophilus somni*, acute bovine interdigital necrobacillosis associated with *Fusobacterium necrophorum* and *Bacteroides melaninogenicus*; and acute metritis associated with bacteria susceptible to ceftiofur. Swine: Treatment and <u>control of swine bacterial respiratory disease associated with Actinobacillus *pleuropneumoniae, Pasturella multocida, Salmonella choleraesuis*, and *Streptococcus suis*.</u>**

FDA File **140-890**
Firm: **Pharmacia & Upjohn Co.**
Use: **Cattle, Swine:** Rx only - **Sterile Injection**
Dosage: **Cattle: Intramuscularly or subcutaneously 1.1 to 2.2 milligrams per kilogram of body weight at 24-hour intervals for 3 to 5 consecutive days. For respiratory diseases 2.2 milligrams per kilogram body weight every other day on days 1 and 3 (48-hour interval). For acute metritis 2.2 milligrams per kilogram body weight daily for 5 days. Swine: Intramuscular use only at 3 to 5 milligrams per kilogram body weight, repeated at 24-hour intervals for a total of 3 consecutive days.**
Purpose: **Cattle: Treatment of bovine respiratory disease and shipping fever. <u>Control of respiratory disease in cattle at high risk</u>**

<u>of developing respiratory disease. Swine: Treatment and control of swine bacterial respiratory disease.</u>

FDA File **140-338**
Firm: **Pharmacia & Upjohn Co.**
Use: **Cattle, Swine, Chickens, Turkeys, Sheep, Goats, Horses, Dogs:** Rx only - **Injection**
Dosage: **Cattle: Intramuscularly or subcutaneously 0.5 to 1.0 milligrams per pound of body weight at 24-hour intervals for 3 days. Treat an additional 2 days if needed. . Day-old chicks: 0.08 to 0.20 milligrams per chick subcutaneously in the neck as a single dose only. Horses: 2.2 to 4.4 milligrams per kilograms body weight intramuscularly. Repeat treatment every 24 hours, continued for 48 hours after clinical signs have disappeared, and not to exceed 10 days. Turkey Poults: 0.17 to 0.5 milligrams per poult subcutaneously in the neck as a single dose only. Dogs: 1.0 milligrams per pound of body weight subcutaneously and repeat at 24-hour intervals, continued for 48 hours after clinical signs have disappeared, for 5 to 14 days. Sheep: Intramuscular use only at 0.5 to 1.0 milligrams per kilogram body weight. Repeat at 24-hour intervals for a total of 3 consecutive days. May be given on days 4 and 5 for sheep that do not show satisfactory response. Goats: Intramuscular injection at 0.5 to 1.0 milligram per pound body weight at 24-hours intervals for a total of 3 consecutive days. Additional treatments may be given on days 4**

and 5 for animals that do not show satisfactory response. Swine: Intramuscular use only at 3 to 5 milligrams per kilogram body weight, repeated at 24-hour intervals for a total of 3 consecutive days.
Purpose: **Cattle: Treatment of bovine respiratory disease and shipping fever. Swine: Treatment and control of swine bacterial respiratory disease. Day-old Chickens: Control of colibacillosis. Day-old turkey Poults: Control of early mortality associated with *E. coil*. Horse: Treatment of respiratory infections. Dogs: Treatment of canine urinary tract infections. Sheep: Treatment of respiratory disease. Goats: Treatment of caprine respiratory disease.**

CEPHAPIRIN (BENZATHINE, SODIUM)

FDA File **108-114**
Firm: **Fort Dodge Animal Health, Div. Of Wyeth**
Use: **Cattle: Intramammary Infusion**
Dosage: **Infuse contents of one syringe (300 milligrams) into each quarter following last milking or at start of dry period.**
Purpose: **Treatment of mastitis caused by susceptible strains of *Streptococcus agalactiae* and *Staphylococcus aureus*, including penicillin resistant strains in dry cows.**

FDA File **097-222**
Firm: **Fort Dodge Animal Health, Div. Of Wyeth**
Use: **Cattle: Intramammary Infusion**
Dosage: **200 milligrams per infected quarter after milking. Repeat only once in 12 hours.**
Purpose: **Treatment of mastitis in lactating cows.**

CHLORAMPHENICOL

FDA File **055-002**
Firm: **Phoenix Scientific, Inc.**
Use: **Dogs:** Rx only **- Injection**
Dosage: **5 to 15 milligrams per pound of body weight every 6 hours.**
Purpose: **Treatment of tonsillitis, enteritis and respiratory and urinary tract infection.**

FDA File **055-007**
Firm: **Evsco Pharmaceuticals**
Use: **Dogs, Cats:** Rx only **- Ophthalmic Ointment**
Dosage: **Apply to the affected eye 4 to 6 times per day for the first 72 hours depending upon the severity of the infection. Continue treatment for 48 hours after animal is asymptomatic. Therapy for cats should not exceed 7 days.**
Purpose: **Treatment of bacterial conjunctivitis.**

FDA File **055-034**
Firm: **Evsco Pharmaceuticals**
Use: **Dogs, Cats:** Rx only **- Ophthalmic Drops**
Dosage: **Apply 1 to 2 drops to the affected eye 4 to 6 times per day for the first 72 hours depending upon the severity of the infection. Intervals between applications may be increased after 2 days. Continue treatment for 48 hours after animal is asymptomatic. Therapy for cats should not exceed 7 days.**

Purpose: **Treatment of bacterial conjunctivitis.**

FDA File **055-047**
Firm: **Fort Dodge Animal Health, Div. Of Wyeth**
Use: **Dogs:** Rx only **- Oral Suspension**
Dosage: **25 milligrams per pound of body weight every 6 hours.**
Purpose: **Treatment of enteritis, bacterial pulmonary infections, bacterial urinary tract, and other infections.**

FDA File **055-051**
Firm: **Fort Dodge Animal Health, Div. Of Wyeth**
Use: **Dogs:** Rx only **- Oral Tablets**
Dosage: **25 milligrams per pound of body weight every 6 hours.**
Purpose: **Treatment of bacterial enteritis, bacterial pulmonary infections, bacterial urinary tract infections and bacterial infections associated with canine distemper.**

FDA File **055-052**
Firm: **Evsco Pharmaceuticals**
Use: **Dogs:** Rx only **- Oral Tablets**
Dosage: **25 milligrams per pound of body weight every 6 hours.**
Purpose: **Treatment of bacterial enteritis, bacterial pulmonary infections, bacterial urinary tract infections and bacterial infections associated with canine distemper.**

FDA File **055-059**
Firm: **Cross Vetpharm Group Ltd.**
Use: **Dogs:** Rx only **- Oral Tablets**
Dosage: **25 milligrams per pound of body weight every 6 hours.**
Purpose: **Treatment of gastroenteritis associated with bacterial**
diarrhea, bacterial pulmonary infections, and bacterial urinary tract infections.

FDA File **065-137**
Firm: **John J. Ferrante**
Use: **Dogs:** Rx only **- Oral Capsules**
Dosage: **25 milligrams per pound of body weight every 6 hours.**
Purpose: **Treatment of bacterial enteritis, bacterial pulmonary infections, bacterial urinary tract infections and bacterial infections associated with canine distemper.**

FDA File **065-149**
Firm: **Fort Dodge Animal Health, Div. Of Wyeth**
Use: **Dogs, Cats:** Rx only **- Ophthalmic Drops**
Dosage: **Apply every 3 hours for 48 hours, after which night instillations may be omitted. Continue treatment for 48 hours after animal is asymptomatic. Therapy for cats should not exceed 7 days.**
Purpose: **Treatment of bacterial conjunctivitis.**

FDA File **065-150**
Firm: **Pharmaceutical Ventures, Ltd.**
Use: **Dogs:** Rx only **- Oral Capsules**
Dosage: **25 milligrams per pound of body weight every 6 hours.**
Purpose: **Treatment of bacterial enteritis, bacterial pulmonary infections, bacterial urinary tract infections and bacterial infections associated with canine distemper.**

FDA File **055-157**
Firm: **Evsco Pharmaceuticals**
Use: **Dogs, Cats:** Rx only **- Ophthalmic Drops**

Dosage: **Apply to the affected eye 4 to 6 times per day for the first 72 hours depending upon the severity of the infection. Continue treatment for 48 hours after animal is asymptomatic. Therapy for cats should not exceed 7 days.**
Purpose: **Treatment of bacterial conjunctivitis.**

FDA File **055-158**
Firm: **Evsco Pharmaceuticals**
Use: **Dogs, Cats:** Rx only **- Ophthalmic Drops**
Dosage: **Apply in the conjunctival sac every 3 hours for the first 48 hours after which night instillations may be omitted. Continue treatment for 48 hours after animal is asymptomatic. Therapy for cats should not exceed 7 days.**
Purpose: **Treatment of bacterial conjunctivitis.**

FDA File **065-241**
Firm: **Pfizer, Inc.**
Use: **Dogs:** Rx only **- Oral Capsules**
Dosage: **25 milligrams per pound of body weight every 6 hours.**
Purpose: **Treatment of gastroenteritis associated with bacterial diarrhea, bacterial pulmonary infections, bacterial urinary tract infections and infections associated with canine distemper.**

FDA File **055-259**
Firm: **Evsco Pharmaceuticals**
Use: **Dogs, Cats:** Rx only **- Ophthalmic Ointment**
Dosage: **Apply to the affected eye 4 to 6 times per day for the first 72 hours depending upon the severity of the infection. Continue treatment for 48 hours after animal is**

asymptomatic. Therapy for cats should not exceed 7 days.**
Purpose: **Treatment of bacterial conjunctivitis.**

FDA File **065-460**
Firm: **Altana, Inc.**
Use: **Dogs, Cats:** Rx only **- Ophthalmic Drops**
Dosage: **Apply in the conjunctival sac every 3 hours for the first 48 hours after which night instillations may be omitted. Continue treatment for 48 hours after animal is asymptomatic. Therapy for cats should not exceed 7 days.**
Purpose: **Treatment of bacterial conjunctivitis.**

FDA File **065-461**
Firm: **Boehringer Ingelheim Vetmedica, Inc.**
Use: **Dogs:** Rx only **- Oral Tablets**
Dosage: **25 milligrams per pound of body weight every 6 hours.**
Purpose: **Treatment of gastroenteritis associated with bacterial diarrhea, bacterial pulmonary infections, bacterial urinary tract infections, and bacterial infections associated with canine distemper.**

FDA File **065-463**
Firm: **Pfizer, Inc.**
Use: **Dogs:** Rx only **- Injection**
Dosage: **5 to 15 milligrams per pound of body weight every 6 hours. In severe infections 4 to 6 hours treatment intervals may be desirable on the first day.**
Purpose: **Treatment of respiratory infections, and bacterial urinary tract infections, enteritis and tonsillitis.**

FDA File **065-489**
Firm: **Pfizer, Inc.**
Use: **Dogs:** Rx only **- Oral Tablets**
Dosage: **25 milligrams per pound of body weight every 6 hours.**
Purpose: **Treatment of bacterial pulmonary infections, bacterial urinary tract infections, enteritis, and bacterial infections associated with canine distemper.**

FDA File **065-491**
Firm: **Boehringer Ingelheim Vet-medica, Inc.**
Use: **Dogs:** Rx only **- Oral Tablets**
Dosage: **25 milligrams per pound of body weight every 6 hours.**
Purpose: **Treatment of bacterial pulmonary infections, bacterial urinary tract infections, enteritis, and bacterial infections associated with canine distemper.**

CHLORHEXIDINE (DIACETATE OR DIHYDROCHLORIDE)

FDA File **009-782**
Firm: **Fort Dodge Animal Health, Div. Of Wyeth**
Use: **Dogs, Cats, Horses: Topical Ointment**
Dosage: **Apply daily.**
Purpose: **Topical antiseptic for surface wounds.**

FDA File **009-809**
Firm: **Fort Dodge Animal Health, Div. Of Wyeth**
Use: **Cattle, Horses: Intrauterine Effervescent**
Dosage: **Contains 1 gram chlorhexidine hydrochloride. Treatment may be repeated in 48 to 72 hours.**
Purpose: **Prevention and treatment of metritis and vaginitis.**

FDA File **200-301**
Firm: **First Priority, Inc.**
Use: **Dogs, Cats, Horses: Topical Ointment**
Dosage: **1 percent chlorhexidine diacetate. Use a topical antiseptic ointment.**
Purpose: **Topical antiseptic for surface wounds.**

FDA File **010-434**
Firm: **Fort Dodge Animal Health, Div. Of Wyeth**
Use: **Cattle, Horses: One tablet or one 28-milliliter syringe. Intra-uterine use.**
Dosage: **Contains 1 gram chlorhexidine hydrochloride. Place 1 or 2 tablets deep in each uterine horn or infuse one syringe into uterus. Treatment may be repeated in 48 to 72 hours.**
Purpose: **Prevention and treatment of metritis and vaginitis.**

CHLOROBUTANOL

FDA File **065-119**
Firm: **Pharmacia & Upjohn Co.**
Use: **Dogs, Cats:** Rx only **- Topical Ointment**
Dosage: **Apply 1 to 3 times daily as necessary.**
Purpose: **Treatment of superficial wounds.**

CHLORTETRACYCLINE (BISUL-PHATE, CALCIUM COMPLEX OR HYDROCHLORIDE)

FDA File **036-361**
Firm: **Alpharma, Inc.**
Use: **Chickens: Feed Additive**
Dosage: **200 grams per ton of feed.**

162

Purpose: **Treatment of chronic respiratory disease.**

FDA File **041-647**
Firm: **Alpharma, Inc.**
Use: **Cattle: Feed Additive**
Dosage: **350 milligrams per head per day for 28 days.**
Purpose: **Maintenance of weight gains in the presence of respiratory disease such as shipping fever.**

FDA File **041-648**
Firm: **Alpharma, Inc.**
Use: **Cattle: Feed Additive**
Dosage: **350 milligrams per head per day for 28 days.**
Purpose: **Maintenance of weight gains in the presence of respiratory disease such as shipping fever.**

FDA File **041-649**
Firm: **Alpharma, Inc.**
Use: **Cattle: Feed Additive**
Dosage: **350 milligrams per head per day for 28 days.**
Purpose: **Maintenance of weight gains in the presence of respiratory disease such as shipping fever.**

FDA File **041-650**
Firm: **Alpharma, Inc.**
Use: **Cattle: Feed Additive**
Dosage: **350 milligrams per head per day for 28 days.**
Purpose: **Maintenance of weight gains in the presence of respiratory disease such as shipping fever.**

FDA File **041-651**
Firm: **Alpharma, Inc.**
Use: **Cattle: Feed Additive**
Dosage: **350 milligrams per head per day for 28 days.**

Purpose: **Maintenance of weight gains in the presence of respiratory disease such as shipping fever.**

FDA File **041-652**
Firm: **Alpharma, Inc.**
Use: **Cattle: Feed Additive**
Dosage: **350 milligrams per head per day for 28 days.**
Purpose: **Maintenance of weight gains in the presence of respiratory disease such as shipping fever.**

FDA File **041-653**
Firm: **Alpharma, Inc.**
Use: **Cattle: Feed Additive**
Dosage: **350 milligrams per head per day for 28 days.**
Purpose: **Maintenance of weight gains in the presence of respiratory disease such as shipping fever.**

FDA File **041-654**
Firm: **Alpharma, Inc.**
Use: **Cattle: Feed Additive**
Dosage: **350 milligrams per head per day for 28 days.**
Purpose: **Maintenance of weight gains in the presence of respiratory disease such as shipping fever.**

FDA File **045-444**
Firm: **Alpharma, Inc.**
Use: **Chickens: Feed Additive**
Dosage: **200 grams per ton of feed for up to 8 weeks.**
Purpose: **Treatment of chronic respiratory disease and for prevention of synovitis.**

FDA File **046-209**
Firm: **Merial Ltd.**
Use: **Chickens: Feed Additive**

Dosage: **200 grams per ton of feed for up to 25 days.**
Purpose: **Prevention of infectious synovitis.**

FDA File **049-287**
Firm: **Pfizer, Inc.**
Use: **Cattle, Swine, Chickens, Turkeys: Feed Additive**
Dosage: **10 to 500 grams per ton of complete feed.**
Purpose: **Increased rate of weight gain and improved feed efficiency and for the control and treatment of various disease conditions.**

FDA File **055-018**
Firm: **Fort Dodge Animal Health, Div. Of Wyeth**
Use: **Cattle: Oral Tablet**
Dosage: **25 milligrams per 5 pounds of body weight every 12 hours for 3 to 5 days.**
Purpose: **Control and treatment of enteritis and pneumonia.**

FDA File **055-040**
Firm: **Alpharma, Inc.**
Use: **Pet Birds: Feed Additive**
Dosage: **22 grams of mix per pound of mash.**
Purpose: **Treatment bacterial diseases in pet birds.**

FDA File **065-222**
Firm: **Hartz-Mountain Products Corp.**
Use: **Pet Birds: Medicated Feed**
Dosage: **Feed exclusively for 15 days.**
Purpose: **Treatment of bacterial diseases in pet birds.**

FDA File **091-647**
Firm: **Trinada, Inc.**
Use: **Chickens: Feed Additive**
Dosage: **10 to 20 grams per ton of complete feed.**
Purpose: **Increase rate of weight gain.**

FDA File **091-668**
Firm: **Alpharma, Inc.**
Use: **Swine: Feed Additive**
Dosage: **100 grams per ton of complete feed.**
Purpose: **Reduction of cervical abscesses, treatment of bacterial enteritis, prevention of enteritis during stress, to increase rate of weight gain and feed efficiency in swine weighing up to 75 pounds and to maintain weight gain in the presence of atrophic rhinitis.**

FDA File **092-507**
Firm: **Alpharma, Inc.**
Use: **Chickens: Feed Additive**
Dosage: **500 grams per ton of complete feed.**
Purpose: **Reduction of mortality due to *E. coli.***

FDA File **138-934**
Firm: **Pennfield Oil Co.**
Use: **Swine: Feed Additive**
Dosage: **100 grams per ton of feed.**
Purpose: **Reduction of cervical abscesses, treatment of bacterial enteritis, prevention of enteritis during stress, to increase rate of weight gain and feed efficiency in swine weighing up to 75 pounds and to maintain weight gain in the presence of atrophic rhinitis.**

FDA File **140-859**
Firm: **Alpharma, Inc.**

Use: **Chickens: Feed Additive**
Dosage: **500 grams per ton of complete feed.**
Purpose: <u>**Reduction of mortality due to E. coli.**</u>

FDA File **140-867**
Firm: **Alpharma, Inc.**
Use: **Chickens: Feed Additive**
Dosage: **500 grams per ton.**
Purpose: <u>**Reduction of mortality due to E. coli.**</u>

FDA File **141-059**
Firm: **Alpharma, Inc.**
Use: **Swine: Feed Additive**
Dosage: **500 grams per ton of complete feed.**
Purpose: <u>**Increase rate of weight gain and improved feed efficiency;**</u> **treatment of bacterial enteritis caused by** *E. coli* **and** *Salmonella choleraesuis* **and bacterial pneumonia caused by** *Pasteurella multocida* <u>**and for control of porcine proliferative enteropathies (ileitis) caused by** *Lawsonia intracellularis.*</u> **Treat for not more than 14 days.**

FDA File **141-147**
Firm: **Alpharma, Inc.**
Use: **Cattle: Feed Additive**
Dosage: **1 gram per 100 pounds body weight.**
Purpose: **Treatment of bacterial enteritis caused by** *E. coli*, **and for treatment of pneumonia caused by** *Pasteurella multocida.* **Treat for not more than 5 days.**

FDA File **141-185**
Firm: **Alpharma, Inc.**
Use: **Cattle: Feed Additive**

Dosage: **1 gram per 100 pounds body weight.**
Purpose: **Treatment of bacterial enteritis caused by** *E. coli*, **and for treatment of pneumonia caused by** *Pasteurella multocida.* **Treat for not more than 5 days.**

FDA File **141-201**
Firm: **Alpharma, Inc.**
Use: **Cattle: Feed Additive**
Dosage: **10 to 350 milligrams per 100 pounds body weight.**
Purpose: <u>**Improved feed efficiency and increased rate of weight gain and for control of bacterial pneumonia caused by** *Pasteurella* **spp.**</u>

FDA File **141-250**
Firm: **Alpharma, Inc.**
Use: **Cattle: Feed Additive**
Dosage: **25 to 4,000 grams per ton of complete feed.**
Purpose: <u>**Increased rate of weight gain and feed efficiency.**</u> **Treatment of bacterial enteritis caused by** *E. coli*, <u>**control of active infections of anaplasmosis,**</u> **and for treatment of pneumonia caused by** *Pasteurella multocida.*

FDA File **200-091**
Firm: **Intervet, Inc.**
Use: **Chickens: Feed Additive**
Dosage: **500 grams per ton.**
Purpose: <u>**Reduction of mortality due to E. coli.**</u>

FDA File **200-095**
Firm: **Intervet, Inc.**
Use: **Chickens: Feed Additive**
Dosage: **500 grams per ton.**
Purpose: <u>**Reduction of mortality due to E. coli.**</u>

FDA File **200-259**
Firm: **Alpharma, Inc.**
Use: **Chickens: Feed Additive**
Dosage: **500 grams per ton.**
Purpose: **Reduction of mortality due to E. coli.**

FDA File **200-260**
Firm: **Alpharma, Inc.**
Use: **Chickens: Feed Additive**
Dosage: **500 grams per ton.**
Purpose: **Reduction of mortality due to E. coli.**

FDA File **200-261**
Firm: **Alpharma, Inc.**
Use: **Chickens: Feed Additive**
Dosage: **500 grams per ton.**
Purpose: **Reduction of mortality due to E. coli.**

FDA File **200-262**
Firm: **Alpharma, Inc.**
Use: **Chickens: Feed Additive**
Dosage: **500 grams per ton.**
Purpose: **Reduction of mortality due to E. coli.**

FDA File **200-263**
Firm: **Alpharma, Inc.**
Use: **Chickens: Feed Additive**
Dosage: **500 grams per ton.**
Purpose: **Reduction of mortality due to E. coli.**

FDA File **200-314**
Firm: **Pennfield Oil Co.**
Use: **Cattle: Feed Additive**
Dosage: **350 milligrams per head per day for 28 days.**
Purpose: **Maintenance of weight gain in the presence of respiratory diseases such as shipping fever.**

FDA File **200-354**
Firm: **Pennfield Oil Co.**
Use: **Chickens: Feed Additive**
Dosage: **500 grams per ton.**
Purpose: **Reduction of mortality due to E. coli.** Feed for not more than 5 days.

FDA File **200-355**
Firm: **Pennfield Oil Co.**
Use: **Chickens: Feed Additive**
Dosage: **500 grams per ton.**
Purpose: **Reduction of mortality due to E. coli.** Feed for not more than 5 days.

FDA File **200-356**
Firm: **Pennfield Oil Co.**
Use: **Swine: Feed Additive**
Dosage: **400 grams per ton.**
Purpose: **Treatment of bacterial enteritis caused by** E. coli **and** Salmonella choleraesuis **and bacterial pneumonia caused by P.** multocida.

FDA File **200-357**
Firm: **Pennfield Oil Co.**
Use: **Chickens: Feed Additive**
Dosage: **500 grams per ton.**
Purpose: **Reduction of mortality due to E. coli.** Feed for not more than 5 days.

FDA File **200-358**
Firm: **Pennfield Oil Co.**
Use: **Swine: Feed Additive**
Dosage: **400 grams per ton.**
Purpose: **Increased rate of weight gains and improved feed efficiency;** treatment of bacterial enteritis caused by E. coli and Salmonella choleraesuis and bacterial pneumonia caused by P. multocida, treatment of porcine proliferative enter-

opathies (ileitis) caused by *Lawsonia intracellularis.*

FDA File **200-359**
Firm: **Pennfield Oil Co.**
Use: **Cattle: Feed Additive**
Dosage: **1 gram per 100 pounds body weight per day for up to 5 days.**
Purpose: **Treatment of bacterial enteritis caused by** *E. coli* **and** *Salmonella choleraesui*s **and bacterial pneumonia caused by** *P. multocida.*

FDA File **055-012**
Firm: **Fort Dodge Animal Health, Div. Of Wyeth**
Use: **Swine: Water Additive**
Dosage: **25 milligrams per gallon for up to 28 days.**
Purpose: **Prevention and treatment of bacterial enteritis, reduction of the incidence of cervical abscesses, and for maintenance of weight gains in the presence of atrophic rhinitis and bacterial enteritis.**

FDA File **055-020**
Firm: **Fort Dodge Animal Health, Div. Wyeth**
Use: **Cattle, Swine, Chickens, Turkeys: Soluble powder**
Dosage: **Cattle and Swine: 10 milligrams per pound of body weight in daily doses as a drench to be use for not more than 5 days. Chickens: 200 to 1000 milligrams per gallon water for up to 14 days. Turkeys: 400 milligrams per gallon water or 15 milligrams per pound body weight daily up to 14 days.**
Purpose: **Cattle, Swine: Treatment of bacterial enteritis and bacterial pneumonia. Chickens: Control of infectious synovitis, chronic respiratory disease, and air-sac infections; control of mortality due to fowl cholera. Turkey: Control of synovitis and bluecomb disease (transmissible enteritis).**

FDA File **065-113**
Firm: **Purina Mill, Inc.**
Use: **Swine: Water Additive**
Dosage: **250 milligrams per gallon for up to 28 days.**
Purpose: **Prevention and treatment of bacterial enteritis, reduction of the incidence of cervical abscesses, and for maintenance of weight gains in the presence of atrophic rhinitis and bacterial enteritis.**

FDA File **065-486**
Firm: **Boehringer Ingelheim Vetmedica, Inc.**
Use: **Cattle, Swine, Chickens, Turkeys: Soluble Powder**
Dosage: **Cattle and Swine: 10 milligrams per pound of body weight in daily doses as a drench to be use for not more than 5 days. Chickens and Turkeys: 200 to 800 milligrams per gallon water for up to 14 days. Turkeys: 400 milligrams per gallon water or 15 milligrams per pound body weight daily up to 14 days.**
Purpose: **Cattle, Swine: Treatment of bacterial enteritis and bacterial pneumonia. Chickens: Control of infectious synovitis, chronic respiratory disease, and air-sac infections; control of mortality due to fowl cholera. Turkey: Control of synovitis and bluecomb disease (transmissible enteritis).**

FDA File **046-699**
Firm: **Alpharma, Inc.**

Use: **Cattle, Sheep, Swine, Chickens, Turkeys: Feed Additive**
Dosage: **10 to 500 grams per ton.**
Purpose: **Cattle, Sheep, Chickens, Turkeys: Treatment or prevention of various diseases. Swine: Control of porcine proliferative enteropathies (ileitis).**

FDA File **048-480**
Firm: **ADM Animal Health & Nutrition Div.**
Use: **Cattle, Swine, Chickens, Turkeys: Feed Additive**
Dosage: **10 to 500 grams per ton. For beef calves feed 400 grams per ton or to provide 10 milligrams per pound of body weight per day.**
Purpose: **For increased weight gain and improved feed efficiency in chickens, turkeys, and calves. For treatment or prevention of various diseases in all species.**

FDA File **048-761**
Firm: **Alpharma, Inc.**
Use: **Cattle, Sheep, Swine, Chickens, Turkeys, Ducks: Feed Additive**
Dosage: **4 to 500 grams per ton or 10 milligrams per pound of body weight per day.**
Purpose: **Chickens, Turkeys, Swine and Sheep: Increased rate of weight gain and improved feed efficiency. Turkeys: Control of hexamitiasis in poults up to 4 weeks of age and reduction of mortality due to paratyphoid. Breeding Swine: Control of porcine proliferative enteropathies (ileitis) and control of leptospirosis by reducing the incidence of abortion and shedding of leptospirae. Chickens: Reduction of mortality due to**

E. coli. **Cattle: Control of active infections of anaplasmosis and bacterial enteritis and bacterial pneumonia.**

FDA File **048-762**
Firm: **Roche Vitamins, Inc.**
Use: **Cattle, Sheep, Swine, Chickens, Turkeys, Ducks, Psittacine Birds (parrots, macaws, cockatoos): Feed Additive**
Dosage: **10 to 500 grams per ton or 10 milligrams per pound of body weight per day.**
Purpose: **Chickens, Turkeys, Swine and Sheep: Increased rate of weight gain and improved feed efficiency. Turkeys: Control of hexamitiasis in poults up to 4 weeks of age and reduction of mortality due to paratyphoid. Breeding Swine: Control of porcine proliferative enteropathies (ileitis) and control of leptospirosis by reducing the incidence of abortion and shedding of leptospirae. Chickens: Reduction of mortality due to *E. coli*. Cattle: Control of active infections of anaplasmosis and bacterial enteritis and bacterial pneumonia. Psittacine Birds: Treatment of birds suspected or known to be infested with psittacosis.**

FDA File **092-286**
Firm: **Phibro Animal Health, Inc.**
Use: **Cattle, Sheep, Swine, Chickens, Turkeys: Feed Additive**
Dosage: **10 to 500 grams per ton or 10 milligrams per pound of body weight per day.**
Purpose: **Chickens, Turkeys, Sheep, Calves: Increased rate of weight gain and improved feed efficiency.**

Cattle, Sheep, Swine, Chickens, Turkeys: Treatment <u>or prevention</u> of various diseases caused by organisms susceptible to chlortetracycline.

FDA File **092-287**
Firm: **Phibro Animal Health, Inc.**
Use: **Cattle, Sheep, Swine, Chickens, Turkeys: Feed Additive**
Dosage: **10 to 500 grams per ton or 10 milligrams per pound of body weight per day.**
Purpose: **Cattle, Sheep, Swine, Chickens, Turkeys: <u>Control or prevention of various diseases caused by organisms susceptible to chlortetracycline.</u>**

FDA File **100-901**
Firm: **Pfizer, Inc.**
Use: **Cattle, Sheep, Swine, Chickens, Turkeys, Horses, Mink: Feed Additive**
Dosage: **10 to 500 grams per ton or 10 milligrams per pound of body weight per day.**
Purpose: **<u>Increased rate of weight gain and improved feed efficiency.</u> Treatment <u>or prevention</u> of various diseases caused by organisms susceptible to chlortetracycline. Increased pelt size in mink.**

FDA File **138-934**
Firm: **Pennfield Oil Co.**
Use: **Swine: Feed Additive**
Dosage: **100 grams per ton.**
Purpose: **<u>Reduction of the incidence of cervical abscesses, treatment of bacterial enteritis and vibrionic dysentery, and for prevention of these diseases during times of stress; maintenance of weight gain in the presence of atrophic rhini-</u>**

<u>tis, and for growth promotion and increased feed efficiency in swine up to 75 pounds body weight.</u>

FDA File **138-935**
Firm: **Pennfield Oil Co.**
Use: **Cattle, Sheep, Swine, Chickens, Turkeys: Feed Additive**
Dosage: **10 to 500 grams per ton or 10 milligrams per pound of body weight per day.**
Purpose: **Treatment <u>or prevention</u> of various diseases caused by organisms susceptible to chlortetracycline.**

FDA File **141-011**
Firm: **Novartis Animal Health US, Inc.**
Use: **Swine: Feed Additive**
Dosage: **400 grams per ton or 10 milligrams per pound of body weight for 14 days.**
Purpose: **Treatment of bacterial enteritis and bacterial pneumonia.**

FDA File **141-059**
Firm: **Alpharma, Inc.**
Use: **Swine: Feed Additive**
Dosage: **400 grams per ton or 10 milligrams per pound of body weight for 14 days.**
Purpose: **<u>Increased rate of weight gain and improved feed efficiency.</u> Treatment of bacterial enteritis and bacterial pneumonia and control of porcine proliferative enteropathies (ileitis).**

FDA File **141-147**
Firm: **Alpharma, Inc.**
Use: **Cattle: Feed Additive**
Dosage: **500 to 20,000 grams per ton or 10 milligrams per pound of**

body weight for not more than 5 days.
Purpose: **Treatment of bacterial enteritis and bacterial pneumonia.**

FDA File **141-185**
Firm: **Alpharma, Inc.**
Use: **Cattle: Feed Additive**
Dosage: **500 to 20,000 grams per ton or 10 milligrams per pound of body weight for not more than 5 days.**
Purpose: **Treatment of bacterial enteritis and bacterial pneumonia.**

FDA File **141-201**
Firm: **Alpharma, Inc.**
Use: **Cattle: Feed Additive**
Dosage: **10 to 350 milligrams per pound of body weight.**
Purpose: **Improved feed efficiency and increased rate of weight gain and for control of bacterial pneumonia associated with shipping fever in cattle fed in confinement for slaughter.**

FDA File **200-091**
Firm: **Intervet, Inc.**
Use: **Chickens: Feed Additive**
Dosage: **500 grams per ton for not more than 5 days.**
Purpose: **Reduction of mortality due to _E. coli._**

FDA File **200-095**
Firm: **Intervet, Inc.**
Use: **Chickens: Feed Additive**
Dosage: **500 grams per ton for not more than 5 days.**
Purpose: **Reduction of mortality due to _E. coli._**

FDA File **200-167**
Firm: **Alpharma, Inc.**

Use: **Swine: Feed Additive**
Dosage: **100 grams per ton.**
Purpose: **Increased rate of weight gain and improved feed efficiency. Treatment of bacterial enteritis or necrotic enteritis, maintenance of weight gains in the presence of atrophic rhinitis. For swine in confinement (dry-lot) or on limited pasture.**

FDA File **200-236**
Firm: **Phoenix Scientific, Inc.**
Use: **Chickens, Turkeys, Swine: Soluble Powder**
Dosage: **200 to 800 milligrams per gallon of drinking water.**
Purpose: **Chickens: Control of infectious synovitis and chronic respiratory disease. Turkeys: Control of infectious synovitis and complicating bacterial organisms associated with bluecomb. Swine: Control and treatment of bacterial enteritis and bacterial pneumonia.**

FDA File **200-242**
Firm: **Alpharma, Inc.**
Use: **Swine: Feed Additive**
Dosage: **400 grams per ton or 10 milligrams per pound of body weight.**
Purpose: **Increased rate of weight gain and improved feed efficiency. Treatment of bacterial enteritis and bacterial pneumonia.**

FDA File **035-688**
Firm: **Alpharma, Inc.**
Use: **Swine: Feed Additive**
Dosage: **100 grams per ton**
Purpose: **Increased rate of weight gain and improved feed efficiency in swine up to 75 pounds body weight. Treatment of bacterial**

enteritis, maintenance of weight gains in the presence of atrophic rhinitis. Reduction in the incidence of cervical abscesses.

FDA File **035-805**
Firm: **Alpharma, Inc.**
Use: **Cattle: Feed Additive**
Dosage: **350 milligrams per head per day.**
Purpose: **Maintenance of weight gains in the presence of respiratory**
diseases such as shipping fever.

FDA File **039-077**
Firm: **Alpharma, Inc.**
Use: **Swine: Feed Additive**
Dosage: **100 grams per ton**
Purpose: **Reduction in the incidence of cervical abscesses,** treatment of bacterial enteritis or necrotic enteritis and vibrionic dysentery, maintenance of weight gains in the presence of atrophic rhinitis, improved rate of weight gain and improved feed efficiency in swine 10 pounds body weight to 6 weeks after weaning. For swine in confinement (dry-lot) or on limited pasture up to 16 weeks after weaning.

FDA File **048-761**
Firm: **Alpharma, Inc.**
Use: **Cattle, Sheep, Swine, Chickens, Turkeys, Ducks: Feed Additive**
Dosage: **10 to 500 grams per ton or 10 milligrams per pound of body weight per day.**
Purpose: **Chickens, Turkeys, Swine and Sheep: Increased weight gain and improved feed efficiency. Ducks: Control and treatment of fowl cholera. Turkeys: Control of**

hexamitiasis, in poults not over 4 weeks of age for reduction of mortality due to paratyphoid. Breeding swine: Control of porcine proliferative enteropathies (ileitis), control of leptospirosis (reducing the incidence of abortion and shedding of leptospirae). Chickens: Reduction of mortality due to _E. coli_. Cattle: Control of active infections of anaplasmosis and bacterial enteritis and bacterial pneumonia.

FDA File **055-039**
Firm: **Fort Dodge Animal Health, Div. Of Wyeth**
Use: **Cattle: Oral bolus.**
Dosage: **500 milligrams per 100 pounds body weight twice per day for 3 to 5 days.**
Purpose: **Treatment of bacterial enteritis and bacterial pneumonia.**

FDA File **065-020**
Firm: **Alpharma, Inc.**
Use: **Swine, Chickens, Turkeys: Feed Additive**
Dosage: **Varies by species: 10 to 500 grams per ton of complete feed for chickens; 50 to 100 grams per ton or 10 milligrams per pound of body weight for swine; 10 to 400 grams per ton of complete feed for turkeys.**
Purpose: **Growth promotion and feed efficiency in chickens, turkeys and swine; prevention of chronic respiratory disease in chickens and infectious, synovitis, bluecomb, hexamitiasis and reduction of mortality due to paratyphoid in turkeys. Maintaining or increasing egg production or hatchability of**

eggs in laying hens. Prevention of early mortality in chicks. Maintenance of weight gain in swine enteritis, reduction of the spread of leptospirosis, and for prevention of bacterial swine enteritis during times of stress.

FDA File **065-071**
Firm: **Fort Dodge Animal Health, Div. Of Wyeth**
Use: **Cattle, Swine, Chickens, Turkeys: Water Additive**
Dosage: **Chickens: 200 to 400 milligrams per gallon of drinking water or 1000 milligrams per gallon, depending on target use. Turkeys: 25 or 400 milligrams per pound of body weight per day, depending on target use. Swine: 10 milligrams per pound of body weight per day in divided doses. Cattle: 10 milligrams per pound of body weight daily in divided doses. Use as a drench in cattle.**
Purpose: **Chickens: Control of infectious synovitis, chronic respiratory disease, air-sac infections and control of mortality due to fowl cholera. Turkeys: Control of infectious synovitis, control of complicating bacterial organisms associated with bluecomb. Swine: Control and treatment of bacterial enteritis and bacterial pneumonia. Cattle: Control and treatment of bacterial enteritis and bacterial pneumonia.**

FDA File **065-078**
Firm: **Boehringer Ingelheim Vetmedica, Inc.**
Use: **Cattle, Swine, Chickens, Turkeys: Water Additive**
Dosage: **Chickens, Turkeys: 200 to 800 milligrams per gallon of**

drinking water. Swine: 10 milligrams per pound of body weight per day in divided doses. Swine, Cattle: 10 milligrams per pound of body weight daily in divided doses. Use as a drench in cattle.
Purpose: **Chickens: Control of infectious synovitis. Turkeys: Control of bluecomb and infectious synovitis: Swine: Control and treatment of bacterial enteritis and bacterial pneumonia. Cattle: Control and treatment of bacterial enteritis and bacterial pneumonia.**

FDA File **065-256**
Firm: **ADM Animal Health & Nutrition Div.**
Use: **Swine, Chickens, Turkeys: Water Additive**
Dosage: **Chickens: 200 to 400 milligrams per gallon of drinking water or 1000 milligrams per gallon, depending on target use. Turkeys: 25 or 400 milligrams per pound of body weight per day, depending on target use. Swine: 10 milligrams per pound of body weight per day in divided doses.**
Purpose: **Chickens: Control of infectious synovitis, chronic respiratory disease, air-sac infections and control of mortality due to fowl cholera. Turkeys: Control of complicating bacterial organisms associated with bluecomb. Swine: Control and treatment of bacterial enteritis and bacterial pneumonia.**

FDA File **065-440**
Firm: **Fort Dodge Animal Health, Div. Of Wyeth**
Use: **Swine, Chickens, Turkeys, Beef Cattle, Dairy Cattle: Water Additive**

Dosage: **Swine: 10 milligrams per pound of body weight. Chickens: 200 to 400 milligrams per gallon for 7 to 14 days. Turkeys: 400 milligrams per gallon. Beef and Dairy cattle: 10 mg per pound of body weight for 3 to 5 days.**
Purpose: **For <u>prevention and</u> treatment of various diseases, depending on the species, dosage, and length of use.**

FDA File **065-480**
Firm: **Pennfield Oil Co.**
Use: **Cattle, Swine: Water Additive**
Dosage: **Swine: 10 milligrams per kilogram of body weight per day. Calves: 10 milligrams per pound of body weight per day. Use for up to 5 days.**
Purpose: **<u>Control and</u> treatment of bacterial enteritis and bacterial pneumonia.**

FDA File **065-481**
Firm: **ADM Animal Health & Nutrition Div.**
Use: **Cattle: Oral Bolus**
Dosage: **250 milligrams per 50 pounds body weight twice daily for 3 to 5 days.**
Purpose: **Treatment of bacterial enteritis and bacterial pneumonia.**

FDA File **121-553**
Firm: **Alpharma, Inc.**
Use: **Chickens: Feed Additive**
Dosage: **500 grams per ton for up to 5 days.**
Purpose: **<u>Reduction of mortality due to *E. coli.*</u>**

FDA File **200-140**
Firm: **Alpharma, Inc.**
Use: **Swine: Feed Additive**

Dosage: **100 grams per ton.**
Purpose: **<u>Reduction in the incidence of cervical abscesses</u>, treatment of bacterial enteritis or necrotic enteritis <u>and maintenance of weight gains in the presence of atrophic rhinitis, improved rate of weight gain and improved feed efficiency.</u>**

FDA File **200-236**
Firm: **Phoenix Scientific, Inc.**
Use: **Chickens, Turkeys, Swine: Water Additive**
Dosage: **Chickens: 200 to 400 milligrams per gallon. Turkeys: 400 to 800 milligrams per gallon. Swine: 10 milligrams per pound of body weight.**
Purpose: **Chickens: <u>Control of infectious synovitis and chronic respiratory disease and air-sac infections. Turkeys: Control of infectious synovitis and complicating bacterial organisms associated with bluecomb.</u> Swine: <u>Control and</u> treatment of bacterial enteritis and bacterial pneumonia.**

FDA File **200-295**
Firm: **Pennfield Oil Co.**
Use: **Cattle, Chickens, Turkeys, Swine: Water Additive**
Dosage: **Chickens: 100 to 200 milligrams per gallon. Turkeys: 400 to 800 milligrams per gallon. Swine: 100 to 600 milligrams per gallon.**
Purpose: **Cattle, Swine: <u>Control of bacterial pneumonia and bacterial enteritis. Chickens: Control of infectious synovitis and chronic respiratory disease, air-sac infections and control of mortality due to fowl cholera. Turkeys: Control of infectious synovitis and compli-</u>**

173

cating bacterial organisms associated with bluecomb.

CLAVULANATE (POTASSIUM)

FDA File **055-099**
Firm: **Pfizer, Inc.**
Use: **Dogs:** Rx only **- Oral Tablets**
Dosage: **1.25 milligrams per pound of body weight twice per day for up to 30 days.**
Purpose: **Treatment of skin and soft tissue infections such as wounds, abscesses, cellulites, superficial juvenile and deep pyoderma. Treatment of periodontal infections.**

FDA File **055-101**
Firm: **Pfizer, Inc.**
Use: **Dogs:** Rx only **- Oral Suspension**
Dosage: **1.25 milligrams per pound of body weight twice per day for up to 30 days.**
Purpose: **Treatment of skin and soft tissue infections such as wounds, abscesses, cellulites, superficial juvenile and deep pyoderma. Treatment of periodontal infections.**

FDA File **055-102**
Firm: **Pfizer, Inc.**
Use: **Dogs, Cats:** Rx only **- Oral Tablets**
Dosage: **12.5 milligrams per pound of body weight twice per day for up to 30 days.**
Purpose: **Treatment of skin and soft tissue infections such as wounds, abscesses, cellulites, superficial juvenile and deep pyoderma.**

Treatment of urinary tract infections.

FDA File **055-103**
Firm: **Pfizer, Inc.**
Use: **Cats:** Rx only **- Oral Suspension**
Dosage: **.5 milligrams per pound of body weight twice per day for up to 30 days.**
Purpose: **Treatment of skin and soft tissue infections such as wounds, abscesses, cellulites, superficial juvenile and deep pyoderma.**

CLINDAMYCIN (HYDROCHLORIDE)

FDA File **120-298**
Firm: **Phoenix Scientific, Inc.**
Use: **Dogs:** Rx only **- Oral Capsules**
Dosage: **2.5 to 15 milligrams per pound of body weight every 12 hours for up to 28 days.**
Purpose: **Treatment of wounds, abscesses, dental infections, and osteomyelitis.**

FDA File **120-316**
Firm: **Virbac Animal Health, Inc.**
Use: **Dogs:** Rx only **- Oral Tablets**
Dosage: **2.5 to 15 milligrams per pound of body weight every 12 hours for up to 28 days.**
Purpose: **Treatment of wounds, abscesses, dental infections, and osteomyelitis.**

FDA File **120-161**
Firm: **Pharmacia & Upjohn Co.**
Use: **Dogs:** Rx only **- Oral Capsules**
Dosage: **2.5 to 15 milligrams per pound of body weight every 12 hours for up to 28 days.**

Purpose: **Treatment of wounds, abscesses, dental infections, and osteomyelitis.**

FDA File **135-940**
Firm: **Pharmacia & Upjohn Co.**
Use: **Dogs, Cats:** Rx only **- Oral Liquid**
Dosage: **Dogs: 2.5 to 15 milligrams per pound of body weight every 12 hours for up to 28 days. For treatment of osteomyelitis 5 to 15 milligrams per pound of body weight per 12 hours for a minimum of 28 days. Cats: 5.0 to 15.0 milligrams per pound of body weight per 24 hours for a maximum of 14 days.**
Purpose: **Dogs: Treatment of wounds, abscesses, dental infections, and osteomyelitis. Cats: Treatment of skin infections, deep wounds and abscesses, and dental infections; treatment of soft tissue infections.**

FDA File **200-193**
Firm: **Phoenix Scientific, Inc.**
Use: **Dogs, Cats:** Rx only **- Oral Liquid**
Dosage: **Dogs: 2.5 to 15 milligrams per pound of body weight every 12 hours for up to 28 days. For osteomyelitis 5 to 15 milligrams per pound of body weight per 12 hours for a minimum of 28 days. Cats: 5.0 to 15.0 milligrams per pound of body weight per 24 hours for a maximum of 14 days.**
Purpose: **Dogs: Treatment of wounds, abscesses, dental infections, and osteomyelitis. Cats: Treatment of skin infections, deep wounds and abscesses, and dental infections; treatment of soft tissue infections.**

FDA File **200-291**
Firm: **Virbac Animal Health, Inc.**
Use: **Dogs, Cats:** Rx only **- Oral Liquid**
Dosage: **Dogs: 2.5 to 15 milligrams per pound of body weight every 12 hours for up to 28 days. For osteomyelitis 5 to 15 milligrams per pound of body weight per 12 hours for a minimum of 28 days. Cats: 5.0 to 10 milligrams per pound of body weight per 24 hours for a maximum of 14 days.**
Purpose: **Dogs: Treatment of skin infections (wounds, abscesses), dental infections, and osteomyelitis. Cats: Treatment of skin infections, deep wounds and abscesses, and dental infections; treatment of soft tissue infections.**

FDA File **200-316**
Firm: **Virbac AH, Inc.**
Use: **Dogs:** Rx only **- Oral Tablets**
Dosage: **2.5 to 15 milligrams per pound of body weight every 12 hours for up to 28 days.**
Purpose: **Treatment of wounds, abscesses, dental infections, and osteomyelitis.**

FDA File **200-383**
Firm: **Novopharm Ltd.**
Use: **Dogs:** Rx only **- Oral Tablets**
Dosage: **2.5 to 15 milligrams per pound of body weight every 12 hours for up to 28 days.**
Purpose: **Treatment of wounds, abscesses, dental infections, and osteomyelitis.**

FDA File **200-398**
Firm: **First Priority, Inc.**

Use: **Dogs, Cats:** Rx only **- Oral Liquid**
Dosage: **Dogs: 2.5 to 15 milligrams per pound of body weight every 12 hours for up to 28 days. For osteomyelitis 5 to 15 milligrams per pound of body weight per 12 hours for a minimum of 28 days. Cats: 5.0 to 15.0 milligrams per pound of body weight per 24 hours for a maximum of 14 days.**
Purpose: **Dogs: Treatment of wounds, abscesses, dental infections, and osteomyelitis. Cats: Treatment of skin infections, deep wounds and abscesses, and dental infections; treatment of soft tissue infections.**

CLOPIDOL

FDA File **034-393**
Firm: **Huvepharma AD**
Use: **Chickens, Turkeys: Feed Additive Premix**
Dosage: **113.5 grams per ton of feed.**
Purpose: **Prevention of coccidiosis.**

FDA File **040-264**
Firm: **Merial Ltd.**
Use: **Chickens: Feed Additive Premix**
Dosage: **113.5 grams per ton of feed.**
Purpose: **Prevention of coccidiosis.**

FDA File **041-541**
Firm: **Merial Ltd.**
Use: **Chickens: Feed Additive Premix**
Dosage: **113.5 grams per ton of feed.**
Purpose: **Prevention of coccidiosis.**

FDA File **044-016**
Firm: **Merial Ltd.**
Use: **Chickens: Feed Additive Premix**
Dosage: **113.5 grams per ton of feed.**
Purpose: **Prevention of coccidiosis.**

FDA File **044-972**
Firm: **Pharmacia & Upjohn Co.**
Use: **Chickens: Feed Additive Premix**
Dosage: **113.5 grams per ton of feed.**
Purpose: **Prevention of coccidiosis.**

FDA File **046-209**
Firm: **Merial Ltd.**
Use: **Chickens: Feed Additive Premix**
Dosage: **113.5 grams per ton of feed.**
Purpose: **Prevention of coccidiosis.**

FDA File **049-934**
Firm: **Merial Ltd.**
Use: **Chickens: Feed Additive Premix**
Dosage: **113.5 grams per ton of feed.**
Purpose: **Prevention of coccidiosis.**

FDA File **099-150**
Firm: **Merial Ltd.**
Use: **Chickens: Feed Additive Premix**
Dosage: **113.5 grams per ton of feed.**
Purpose: **Prevention of coccidiosis.**

FDA File **200-207**
Firm: **Alpharma, Inc.**
Use: **Chickens: Feed Additive Premix**

Dosage: **113.5 grams per ton of feed.**
Purpose: **Prevention of coccidiosis.**

FDA File **200-218**
Firm: **Alpharma, Inc.**
Use: **Chickens: Feed Additive Premix**
Dosage: **113.5 grams per ton of feed.**
Purpose: **Prevention of coccidiosis.**

CLOXACILLIN (BENZATHINE OR SODIUM)

FDA File **055-058**
Firm: **Fort Dodge Animal Health, Div. Of Wyeth**
Use: **Cattle:** Rx only **- Intramammary Infusion**
Dosage: **500 milligrams per quarter.**
Purpose: **Treatment of mastitis.**

FDA File **055-068**
Firm: **Norbrook Laboratories**
Use: **Cattle:** Rx only **- Intramammary Infusion**
Dosage: **500 milligrams per quarter.**
Purpose: **Treatment of mastitis in dry cows.**

FDA File **055-069**
Firm: **Schering-Plough Animal Health**
Use: **Cattle:** Rx only **- Intramammary Infusion**
Dosage: **500 milligrams per quarter.**
Purpose: **Treatment of mastitis in dry cows.**

FDA File **055-070**
Firm: **Schering-Plough Animal Health**

Use: **Cattle: Intramammary Infusion**
Dosage: **10 ml (200 milligrams) per infected quarter after milking, cleaning, and disinfecting. Repeat at 12 hour intervals.**
Purpose: **Treatment of mastitis in lactating cows.**

COPPER NAPHTHENATE

FDA File **012-991**
Firm: **Fort Dodge Animal Health, Div. Of Wyeth**
Use: **Horses: Topical Solution**
Dosage: **Apply 37.5 percent solution to hoof.**
Purpose: **Treatment of degenerative hoof disease (thrush).**

FDA File **100-616**
Firm: **Farnam Companies, Inc.**
Use: **Horses: Topical Solution**
Dosage: **Apply 37.5 percent solution to hoof**
Purpose: **Treatment of degenerative hoof disease (thrush).**

FDA File **200-304**
Firm: **First Priority, Inc.**
Use: **Horses: Topical Solution**
Dosage: **Apply 37.5 percent solution to hoof.**
Purpose: **Treatment of degenerative hoof disease (thrush).**

CUPRIMYXIN (6-methoxy-1-phenazinol 5, 10 dioxide, cupric complex)

FDA File **093-029**
Firm: **Roche Vitamins, Inc.**
Use: **Dogs, Cats, Horses:** Rx only **- Topical Cream**

Dosage: **Apply cream containing 0.5 percent cuprimyxin to skin, hair and external mucosa.**
Purpose: **Treatment of superficial infections caused by gram-positive and gram-negative bacteria.**

CYCLOSPORINE

FDA File **141-052**
Firm: **Schering-Plough Animal Health**
Use: **Dogs:** Rx only **- Ophthalmic Ointment**
Dosage: **Apply a one-quarter inch strip of ointment containing 2 mg per gram to affected eye(s) every 12 hours.**
Purpose: **Management of chronic keratoconjunctivitis sicca and chronic superficial keratitis.**

FDA File **141-218**
Firm: **Novartis Animal Health US, Inc.**
Use: **Dogs:** Rx only **- Oral Capsules**
Dosage: **5 milligrams per kilogram of body weight daily for 30 days.**
Purpose: **Control of atopic dermatitis.**

DANOFLOXACIN (MESYLATE)

FDA File **141-207**
Firm: **Pfizer, Inc.**
Use: **Cattle:** Rx only **- Injection**
Dosage: **6 milligrams per kilogram of body weight by subcutaneous injection and repeat in 48 hours.**
Purpose: **Treatment of bovine respiratory disease.**

DECOQUINATE

FDA File **039-417**
Firm: **Alpharma, Inc.**
Use: **Cattle, Chickens, Sheep, Goats: Feed additive premix**
Dosage: **Chickens: 27.2 grams per ton of complete feed; Cattle, Sheep, Goats: 22.7 milligrams per 100 pounds body weight; Dry milk replacer: 0.0015 to 0.059 percent.**
Purpose: **Prevention of coccidiosis.**

FDA File **040-435**
Firm: **Alpharma, Inc.**
Use: **Chickens: Feed Additive Premix**
Dosage: **Chickens: 27.2 grams per ton of complete feed.** Purpose: **Prevention of coccidiosis.**

FDA File **045-348**
Firm: **Alpharma, Inc.**
FDA File **045-444**
Firm: **Alpharma, Inc.**
Use: **Chickens: Feed Additive**
Dosage: **Chickens: 27.2 grams per ton of complete feed for up to 8 weeks.**
Purpose: **Prevention of coccidiosis.**

FDA File **047-261**
Firm: **Pharmacia & Upjohn Co.**
Use: **Chickens: Feed Additive**
Dosage: **Chickens: 27.2 grams per ton of complete feed.** Purpose: **Prevention of coccidiosis.**

FDA File **047-262**
Firm: **Alpharma, Inc.**
Use: **Chickens: Feed Additive**
Dosage: **Chickens: 27.2 grams per ton of complete feed.**

Purpose: **Prevention of coccidiosis.**

FDA File **091-326**
Firm: **Alpharma, Inc.**
Use: **Chickens: Feed Additive**
Dosage: **Chickens: 27.2 grams per ton of complete feed.** Purpose: **Prevention of coccidiosis.**

FDA File **141-060**
Firm: **Alpharma, Inc.**
Use: **Calves: Milk Additive**
Dosage: **22.7 milligrams per 100 pounds body weight per day for 28 days.**
Purpose: **Prevention of coccidiosis.**

FDA File **141-100**
Firm: **Alpharma, Inc.**
Use: **Chickens: Feed Additive**
Dosage: **Chickens: 27.2 grams per ton of complete feed.** Purpose: **Prevention of coccidiosis.**

FDA File **141-102**
Firm: **Alpharma, Inc.**
Use: **Chickens: Feed Additive**
Dosage: **Chickens: 27.2 grams per ton of complete feed.** Purpose: **Prevention of coccidiosis.**

FDA File **141-147**
Firm: **Alpharma, Inc.**
Use: **Cattle: Feed Additive**
Dosage: **12.9 to 90.8 grams per ton of complete feed and 90.0 to 535.7 grams per ton in feed supplements.**
Purpose: **Prevention of coccidiosis.**

FDA File **141-148**
Firm: **Alpharma, Inc.**
Use: **Cattle: Feed Additive**

Dosage: **12.9 to 90.8 grams per ton of complete feed for at least 28 days.**
Purpose: **Prevention of coccidiosis.**

FDA File **141-149**
Firm: **Alpharma, Inc.**
Use: **Cattle: Feed Additive**
Dosage: **13.6 to 27.2 grams per ton of complete feed to achieve 22.7 milligrams per 100 pounds of body weight per day for at least 28 days.**
Purpose: **Prevention of coccidiosis.**

FDA File **141-185**
Firm: **Alpharma, Inc.**
Use: **Cattle: Feed Additive**
Dosage: **12.9 to 90.8 grams per ton of complete feed to achieve 22.7 milligrams per 100 pounds of body weight per day for 28 days. In feed supplements, 90.0 to 535.7 grams per ton.**
Purpose: **Prevention of coccidiosis.**

FDA File **200-206**
Firm: **Alpharma, Inc.**
Use: **Chickens: Feed Additive**
Dosage: **Chickens: 27.2 grams per ton of complete feed.** Purpose: **Prevention of coccidiosis.**

FDA File **200-213**
Firm: **Alpharma, Inc.**
Use: **Chickens: Feed Additive**
Dosage: **Chickens: 27.2 grams per ton of complete feed.** Purpose: **Prevention of coccidiosis.**

FDA File **200-359**
Firm: **Pennfield Oil Co.**
Use: **Cattle: Feed Additive**
Dosage: **12.9 to 90.8 grams per ton of complete feed to achieve 22.7**

milligrams per 100 pounds of body weight per day for 28 days.
Purpose: **Prevention of coccidiosis.**

DICLAZURIL

FDA File **140-951**
Firm: **Huvepharma AD**
Use: **Chickens, Turkeys: Feed Additive**
Dosage: **Chickens and Turkeys: Administer at the rate of 1 part per million of complete feed.**
Purpose: **Prevention of coccidiosis.**

FDA File **141-090**
Firm: **Huvepharma AD**
Use: **Chickens: Feed Additive**
Dosage: **Chickens: Administer 0.91 grams per ton of complete feed.**
Purpose: **Prevention of coccidiosis.**

FDA File **141-153**
Firm: **Huvepharma AD**
Use: **Chickens: Feed Additive**
Dosage: **Chickens: Administer 0.91 grams per ton of complete feed.**
Purpose: **Prevention of coccidiosis.**

FDA File **141-158**
Firm: **Huvepharma AD**
Use: **Chickens: Feed Additive**
Dosage: **Chickens: Administer 0.91 grams per ton of complete feed.**
Purpose: **Prevention of coccidiosis.**

FDA File **141-190**
Firm: **Huvepharma AD**
Use: **Chickens: Feed Additive**
Dosage: **Chickens: Administer 1 part per million of complete feed.**
Purpose: **Prevention of coccidiosis.**

FDA File **141-194**
Firm: **Huvepharma AD**
Use: **Turkeys: Feed Additive**
Dosage: **Turkeys: Administer 0.91 grams per ton of complete feed.**
Purpose: **Prevention of coccidiosis.**

FDA File **141-195**
Firm: **Huvepharma AD**
Use: **Turkeys: Feed Additive**
Dosage: **Turkeys: Administer 0.91 grams per ton of complete feed.**
Purpose: **Prevention of coccidiosis.**

FDA File **140-951**
Firm: **Huvepharma AD**
Use: **Chickens, Turkeys: Feed Additive**
Dosage: **Chickens and Turkeys: Administer at the rate of 1 part per million of complete feed.**
Purpose: **Prevention of coccidiosis.**

FDA File **141-090**
Firm: **Huvepharma AD**
Use: **Chickens: Feed Additive**
Dosage: **Chickens: Administer 0.91 grams per ton of complete feed.**
Purpose: **Prevention of coccidiosis.**

FDA File **141-153**
Firm: **Huvepharma AD**
Use: **Chickens: Feed Additive**
Dosage: **Chickens: Administer 0.91 grams per ton of complete feed.**
Purpose: **Prevention of coccidiosis.**

FDA File **141-158**
Firm: **Huvepharma AD**
Use: **Chickens: Feed Additive**
Dosage: **Chickens: Administer 0.91 grams per ton of complete feed.**

Purpose: **Prevention of coccidiosis.**

FDA File **141-194**
Firm: **Huvepharma AD**
Use: **Turkeys: Feed Additive**
Dosage: **Turkeys: Administer 0.91 grams per ton of complete feed.**
Purpose: **Prevention of coccidiosis.**

FDA File **141-195**
Firm: **Huvepharma AD**
Use: **Turkeys: Feed Additive**
Dosage: **Turkeys: Administer 0.91 grams per ton of complete feed.**
Purpose: **Prevention of coccidiosis.**

DICLOXACILLIN (SODIUM, MONOHYDRATE)

FDA File **055-032**
Firm: **Fort Dodge Animal Health, Div. Of Wyeth**
Use: **Dogs:** Rx only **- Oral Capsules**
Dosage: **5 to 10 milligrams per pound of body weight three times per day for 24 to 48 hours. In severe cases increase to 25 milligrams per pound.**
Purpose: **Treatment of pyoderma (pyrogenic dermatitis) caused by penicillinase-producing staphylococci shown to be sensitive to the drug.**

DIFLOXACIN (HYDROCHLORIDE)

FDA File **141-096**
Firm: **Fort Dodge Animal Health, Div. Of Wyeth**
Use: **Dogs:** Rx only **- Oral Tablets**
Dosage: **5 to 10 milligrams per kilogram of body weight once a day for 2 to 3 days beyond cessation** of clinical signs of disease up to a maximum of **30 days.**
Purpose: **Management of diseases of dogs associated with bacteria susceptible to difloxacin.**

DIHYDROSTREPTOMYCIN (SULFATE)

FDA File **055-028**
Firm: **West Chemical Products, Inc.**
Use: **Cattle:** Rx only **- Intramammary Infusion**
Dosage: **One 10 milliliter syringe containing 1 million units of penicillin g and 1 gram of streptomycin infused into each quarter after last milking prior to drying off.**
Purpose: **Reduce the frequency of existing infections and to prevent new infections in dry cows.**

FDA File **055-097**
Firm: **Boehringer Ingelheim Vetmedica, Inc.**
Use: **Cattle: Intramammary Infusion**
Dosage: **One 10 milliliter syringe containing 200,000 units of penicillin g and 300 milligrams of streptomycin infused into each quarter after last milking prior to drying off.**
Purpose: **Treatment of subclinical mastitis at the time of drying off.**

FDA File **065-013**
Firm: **Norbrook Laboratories**
Use: **Dogs, Cattle, Swine, Horses:** Rx only **- Injection.**
Dosage: **5 milligrams per pound of body weight every 12 hours for at least 3 to 5 days, or until urine is free of *leptospira* for 72 hours.**

Purpose: **Treatment of leptospirosis.**

FDA File **065-483**
Firm: **Pfizer, Inc.**
Use: **Dogs, Cattle, Swine, Horses:** Rx only **- Injection**
Dosage: **5 milligrams per pound of body weight every 12 hours for 3 to 5 days or until urine is free of** *leptospira.*
Purpose: **Treatment of leptospirosis.**

DOXYCYCLINE (HYCLATE)

FDA File **141-082**
Firm: **Pharmacia & Upjohn Co.**
Use: **Dogs:** Rx only **- Solution**
Dosage: **Apply 8.5 percent solution subgingivally to periodontal pockets of affected teeth.**
Purpose: **Treatment and control of periodontal disease.**

ENROFLOXACIN

FDA File **140-441**
Firm: **Bayer Healthcare LLC, Animal Health**
Use: **Dogs, Cats:** Rx only **- Oral Tablets**
Dosage: **5 to 20 milligrams per kilogram of body weight at 12 hour intervals daily for at least 2 to 3 days beyond cessation of clinical symptoms, for a maximum of 30 days.**
Purpose: **Management of diseases associated with bacteria susceptible to enrofloxacin.**

FDA File **140-828**
Firm: **Bayer Healthcare LLC, Animal Health**
Use: **Dogs, Cats:** Rx only **- Oral Tablets**
Dosage: **5 to 20 milligrams per kilogram of body weight at 12 hour intervals daily for at least 2 to 3 days beyond cessation of clinical symptoms, for a maximum of 30 days.**
Purpose: **Management of diseases associated with bacteria susceptible to enrofloxacin.**

FDA File **140-913**
Firm: **Bayer Healthcare LLC, Animal Health**
Use: **Dogs:** Rx only **- Injectable Solution**
Dosage: **2.5 milligrams per kilogram of body weight as a single initial dose followed by use of enrofloxacin tablets twice daily for 2 to 3 days beyond cessation of clinical signs up to a maximum of 10 days.**
Purpose: **Management of diseases associated with bacteria susceptible to enrofloxacin.**

FDA File **141-068**
Firm: **Bayer Healthcare LLC, Animal Health**
Use: **Cattle, Swine:** Rx only **- Injectable Solution**
Dosage: **Cattle: 7.5 to 12.5 milligrams per kilogram of body weight. For multiple-day therapy administer 2.5 to 5.0 milligrams per kilogram of body weight once daily for 3 to 5 days. Swine: 7.5 mg/kg body weight once.**

Purpose: **Treatment of bovine respiratory disease and treatment and control of swine respiratory disease.**

FDA File **141-176**
Firm: **Bayer Healthcare LLC, Animal Health**
Use: **Dogs:** Rx only - **Otic Emulsion**
Dosage: **Contains 5 milligrams enrofloxacin per milliliter: Administer 5 to 10 drops for dogs 35 pounds body weight or less and 10 to 15 drops for dogs greater than 35 pounds body weight. Apply twice daily for 14 days.**
Purpose: **Treatment of otitis externa.**

ERYTHROMYCIN (BASE, PHOSPHATE OR THIOCYANATE)

FDA File **010-092**
Firm: **Cross Vetpharm Group LTD**
Use: **Chickens, Turkeys, Cattle, Swine: Feed Additive**
Dosage: **4.6 to 185 grams per ton of complete feed.**
Purpose: **Chickens and Turkeys: Growth promotion, increased egg production and feed efficiency and prevention and treatment of chronic respiratory disease; Cattle: Increased rate of weight gain and improved feed efficiency; Swine: Increased rate of weight gain and improved feed efficiency.**

FDA File **012-123**
Firm: **Cross Vetpharm Group LTD**
Use: **Cattle: Injection**
Dosage: **4 milligrams per pound of body weight as an intramuscular injection once daily for up to 5 days.**

Purpose: **Treatment of bovine respiratory disease.**

FDA File **035-157**
Firm: **Cross Vetpharm Group LTD**
Use: **Chickens, Turkeys: Water Additive**
Dosage: **Chickens: Administer 0.5 milligrams per gallon of drinking water for 5 days for respiratory disease and 7 days for coryza. Turkeys: Administer same dose for 7 days.**
Purpose: **Chickens: Control of chronic respiratory disease and infectious coryza. Turkeys: Control of bluecomb.**

FDA File **035-455**
Firm: **Cross Vetpharm Group LTD**
Use: **Cattle: Intramammary Solution**
Dosage: **Infuse one 6-milliliter syringe containing 300 miligrams into each infected quarter of lactating cows and repeat treatment after each milking for 3 consecutive infusions. Dry cows: Infuse one 12-milliliter syringe containing 600 milligrams into each quarter.**
Purpose: **Treatment of mastitis.**

FDA File **035-456**
Firm: **Cross Vetpharm Group LTD**
Use: **Cattle: Sterile Intramammary Solution**
Dosage: **Infuse one 6-milliliter syringe containing 300 miligrams into each infected quarter of lactating cows and repeat treatment after each milking for 3 consecutive infusions. Dry cows: Infuse one 12-milliliter syringe contain-**

ing 600 milligrams into each quarter.
Purpose: **Treatment of mastitis.**

FDA File **037-586**
Firm: **Fort Dodge Animal Health, Div. Of Wyeth**
Use: **Cattle: Intramammary Solution**
Dosage: **300 milligrams erythromycin into each infected quarter of lactating cows and repeat treatment after each milking for 3 consecutive infusions. Dry cows: 600 milligrams into each infected quarter 10 to 14 days after drying off.**
Purpose: **Treatment of mastitis.**

FDA File **038-241**
Firm: **Cross Vetpharm Group LTD**
Use: **Chickens: Feed Additive**
Dosage: **4.6 to 185 grams per ton of complete feed. .**
Purpose: **Growth promotion and feed efficiency.**

FDA File **038-242**
Firm: **Cross Vetpharm Group LTD**
Use: **Chickens: Feed Additive**
Dosage: **4.6 to 18.5 grams per ton of feed.**
Purpose: **Growth promotion and feed efficiency.**

FDA File **038-624**
Firm: **Cross Vetpharm Group LTD**
Use: **Chickens: Feed Additive**
Dosage: **4.6 to 18.5 or 92.5 or 185 grams per ton of feed depending on intended effect.**
Purpose: **Growth promotion and feed efficiency; prevention of infectious coryza, chronic respiratory disease and reduction of le-**sions; lower the severity of chronic respiratory disease.

FDA File **041-955**
Firm: **Cross Vetpharm Group LTD**
Use: **Swine: Feed Additive**
Dosage: **9.25 to 64.75 grams per ton of feed.**
Purpose: **Growth promotion and feed efficiency.**

FDA File **101-690**
Firm: **Cross Vetpharm Group LTD**
Use: **Dogs, Cats:** Rx only - **Injection**
Dosage: **3 to 5 milligrams per pound of body weight 2 to 3 times per day for up to 5 days.**
Purpose: **Dogs: Treatment of bacterial pneumonia, upper respiratory and bacterial wound infections; endometritis and metritis. Cats: Treatment of secondary infections associated with panleukopenia.**

ETHOPABATE

FDA File **013-461**
Firm: **Huvepharma AD**
Use: **Chickens: Feed Additive Premix**
Dosage: **3.6 grams per ton of feed.**
Purpose: **Prevention of coccidiosis.**

FDA File **036-304**
Firm: **Merial LTD.**
Use: **Chickens: Feed Additive**
Dosage: **36.3 grams per ton of feed.**
Purpose: **Prevention of coccidiosis where severe exposure is likely.**
FDA File **013-461**
Firm: **Merial LTD.**
Use: **Chickens: Feed Additive**
Dosage: **3.6 grams per ton of feed.**
Purpose: **Prevention of coccidiosis.**

FDA File **038-242**
Firm: **Cross Vetpharm Group LTD.**
Use: **Chickens: Feed Additive**
Dosage: **36.3 grams per ton of feed.**
Purpose: **Prevention of coccidiosis.**

FDA File **039-284**
Firm: **Swisher Feed Division**
Use: **Chickens: Feed Additive**
Dosage: **36.3 grams per ton of feed.**
Purpose: **Prevention of coccidiosis where severe exposure is likely.**

FDA File **042-178**
Firm: **Pharmacia & Upjohn Co.**
Use: **Chickens: Feed Additive**
Dosage: **3.6 grams per ton of feed.**
Purpose: **Prevention of coccidiosis.**

FDA File **044-820**
Firm: **Pharmacia & Upjohn Co.**
Use: **Chickens: Feed Additive**
Dosage: **3.6 grams per ton of feed.**
Purpose: **Prevention of coccidiosis.**

FDA File **049-179**
Firm: **Merial LTD.**
Use: **Chickens: Feed Additive**
Dosage: **3.6 grams per ton of feed.**
Purpose: **Prevention of coccidiosis.**

FDA File **049-180**
Firm: **Merial LTD.**
Use: **Chickens: Feed Additive**
Dosage: **36.3 grams per ton of feed.**
Purpose: **Prevention of coccidiosis.**

FDA File **091-647**
Firm: **Trinada, Inc.**
Use: **Chickens: Feed Additive**
Dosage: **3.6 grams per ton of feed.**
Purpose: **Prevention of coccidiosis in floor raised broilers.**

FDA File **095-543**
Firm: **Intervet, Inc.**
Use: **Chickens: Feed Additive**
Dosage: **36.3 grams per ton of feed.**
Purpose: **Prevention of coccidiosis under conditions of severe exposure.**

FDA File **095-547**
Firm: **Intervet, Inc.**
Use: **Chickens: Feed Additive**
Dosage: **36.3 grams per ton of feed.**
Purpose: **Prevention of coccidiosis under conditions of severe exposure.**

FDA File **095-549**
Firm: **Intervet, Inc.**
Use: **Chickens: Feed Additive**
Dosage: **36.3 grams per ton of feed.**
Purpose: **Prevention of coccidiosis under conditions of severe exposure.**

FDA File **105-758**
Firm: **Alpharma, Inc.**
Use: **Chickens: Feed Additive**
Dosage: **36.3 grams per ton of feed.**
Purpose: **Prevention of coccidiosis.**

FDA File **114-794**
Firm: **Alpharma, Inc.**
Use: **Chickens: Feed Additive**
Dosage: **36.3 grams per ton of feed.**
Purpose: **Prevention of coccidiosis.**

FDA File **122-822**
Firm: **Phibro Animal Health, Inc.**
Use: **Chickens: Feed Additive**
Dosage: **36.3 grams per ton of feed.**
Purpose: **Prevention of coccidiosis.**

FDA File **200-205**
Firm: **Alpharma, Inc.**
Use: **Chickens: Feed Additive**
Dosage: **36.3 grams per ton of feed.**
Purpose: **Prevention of coccidiosis.**

FDA File **200-214**
Firm: **Alpharma, Inc.**
Use: **Chickens: Feed Additive**
Dosage: **3.6 grams per ton of feed.**
Purpose: **Prevention of coccidiosis.**

FDA File **200-217**
Firm: **Alpharma, Inc.**
Use: **Chickens: Feed Additive**
Dosage: **36.3 grams per ton of feed.**
Purpose: **Prevention of coccidiosis where severe exposure is likely.**

FLORFENICOL

FDA File **141-063**
Firm: **Schering-Plough Animal Health**
Use: **Cattle:** Rx only **- Injection-Intramuscular or Subcutaneous**
Dosage: **20 milligrams per kilogram of body weight followed by a second intramuscular injection 48 hours later or a single subcutaneous dose of 40 milligrams per kilogram for treatment or control of respiratory disease.**
Purpose: **Treatment of respiratory disease, control of respiratory disease, and for treatment of interdigital phlegmon.**

FDA File **141-206**
Firm: **Schering-Plough Animal Health**
Use: **Swine:** Rx only **- Water Additive Solution**

Dosage: **400 milligrams per gallon of drinking water for 5 days.**
Purpose: **Treatment of respiratory disease.**

FDA File **141-246**
Firm: **Schering-Plough Animal Health**
Use: **Catfish, Salmonids:** Rx (VFD) only **- Feed Additive**
Dosage: **Administer 10 mg/kg of catfish and freshwater-reared salmonids daily for 10 consecutive days.**
Purpose: **Control of mortality due to enteric septicemia of catfish associated with *Edwardsiella ictaluri*, freshwater-reared salmonids due to coldwater disease associated with *Flavobacterium psychrophilum*, and furunculosis associated with *Aeromonas salmonicida*.**

FDA File **141-259**
Firm: **Schering-Plough Animal Health**
Use: **Catfish:** Rx (VFD) only **- Feed Additive**
Dosage: **Administer 182 to 1816 grams florfenicol per ton of feed as a sole ration for 10 days.**
Purpose: **Control of mortality due to columnaris disease associated with *Flavobacterium columnare*.**

FDA File **141-264**
Firm: **Schering-Plough Animal Health**
Use: **Swine:** Rx (VFD) only **- Feed Additive**
Dosage: **182 grams per ton of feed continuously as the sole ration for 5 days.**

Purpose: **Control of respiratory disease in groups of swine in buildings experiencing an outbreak of swine respiratory disease.**

FDA File **141-265**
Firm: **Schering-Plough Animal Health**
Use: **Cattle:** Rx only – **Injection-Intramuscular or subcutaneous.**
Dosage: **20 or 40 milligrams depending on indication.**
Purpose: **Treatment of respiratory disease and for treatment of interdigital phlegmon necrobacillosis, infectious pododermatitis and for control of respiratory disease in cattle at high risk of developing respiratory disease.**

FORMALIN (also known as "formaldehyde")

FDA File **137-687**
Firm: **Natchez Animal Supply Co.**
Use: **Salmon, Trout, Catfish, Largemouth Bass, Bluegill, Shrimp, Esocid Eggs: Water Additive Solution**
Dosage: **Holding Tanks: Up to 170 µL/L (parts per million) in water below 50 degrees Fahrenheit; up to 250 µL/L in water above 50 degrees Fahrenheit for up to one hour daily. Earthen Ponds: 15 to 25 µL/L per day until control is achieved. Ponds may be repeated in 5 to 10 days. For fungi on trout, esocid eggs, and salmon apply in constant flow water supply for 15 minutes at 1000 to 2000 µL/L as often as necessary.**
Purpose: **Control external parasites and fungi in holding tanks, ponds and constant flow water supplies (raceways).**

FDA File **140-831**
Firm: **Argent Laboratories**
Use: **Salmon, Trout, Catfish, Largemouth Bass, Bluegill, Shrimp, Esocid Eggs: Water Additive Solution (37%)**
Dosage: **Holding Tanks: Up to 170 µL/L (ppm) in water below 50 degrees Fahrenheit for up to one hour daily; up to 250 µL/L in water above 50 degrees Fahrenheit for up to one hour daily. Earthen Ponds: 15 to 25 µL/L per day until control is achieved. Ponds may be repeated in 5 to 10 days. For fungi on trout, esocid eggs, and salmon apply in constant flow water supply for 15 minutes at 1000 to 2000 µL/L as often as necessary.**
Purpose: **Control external parasites and fungi in holding tanks, ponds and constant flow water supplies (raceways).**

FDA File 140-989
Firm: **Western Chemical, Inc.**
Use: **Salmon, Trout, Catfish, Largemouth Bass, Bluegill, Shrimp, Esocid Eggs: Water Additive Solution (37%)**
Dosage: **Holding Tanks: Up to 170 µL/L (ppm) in water below 50 degrees Fahrenheit for up to one hour daily; up to 250 µL/L in water above 50 degrees Fahrenheit for up to one hour daily. Earthen Ponds: 15 to 25 µL/L per day until control is achieved. Ponds may be repeated in 5 to 10 days. For fungi on trout, esocid eggs, and salmon apply in constant flow water supply for 15 minutes at 1000 to 2000 µL/L as often as necessary.**
Purpose: **Control external parasites and fungi in holding tanks, ponds**

and constant flow water supplies (raceways).

FURAZOLIDONE

FDA File **032-319**
Firm: **Fort Dodge Animal Health, Div. Of Wyeth**
Use: **Dogs, Horses: Topical Spray**
Dosage: **Contains 10 percent furazolidone. Apply once or twice daily and repeat as required.**
Purpose: **Treatment of superficial wounds, abrasions, lacerations.**

FDA File **111-104**
Firm: **Farnam Companies, Inc.**
Use: **Horses: Topical Spray**
Dosage: **Contains 4 percent furazolidone. Apply once or twice daily and repeat as required.**
Purpose: **Treatment of superficial wounds, abrasions, lacerations.**

GENTAMICIN (SULFATE)

FDA File **034-267**
Firm: **Schering-Plough Animal Health**
Use: **Dogs:** Rx only **- Ophthalmic Drops**
Dosage: **Contains 3 milligrams per milliliter gentamicin. Instill 1 to 2 drops in the conjunctival sac 3 to 4 times per day. In chronic conditions withdraw slowly by gradually reducing dosage.**
Purpose: **Treatment of bacterial infections of the eye (conjunctiva and cornea).**

FDA File **038-292**
Firm: **Schering-Plough Animal Health**

Use: **Dogs, Cats:** Rx only **- Injection**
Dosage: **2 milligrams per pound of body weight twice the first day, then once per day thereafter for up to 7 days.**
Purpose: **Treatment of bacterial infections or the urinary tract, cystitis, nephritis, respiratory tract infections and infections of skin and soft tissue.**

FDA File **046-724**
Firm: **Schering-Plough Animal Health**
Use: **Horses:** Rx only **- Intrauterine**
Dosage: **2 to 2.5 grams per day for 3 to 5 days during estrus.**
Purpose: <u>**Control of bacterial infections of the uterus (metritis) and improving conception.**</u>

FDA File **046-821**
Firm: **Schering-Plough Animal Health**
Use: **Dogs, Cats:** Rx only **- Otic and Topical Solution**
Dosage: **Contains 3 milligrams gentamicin per milliliter of solution. Three to eight drops into the ear canal twice per day for 7 to 14 days. For superficial lesions remove excessive hair and cover the affected area twice per day for 7 to 14 days.**
Purpose: **Treatment of acute and chronic otitis external and superficial infected lesions.**

FDA File **091-191**
Firm: **Schering-Plough Animal Health**
Use: **Swine: Water Additive.**
Dosage: **0.5 milligrams per pound of body weight per day for three**

days for colibacillosis; 1.0 milligram per pound of body weight per day for three days for swine dysentery. Repeat if necessary.
Purpose: **Control and treatment of colibacillosis and for control and treatment of swine dysentery.**

FDA File **092-523**
Firm: **Schering-Plough Animal Health**
Use: **Turkey Eggs: Dip**
Dosage: **Dip solution to contain 250 to 1000 parts per million.**
Purpose: **Reduction or elimination of specified bacteria from hatching eggs.**

FDA File **098-989**
Firm: **Schering-Plough Animal Health**
Use: **Dogs, Cats:** Rx only **- Ophthalmic Ointment**
Dosage: **3 milligrams two to four times per day**
Purpose: **Treatment of conjunctivitis.**

FDA File **099-008**
Firm: **Schering-Plough Animal Health**
Use: **Dogs, Cats:** Rx only **- Ophthalmic Solution**
Dosage: **Contains 3 milligrams gentamicin per milliliter drop. Instill 1 to 2 drops in the conjunctival sac 2 to 4 times per day.**
Purpose: **Treatment of conjunctivitis.**

FDA File **101-862**
Firm: **Schering-Plough Animal Health**
Use: **Chickens, Turkeys: Injection**

Dosage: **Chickens: 0.2 milligrams injected subcutaneously in the neck; Turkeys: 1 Milligram injected subcutaneously in the neck.**
Purpose: **Prevention of early mortality caused by specific bacteria.**

FDA File **103-037**
Firm: **Schering-Plough Animal Health**
Use: **Swine: Inject piglets up to 3 days old.**
Dosage: **5 milligrams injected intramuscularly one time.**
Purpose: **Treatment of porcine colibacillosis.**

FDA File **113-231**
Firm: **Schering-Plough Animal Health**
Use: **Dogs:** Rx only **- Otic Ointment**
Dosage: **Contains 3 milligrams per gram gentamicin. Install 3 to 8 drop into the ear canal twice per day for 7 days. For superficial lesions cover the area twice per day for 7 to 14 days.**
Purpose: **Treatment of acute and chronic otitis externa and infected superficial lesions.**

FDA File **130-464**
Firm: **Schering-Plough Animal Health**
Use: **Swine: Oral Liquid.**
Dosage: **Administer 5 milligrams per piglet 1 to 3 days of age by hand-operated pump.**
Purpose: **Treatment of porcine colibacillosis.**

FDA File **130-952**
Firm: **Schering-Plough Animal Health**

Use: **Beef Cattle, Dairy Cattle: Ophthalmic Solution**
Dosage: **Hand operated pump delivers 0.75 milligrams per actuation. Spray onto eye once per day.**
Purpose: **Treatment of pink eye (keratoconjunctivitis).**

FDA File **132-338**
Firm: **Schering-Plough Animal Health**
Use: **Dogs:** Rx only **- Topical Spray**
Dosage: **Contains 0.57 milligrams per milliliter. Administer 0.7 milliliters 2 to 4 times per day for 7 days.**
Purpose: **Treatment of superficial infected lesions.**

FDA File **133-836**
Firm: **Schering-Plough Animal Health**
Use: **Swine: Water Additive**
Dosage: **Colibacillosis: 0.5 milligram per kilogram of body weight per day in drinking water for 3 days. Swine dysentery: 1 milligram per day for 3 days. Repeat treatment if dysentery recurs.**
Purpose: **Treatment of porcine colibacillosis. Control and treatment of swine dysentery.**

FDA File **137-310**
Firm: **Boehringer Ingelheim Vetmedica, Inc.**
Use: **Dogs:** Rx only **- Injectable Solution**
Dosage: **Inject intramuscularly or subcutaneously 2 milligrams per pound of body weight twice on the first day, then once daily for up to 7 days.**
Purpose: **Treatment of urinary tract infections.**

FDA File **140-896**
Firm: **Schering-Plough Animal Health**
Use: **Dogs:** Rx only **- Otic Ointment**
Dosage: **Each gram contains 3 milligrams gentamicin sulfate. Apply to ear canal at the rate of 2 to 8 drops (depending on body weight) twice per day for 7 consecutive days.**
Purpose: **Treatment of otitis externa.**

FDA File **141-177**
Firm: **Schering-Plough Animal Health**
Use: **Dogs:** Rx only **- Otic Suspension**
Dosage: **Each gram contains 3 milligrams gentamicin sulfate. Apply to ear canal at the rate of 2 to 8 drops (depending on body weight) twice per day for 7 consecutive days.**
Purpose: **Treatment of otitis externa.**

FDA File **200-023**
Firm: **Boehringer Ingelheim Vetmedica, Inc.**
Use: **Horse:** Rx only **- Intrauterine Solution**
Dosage: **2 to 2.5 grams gentamicin per day for 3 to 5 days during estrus by intrauterine infusion.**
Purpose: **Control of bacterial infections and aid in improving conception.**

FDA File **200-037**
Firm: **Agri-Laboratories, Ltd.**
Use: **Horse:** Rx only **- Intrauterine Solution**
Dosage: **2 to 2.5 grams gentamicin per day for 3 to 5 days during estrus by intrauterine infusion.**

Purpose: **Control of bacterial infections and aid in improving conception.**

FDA File **200-102**
Firm: **Fort Dodge Animal Health, Div. Of Wyeth**
Use: **Horse:** Rx only **- Intrauterine Solution**
Dosage: **2 to 2.5 grams gentamicin per day for 3 to 5 days by intra-uterine infusion.**
Purpose: **Control of bacterial infections and aid in improving conception.**

FDA File **200-115**
Firm: **Cross Vetpharm Group, Ltd.**
Use: **Horse:** Rx only **- Intrauterine Solution**
Dosage: **2 to 2.5 grams gentamicin per day for 3 to 5 days by intra-uterine infusion.**
Purpose: **Control of bacterial infections and aid in improving conception.**

FDA File **200-137**
Firm: **Phoenix Scientific, Inc.**
Use: **Horse:** Rx only **- Intrauterine Solution**
Dosage: **2 to 2.5 grams gentamicin per day for 3 to 5 days by intra-uterine infusion.**
Purpose: **Control of bacterial infections and aid in improving conception.**

FDA File **200-147**
Firm: **Phoenix Scientific, Inc.**
Use: **Chickens, Turkeys: Injection**
Dosage: **Chickens: 0.2 milligrams injected subcutaneously in the neck; Turkeys: 1 Milligram inject-**ed subcutaneously in the neck at 1 to 3 days of age.
Purpose: **Prevention of early mortality caused by specified bacteria.**

FDA File **200-174**
Firm: **Phoenix Scientific, Inc.**
Use: **Swine: Oral Pump**
Dosage: **5 milligrams per pig.**
Purpose: **Control and treatment of colibacillosis in pigs 1 to 3 days of age.**

FDA File **200-183**
Firm: **Med-Pharmex, Inc.**
Use: **Dogs, Cats:** Rx only **- Otic Solution**
Dosage: **3 to 8 drops containing 3 milligrams gentamicin base per milliliter into the ear canal twice per day for 7 to 14 days. For superficial lesions, cover affected area twice per day for 7 to 14 days.**
Purpose: **Treatment of acute and chronic otitis externa and superficial infected lesions.**

FDA File **200-185**
Firm: **Agri-Laboratories, Ltd.**
Use: **Swine: Water Additive**
Dosage: **Colibacillosis: 0.5 Milligram per kilogram of body weight per day in drinking water for 3 days. Swine dysentery: 1 Milligram per day for 3 days. Repeat treatment if dysentery recurs.**
Purpose: **Treatment of porcine colibacillosis. Control and treatment of swine dysentery.**

FDA File **200-188**
Firm: **Med-Pharmex, Inc.**
Use: **Dogs:** Rx only **- Topical Spray**
Dosage: **Contains 0.57 milligrams per milliliter. Administer 0.7 mil-**

liliters 2 to 4 times per day for 7 days.
Purpose: **Treatment of superficial infected lesions.**

FDA File **200-190**
Firm: **Med-Pharmex, Inc.**
Use: **Swine: Water Additive**
Dosage: **Colibacillosis: 0.5 Milligram per kilogram of body weight per day in drinking water for 3 days. Swine dysentery: 1 Milligram per day for 3 days. Repeat treatment if dysentery recurs.**
Purpose: **Treatment of porcine colibacillosis. Control and treatment of swine dysentery.**

FDA File **200-191**
Firm: **Med-Pharmex, Inc.**
Use: **Turkey Eggs: Dip**
Dosage: **Dip solution to contain 250 to 1000 parts per million.**
Purpose: **Reduction or elimination of specified bacteria from hatching eggs.**

FDA File **200-229**
Firm: **Med-Pharmex, Inc.**
Use: **Dogs:** Rx only **- Otic Ointment**
Dosage: **Each gram contains 3 milligrams gentamicin sulfate. Apply to ear canal at the rate of 2 to 8 drops (depending on body weight) twice per day for 7 consecutive days.**
Purpose: **Treatment of otitis externa.**

FDA File **200-415**
Firm: **First Priority, Inc.**
Use: **Dogs:** Rx only **- Topical Spray**
Dosage: **Contains 0.57 milligrams per milliliter. Administer 0.7 milliliters 2 to 4 times per day for 7 days.**

Purpose: **Treatment of superficial infected lesions.**

FDA File **200-273**
Firm: **Altana, Inc.**
Use: **Dogs, Cats:** Rx only **- Ophthalmic Ointment**
Dosage: **3 milligrams to the affected eye 2 to 4 times per day**
Purpose: **Treatment of conjunctivitis.**

FDA File **200-283**
Firm: **Altana, Inc.**
Use: **Dogs:** Rx only **- Otic Ointment**
Dosage: **Each gram contains 3 milligrams gentamicin sulfate. Apply to ear canal at the rate of to 8 drops (depending on body weight) twice per day for 7 consecutive days.**
Purpose: **Treatment of otitis externa.**

FDA File **200-287**
Firm: **Ivx Animal Health**
Use: **Dogs:** Rx only **- Otic Ointment**
Dosage: **Each gram contains 3 milligrams gentamicin sulfate. Apply to ear canal at the rate of to 8 drops (depending on body weight) twice per day for 7 consecutive days.**
Purpose: **Treatment of acute and chronic otitis externa.**

FDA File **200-394**
Firm: **Sparhawk Laboratories, Inc.**
Use: **Swine: Injection**
Dosage: **Administer 5 milligrams as a single imtramuscular injection in pigs up to 3 days old only.**
Purpose: **Treatment of colibacillosis.**

FDA File **200-395**
Firm: **Sparhawk Laboratories, Inc.**

Use: **Horses:** Rx only - **Intrauterine**
Dosage: **2 to 2.5 grams per day for 3 to 5 days during estrus.**
Purpose: **Control of bacterial infections of the uterus (metritis) and improving conception.**

HALOFUGINONE (HYDROBROMIDE)

FDA File **130-951**
Firm: **Intervet, Inc.**
Use: **Chickens: Feed Additive**
Dosage: **2.72 Grams per ton of feed for 16 to 20 weeks.**
Purpose: **Prevention of coccidiosis.**

FDA File **137-483**
Firm: **Intervet, Inc.**
Use: **Chickens: Feed Additive**
Dosage: **3 parts per million of feed for 16 to 20 weeks.**
Purpose: **Prevention of coccidiosis.**

FDA File **139-473**
Firm: **Intervet, Inc.**
Use: **Chickens: Feed Additive**
Dosage: **3 parts per million of feed.**
Purpose: **Prevention of coccidiosis.**

FDA File **140-340**
Firm: **Intervet, Inc.**
Use: **Chickens: Feed Additive**
Dosage: **3 parts per million of feed.**
Purpose: **Prevention of coccidiosis.**

FDA File **140-533**
Firm: **Intervet, Inc.**
Use: **Chickens: Feed Additive**
Dosage: **3 parts per million of feed.**
Purpose: **Prevention of coccidiosis.**

FDA File **140-584**
Firm: **Intervet, Inc.**

Use: **Chickens: Feed Additive**
Dosage: **2.72 Grams per ton of feed for 16 to 20 weeks.**
Purpose: **Prevention of coccidiosis.**

FDA File **140-824**
Firm: **Intervet, Inc.**
Use: **Turkeys: Feed Additive**
Dosage: **1.36 to 2.72 grams per ton of feed used continuously.**
Purpose: **Prevention of coccidiosis.**

FDA File **140-918**
Firm: **Intervet, Inc.**
Use: **Turkeys: Feed Additive**
Dosage: **1.36 to 2.72 grams per ton of feed used continuously.**
Purpose: **Prevention of coccidiosis.**

FDA File **140-919**
Firm: **Intervet, Inc.**
Use: **Turkeys: Feed Additive**
Dosage: **1.36 to 2.72 grams per ton of feed used continuously.**
Purpose: **Prevention of coccidiosis.**

FDA File **141-157**
Firm: **Intervet, Inc.**
Use: **Chickens: Feed Additive**
Dosage: **2.72 Grams per ton of feed for 16 to 20 weeks.**
Purpose: **Prevention of coccidiosis.**

HETACILLIN (POTASSIUM)

FDA File **055-021**
Firm: **Fort Dodge Animal Health, Div. Of Wyeth**
Use: **Dogs, Cats:** Rx only - **Oral Capsule**
Dosage: **Dogs: 5 to 20 milligrams per pound of body weight 2 to 3 times per day; Cats: 50 milligrams per pound of body weight per day.**

SUPERBUGS

Treat until 72 hours after animal is
asymptomatic.
Purpose: **Treatment of respiratory,
urinary, gastrointestinal, skin, soft
tissue, and postoperative infections.**

FDA File **055-022**
Firm: **Fort Dodge Animal Health,
Div. Of Wyeth**
Use: **Dogs, Cats:** Rx only **- Oral
Tablet**
Dosage: **Dogs: 5 to 20 milligrams
per pound of body weight 2 to 3
times per day; Cats: 50 milligrams
per pound of body weight per day.
Treat until 72 hours after animal is
asymptomatic.**
Purpose: **Treatment of respiratory,
urinary, gastrointestinal, skin, soft
tissue, and postoperative infections.**

FDA File **055-048**
Firm: **Fort Dodge Animal Health,
Div. Of Wyeth**
Use: **Dogs, Cats:** Rx only **- Oral
Liquid**
Dosage: **Dogs: 5 to 20 milligrams
per pound of body weight 2 to 3
times per day; Cats: 50 milligrams
per pound of body weight per day.
Treat until 72 hours after animal is
asymptomatic.**
Purpose: **Treatment of respiratory,
urinary, gastrointestinal, skin, soft
tissue, and postoperative infections.**

FDA File **055-054**
Firm: **Fort Dodge Animal Health,
Div. Of Wyeth**
Use: **Cattle:** Rx only **- Intramam-
mary Infusion**

Dosage: **62.5 milligrams per quarter repeated at 24 hours for three
treatments.**
Purpose: **Treatment of acute, chronic or subclinical mastitis.**

HYDROGEN PEROXIDE

FDA File **141-255**
Firm: **EKA Chemicals, Inc.**
Use: **Finfish, Fish Eggs, Salmon,
Catfish, Trout: Water Additive**
Dosage: **500 to 1000 milligrams per
liter of culture water for 15 minutes for fresh-water reared finfish
eggs. For all coldwater and coolwater species of freshwater reared
finfish fingerlings and adults and
channel catfish fingerlings and
adults use 50 to 75 milligrams per
liter for 60 minutes once per day
on alternate days for three treatments.**
Purpose: **Control of mortality in
freshwater-reared finfish eggs due
to saprolegniasis; for control of
mortality in freshwater-reared
salmonids due to bacterial gill
disease and for control of mortality in freshwater-reared coolwater
finfish and channel catfish due to
external columnaris disease.**

IODOCHLORHYDROXYQUIN

FDA File **031-448**
Firm: **Fort Dodge Animal Health,
Div. Of Wyeth**
Use: **Horses:** Rx only **- Oral Bolus**
Dosage: **10 Grams per 1000 pounds
of body weight until feces becomes
formed, then lower dosage and
give on alternate days.**
Purpose: **Treatment of diarrhea.**

KANAMYCIN (SULFATE)

FDA File **041-836**
Firm: **Fort Dodge Animal Health, Div. Of Wyeth**
Use: **Dogs, Cats:** Rx only - **Injection**
Dosage: **5 milligrams per pound of body weight for up to 5 days.**
Purpose: **Treatment of bacterial infections.**

FDA File **042-548**
Firm: **Fort Dodge Animal Health, Div. Of Wyeth**
Use: **Dogs, Cats:** Rx only - **Oral Suspension**
Dosage: **One to 3 teaspoonfuls 100 to 300 milligrams per 20 pounds of body weight every 8 hours.**
Purpose: **Treatment of acute bacterial diarrhea.**

FDA File **042-661**
Firm: **Fort Dodge Animal Health, Div. Of Wyeth**
Use: **Dogs:** Rx only - **Ophthalmic Ointment**
Dosage: **Contains 3.5 milligrams per gram: Apply thin film to eye 3 to 4 times daily or as indicated for at least 18 hours after eye is asymptomatic.**
Purpose: **Treatment of eye infections.**

FDA File **042-841**
Firm: **Fort Dodge Animal Health, Div. Of Wyeth**
Use: **Dogs:** Rx only - **Oral Tablet**
Dosage: **One tablet (100 milligrams) per 20 pounds body weight every 8 hours (not to exceed 3 tablets each 8 hours). Initial dose may be doubled.**
Purpose: **Treatment of bacterial enteritis and associated diarrhea.**

FDA File **042-883**
Firm: **Fort Dodge Animal Health, Div. Of Wyeth**
Use: **Dogs:** Rx only - **Ophthalmic Solution**
Dosage: **Contains 10 milligrams per milliliter: Administer as often as possible for first 48 hours and continue treatment until eyes are asymptomatic.**
Purpose: **Treatment of eye infections.**

FDA File **043-784**
Firm: **Fort Dodge Animal Health, Div. Of Wyeth**
Use: **Dogs:** Rx only - **Topical Ointment**
Dosage: **Contains 5.0 milligrams per gram: Apply at least twice daily, reducing frequency as conditions improve, for up to 7 days.**
Purpose: **For treatment of conditions such as acute otitis externa, furunculosis, folliculitis, pruritis, anal gland infections, erythema, decubital ulcers, superficial wounds, and superficial abscesses.**

FDA File **047-997**
Firm: **Fort Dodge Animal Health, Div. Of Wyeth**
Use: **Dogs:** Rx only - **Otic Cream**
Dosage: **Contains 5.0 milligrams per gram: Apply to affected area at least twice daily initially, reducing dosage as conditions improve for up to 7 days.**
Purpose: **Treatment of acute otitis externa and topical infections such as folliculitis, anal gland infections, superficial wounds, etc.**

LAIDLOMYCIN (PROPIONATE, SODIUM, POTASSIUM)

FDA File **141-025**
Firm: **Alpharma, Inc.**
Use: **Cattle: Feed Additive**
Dosage: **30 to 150 milligrams per head per day.**
Purpose: **Improved feed efficiency and increased rate of weight gain.**

FDA File **141-201**
Firm: **Alpharma, Inc.**
Use: **Cattle: Feed Additive**
Dosage: **5 to 150 grams per ton of feed.**
Purpose: **Improved feed efficiency and increased rate of weight gain.**

FDA File **096-298**
Firm: **Alpharma, Inc.**
Use: **Cattle, Chickens, Turkeys, Chukar Partridge, Sheep, Rabbit: Feed Additive**
Dosage: **Cattle: 60 to 300 milligrams per head per day. All other species: 68 to 113 grams per ton of feed.**
Purpose: **Cattle: Improved feed efficiency and increased rate of weight gain. Calves: Improved feed efficiency, increased rate of weight gains and for control of coccidiosis. Sheep, Chickens, Turkeys, Chukar Partridges and Rabbits: Prevention of coccidiosis.**

FDA File **101-689**
Firm: **Pharmacia & Upjohn Co.**
Use: **Chickens: Feed Additive**
Dosage: **68 grams per ton of feed. Use continuously in broiler chickens.**

Purpose: **Prevention of coccidiosis.**

FDA File **102-489**
Firm: **Alpharma, Inc.**
Use: **Chickens: Feed Additive**
Dosage: **68 to 113 grams per ton of feed. Administer continuously in broiler chickens.**
Purpose: **Prevention of coccidiosis.**

FDA File **107-996**
Firm: **Alpharma, Inc.**
Use: **Chickens: Feed Additive**
Dosage: **68 to 113 grams per ton of feed. Use continuously in broiler chickens.**
Purpose: **Prevention of coccidiosis.**

FDA File **112-661**
Firm: **Alpharma, Inc.**
Use: **Chickens: Feed Additive**
Dosage: **68 to 113 grams per ton of feed. Use continuously in broiler chickens.**
Purpose: **Prevention of coccidiosis.**

FDA File **112-687**
Firm: **Alpharma, Inc.**
Use: **Chickens: Feed Additive**
Dosage: **68 to 113 grams per ton of feed. Use continuously in broiler chickens.**
Purpose: **Prevention of coccidiosis.**

FDA File **116-082**
Firm: **Alpharma, Inc.**
Use: **Chickens: Feed Additive**
Dosage: **68 to 113 grams per ton of feed. Use continuously in broiler chickens.**
Purpose: **Prevention of coccidiosis.**

FDA File **122-608**
Firm: **Phibro Animal Health, Inc.**

Use: **Chickens: Feed Additive**
Dosage: **68 to 113 grams per ton of feed. Use continuously in broiler chickens.**
Purpose: **Prevention of coccidiosis.**

FDA File **126-052**
Firm: **Alpharma, Inc.**
Use: **Chickens: Feed Additive**
Dosage: **68 to 113 grams per ton of feed. Use continuously in broiler chickens.**
Purpose: **Prevention of coccidiosis.**

FDA File **131-894**
Firm: **Alpharma, Inc.**
Use: **Chickens: Feed Additive**
Dosage: **68 to 113 grams per ton of feed. Use continuously in broiler chickens.**
Purpose: **Prevention of coccidiosis.**

FDA File **138-904**
Firm: **Pharmacia & Upjohn Co.**
Use: **Cattle: Feed Additive**
Dosage: **10 to 30 grams per ton of feed.**
Purpose: **Prevention of coccidiosis, increased rate of weight gain, and improved feed efficiency.**

FDA File **138-992**
Firm: **Pharmacia & Upjohn Co.**
Use: **Cattle: Feed Additive-Liquid Feed**
Dosage: **10 to 30 grams per ton of feed for heifers fed in confinement for slaughter.**
Purpose: **Increased rate of weight gain and improved feed efficiency; reduced incidence of liver abscesses.**

FDA File **138-993**
Firm: **ADM Alliance Nutrition, Inc.**

Use: **Cattle: Feed Additive**
Dosage: **1.06 percent in feed.**
Purpose: **Increased rate of weight gain.**

FDA File **139-876**
Firm: **Pharmacia & Upjohn Co.**
Use: **Cattle: Feed Additive**
Dosage: **100 to 360 milligrams per head per day for heifers fed in confinement for slaughter.**
Purpose: **Increased rate of weight gain, and improved feed efficiency.**

FDA File **140-288**
Firm: **Pharmacia & Upjohn Co.**
Use: **Cattle: Feed Additive**
Dosage: **10 to 30 grams per ton of feed for heifers fed in confinement for slaughter.**
Purpose: **Increased rate of weight gain, and improved feed efficiency.**

FDA File **140-579**
Firm: **Alpharma, Inc.**
Use: **Cattle: Feed Additive**
Dosage: **10 to 30 grams per ton of feed for heifers fed in confinement for slaughter.**
Purpose: **Increased rate of weight gain, and improved feed efficiency.**

FDA File **141-083**
Firm: **Alpharma, Inc.**
Use: **Chickens: Feed Additive**
Dosage: **68 to 113 grams per ton of feed. Use continuously in broiler chickens.**
Purpose: **Prevention of coccidiosis.**

FDA File **141-109**
Firm: **Alpharma, Inc.**
Use: **Turkey: Feed Additive**

Dosage: **68 to 113 grams per ton of feed. Use continuously as sole ration.**
Purpose: **Prevention of coccidiosis.**

FDA File **141-129**
Firm: **Alpharma, Inc.**
Use: **Chickens: Feed Additive**
Dosage: **68 to 113 grams per ton of feed. Use continuously in broiler chickens.**
Purpose: **Prevention of coccidiosis.**

FDA File **141-150**
Firm: **Alpharma, Inc.**
Use: **Turkey: Feed Additive**
Dosage: **68 to 113 grams per ton of feed. Use continuously as sole ration.**
Purpose: **Prevention of coccidiosis.**

FDA File **141-171**
Firm: **Purina Mills, Inc.**
Use: **Cattle: Feed Additive**
Dosage: **60 to 300 milligrams per head per day.**
Purpose: **Increased rate of weight gain.**

FDA File **141-179**
Firm: **Alpharma, Inc.**
Use: **Turkey: Feed Additive**
Dosage: **68 to 113 grams per ton of feed. Use continuously as sole ration.**
Purpose: **Prevention of coccidiosis.**

FDA File **141-181**
Firm: **Alpharma, Inc.**
Use: **Turkey: Feed Additive**
Dosage: **68 to 113 grams per ton of feed. Use continuously as sole ration.**
Purpose: **Prevention of coccidiosis.**

FDA File **141-187**
Firm: **Ridley Block Operations Inc.**
Use: **Cattle: Feed Additive**
Dosage: **60 milligrams per head per day or higher.**
Purpose: **Increased rate of weight gain in pasture cattle.**

FDA File **200-208**
Firm: **Alpharma, Inc.**
Use: **Chickens: Feed Additive**
Dosage: **68 to 113 grams per ton of feed. Use continuously in broiler chickens.**
Purpose: **Prevention of coccidiosis.**

FDA File **200-451**
Firm: **Ivy Laboratories**
Use: **Cattle: Feed Additive**
Dosage: **10 to 30 grams per ton of feed for heifers fed in confinement for slaughter.**
Purpose: **Increased rate of weight gain, and improved feed efficiency.**

LASALOCID (SODIUM)

FDA File **096-298**
Firm: **Alpharma, Inc.**
Use: **Cattle, Chickens, Turkeys, Chukar Partridge, Sheep, Rabbit: Feed Additive**
Dosage: **Cattle: 100 to 360 milligrams per head per day for feed efficiency or 250 to 360 milligrams per head per day for improved feed efficiency and increased rate of weight gain in cattle fed in confinement for slaughter. In pasture cattle: 60 to 250 milligrams per head per day or free choice at 60 to 300 milligrams per head per day. Same for replacement calves for increased rate of weight gain. Chickens: 68 to 113 grams per ton of complete feed. Sheep in confine-**

ment: 15 to 70 grams per head per day. Turkeys: 68 to 113 grams per ton of complete feed. Rabbits: 113 grams per ton of complete feed up to 6 and ½ weeks of age.
Purpose: **Increased rate of weight gain and improved feed efficiency.**

LINCOMYCIN (BASE, HYDRO-CHLORIDE, HYDROCHLORIDE MONOHYDRATE)

FDA File **047-262**
Firm: **Alpharma, Inc.**
Use: **Chickens: Feed Additive**
Dosage: **2 Grams per ton of feed. Use continuously in broiler chickens.**
Purpose: **Increased rate of weight gain and improved feed efficiency.**

FDA File **047-261**
Firm: **Pharmacia & Upjohn Co.**
Use: **Chickens: Feed Additive**
Dosage: **2 Grams per ton of feed. Use continuously in broiler chickens.**
Purpose: **Increased rate of weight gain and improved feed efficiency.**

FDA File **137-537**
Firm: **Roche Vitamins, Inc.**
Use: **Chickens: Feed Additive**
Dosage: **2 to 4 grams per ton of feed. Use continuously in broiler chickens.**
Purpose: **Improved feed efficiency.**

FDA File **140-947**
Firm: **Elanco Animal Health, Div. Eli Lilly & Co.**
Use: **Chickens: Feed Additive**
Dosage: **2 to 4 grams per ton of feed. Use continuously in broiler chickens.**

Purpose: **Improved feed efficiency.**

FDA File **140-954**
Firm: **Intervet, Inc.**
Use: **Swine: Feed Additive**
Dosage: **20 to 200 grams per ton of feed. Use in swine up to 250 pounds body weight.**
Purpose: **Increased rate of weight gain in growing-finishing swine; treatment and control of swine dysentery, and for reduction in the severity of swine mycoplasmal pneumonia.**

FDA File **141-054**
Firm: **Merial Ltd.**
Use: **Swine: Feed Additive**
Dosage: **40 to 200 grams per ton of feed. Use in swine up to 250 pounds body weight.**
Purpose: **Increased rate of weight gain in growing-finishing swine; treatment and control of swine dysentery, and for reduction in the severity of swine mycoplasmal pneumonia.**

FDA File **200-090**
Firm: **Intervet, Inc.**
Use: **Chickens: Feed Additive**
Dosage: **2 grams per ton of feed. Use continuously in broiler chickens.**
Purpose: **Improved feed efficiency.**

FDA File **200-093**
Firm: **Intervet, Inc.**
Use: **Chickens: Feed Additive**
Dosage: **2 to 4 grams per ton of feed. Use continuously in broiler chickens.**
Purpose: **Improved feed efficiency.**

FDA File **200-170**
Firm: **Planalquimica Industrial Ltd.**
Use: **Chickens: Feed Additive**
Dosage: **2 Grams per ton of feed. Use continuously in broiler chickens.**
Purpose: **Increased rate of weight gain.**

FDA File **200-171**
Firm: **Planalquimica Industrial Ltd.**
Use: **Chickens: Feed Additive**
Dosage: **2 Grams per ton of feed. Use continuously in broiler chickens.**
Purpose: **Increased rate of weight gain.**

FDA File **200-274**
Firm: **Alpharma, Inc.**
Use: **Swine: Injectable Solution**
Dosage: **5 milligrams per pound of body weight once daily for 3 to 7 days.**
Purpose: **Treatment of infectious arthritis and mycoplasma pneumonia.**

FDA File **200-315**
Firm: **Sparhawk Laboratories, Inc.**
Use: **Swine: Injectable Solution**
Dosage: **5 milligrams per pound of body weight once daily for 3 to 7 days.**
Purpose: **Treatment of infectious arthritis and mycoplasma pneumonia.**

FDA File **200-351**
Firm: **Phoenix Scientific, Inc.**
Use: **Swine: Injectable Solution**

Dosage: **5 milligrams per pound of body weight once daily for 5 to 7 days.**
Purpose: **Treatment of infectious arthritis and mycoplasma pneumonia.**

FDA File **092-482**
Firm: **Pharmacia & Upjohn Co.**
Use: **Chickens: Feed Additive**
Dosage: **2 Grams per ton of feed. Use continuously in broiler chickens.**
Purpose: **Increased rate of weight gain and improved feed efficiency.**

FDA File **200-171**
Firm: **Pharmacia & Upjohn Co.**
Use: **Chickens: Feed Additive**
Dosage: **2 Grams per ton of feed. Use continuously in broiler chickens.**
Purpose: **Increased rate of weight gain and improved feed efficiency.**

FDA File **093-106**
Firm: **Pharmacia & Upjohn Co.**
Use: **Chickens: Feed Additive**
Dosage: **2 Grams per ton of feed. Use continuously in broiler chickens.**
Purpose: **Increased rate of weight gain and improved feed efficiency.**

FDA File **101-689**
Firm: **Pharmacia & Upjohn Co.**
Use: **Chickens: Feed Additive**
Dosage: **2 Grams per ton of feed. Use continuously in broiler chickens.**
Purpose: **Increased rate of weight gain and improved feed efficiency.**

FDA File **107-997**
Firm: **Phibro Animal Health, Inc.**
Use: **Chickens: Feed Additive**
Dosage: **2 Grams per ton of feed.
Use continuously in broiler chickens.**
Purpose: **Increased rate of weight gain.**

FDA File **108-116**
Firm: **Phibro Animal Health, Inc.**
Use: **Chickens: Feed Additive**
Dosage: **2 Grams per ton of feed.
Use continuously in broiler chickens.**
Purpose: **Increased rate of weight gain.**

FDA File **112-661**
Firm: **Alpharma, Inc.**
Use: **Chickens: Feed Additive**
Dosage: **2 Grams per ton of feed.
Use continuously in broiler chickens.**
Purpose: **Increased rate of weight gain and improved feed efficiency.**

FDA File **132-923**
Firm: **International Nutrition, Inc.**
Use: **Swine: Feed Additive**
Dosage: **100 Grams per ton of feed.**
Purpose: **Control and treatment of swine dysentery.**

FDA File **140-340**
Firm: **Intervet, Inc.**
Use: **Chickens: Feed Additive**
Dosage: **2 to 4 grams per ton of feed. Use continuously as the sole ration in broiler chickens.**
Purpose: **Improved feed efficiency.**

FDA File **140-581**
Firm: **Alpharma, Inc.**
Use: **Chickens: Feed Additive**
Dosage: **2 Grams per ton of feed.
Use continuously as the sole ration in broiler chickens.**
Purpose: **Improved feed efficiency.**

FDA File **200-189**
Firm: **Alpharma, Inc.**
Use: **Chickens, Swine: Water Soluble Powder**
Dosage: **Chickens: 64 milligrams per gallon of water for 7 consecutive days; Swine up to 250 pounds body weight: 3.8 milligrams per pound of body weight per day for up to 10 days.**
Purpose: **Chickens: Control of necrotic enteritis; Swine: Treatment of swine dysentery.**

FDA File **200-233**
Firm: **Alpharma, Inc.**
Use: **Chickens, Swine: Water Soluble Powder**
Dosage: **Chickens: 64 milligrams per gallon of water for 7 consecutive days; Swine up to 250 pounds body weight: 3.8 milligrams per pound of body weight per day for up to 10 days.**
Purpose: **Chickens: Control of necrotic enteritis; Swine: Treatment of swine dysentery.**

FDA File **200-241**
Firm: **Med-Pharmex, Inc.**
Use: **Chickens, Swine: Water Soluble Powder**
Dosage: **Chickens: 64 milligrams per gallon of water for 7 consecutive days; Swine up to 250 pounds body weight: 3.8 milligrams per pound of body weight per day for up to 10 days.**

Purpose: **Chickens: <u>Control of ne-crotic enteritis</u>; Swine: Treatment of swine dysentery.**

FDA File **200-303**
Firm: **Phoenix Scientific, Inc.**
Use: **Chickens, Swine: Water Soluble Powder**
Dosage: **Chickens: 64 milligrams per gallon of water for 7 consecutive days; Swine up to 250 pounds body weight: 3.8 milligrams per pound of body weight per day for up to 10 days.**
Purpose: **Chickens: <u>Control of ne-crotic enteritis</u>; Swine: Treatment of swine dysentery.**

FDA File **034-025**
Firm: **Pharmacia & Upjohn Co.**
Use: **Dogs, Cats, Swine:** Rx only **- Injectable Solution**
Dosage: **Dogs, Cats: 10 milligrams per pound of body weight twice per day or 5 to 10 milligrams per pound of body weight every 8 hours for up to 12 days; Swine: 5 milligrams per pound of body weight per day as a single dose for 3 to 7 days.**
Purpose: **Dogs, Cats: Treatment of infections caused by gram-positive organisms sensitive to lincomycin. Swine: treatment of infectious arthritis and mycoplasma pneumonia.**

FDA File **200-368**
Firm: **Cross Vetpharm Group Ltd.**
Use: **Swine: Injectable Solution**
Dosage: **5 milligrams per pound of body weight per day as a single dose for 3 to 7 days.**

Purpose: **Treatment of infectious arthritis and mycoplasma pneumonia.**

FDA File **034-085**
Firm: **Pharmacia & Upjohn Co.**
Use: **Chickens: Feed Additive**
Dosage: **2 to 4 grams per ton of feed. Use continuously in broiler chickens.**
Purpose: **<u>Increased rate of weight gain and improved feed efficiency.</u>**

FDA File **040-587**
Firm: **Pharmacia & Upjohn Co.**
Use: **Dogs, Cats:** Rx only **- Liquid**
Dosage: **10 milligrams per pound of body weight every 12 hours or 7 milligrams per pound of body weight every 8 hours for up to 12 days.**
Purpose: **Treatment of infections caused by organisms sensitive to lincomycin.**

FDA File **041-178**
Firm: **Pharmacia & Upjohn Co.**
Use: **Chickens: Feed Additive**
Dosage: **2 to 4 grams per ton of feed. Use continuously in broiler chickens.**
Purpose: **<u>Increased rate of weight gain and improved feed efficiency.</u>**

FDA File **044-820**
Firm: **Pharmacia & Upjohn Co.**
Use: **Chickens: Feed Additive**
Dosage: **2 to 4 grams per ton of feed. Use continuously in broiler chickens.**
Purpose: **<u>Increased rate of weight gain and improved feed efficiency.</u>**

FDA File **044-972**
Firm: **Pharmacia & Upjohn Co.**
Use: **Chickens: Feed Additive**
Dosage: **2 to 4 grams per ton of feed. Use continuously in broiler chickens.**
Purpose: **Increased rate of weight gain and improved feed efficiency.**

FDA File **045-738**
Firm: **Pharmacia & Upjohn Co.**
Use: **Chickens: Feed Additive**
Dosage: **2 to 4 grams per ton of feed. Use continuously in broiler chickens.**
Purpose: **Increased rate of weight gain and improved feed efficiency.**

FDA File **046-109**
Firm: **Pharmacia & Upjohn Co.**
Use: **Chickens: Water Soluble Powder**
Dosage: **Chickens: 2 grams per gallon of drinking water for the first 5 to 7 days of life.**
Purpose: **Chickens: Control of airsacculitis and complicated respiratory disease.**

FDA File **047-261**
Firm: **Pharmacia & Upjohn Co.**
Use: **Chickens: Feed Additive**
Dosage: **2 grams per ton of feed. Use continuously in broiler chickens.**
Purpose: **Increased rate of weight gain and improved feed efficiency.**

FDA File **048-954**
Firm: **Pharmacia & Upjohn Co.**
Use: **Chickens: Feed Additive**
Dosage: **2 grams per ton of feed. Use continuously in broiler chickens.**

Purpose: **Increased rate of weight gain and improved feed efficiency.**

FDA File **097-505**
Firm: **Pharmacia & Upjohn Co.**
Use: **Chickens, Swine: Feed Additive**
Dosage: **Chickens: 2 to 4 grams per ton of feed. Use continuously in broiler chickens. Swine: 20, 40, 100 or 200 grams per ton of feed.**
Purpose: **Chickens: Increased rate of weight gain and improved feed efficiency and control of necrotic enteritis. Swine: Increased rate of weight gain in growing/finishing swine, for treatment and control of swine dysentery, control of porcine proliferative enteropathies (illeitis) and for reduction in severity of swine mycoplasmal pneumonia.**

FDA File **111-636**
Firm: **Pharmacia & Upjohn Co.**
Use: **Swine, Chickens: Water Soluble Powder**
Dosage: **Chickens: 64 milligrams per gallon of drinking water for 7 days; Swine: 3.8 milligrams per pound of body weight per day for up to 10 days.**
Purpose: **Swine: Treatment of swine dysentery; Chickens: Control of necrotic enteritis.**

FDA File **116-044**
Firm: **Phibro Animal Health, Inc.**
Use: **Swine: Feed Additive**
Dosage: **40 to 100 grams per ton of complete feed.**
Purpose: **Treatment of swine dysentery in swine up to 250 pounds body weight.**

FDA File **132-574**
Firm: **Virbac AH, Inc.**
Use: **Swine: Feed Additive**
Dosage: **40 to 100 grams per ton of complete feed.**
Purpose: **Treatment <u>and/or control</u> of dysentery <u>and reduction of severity of mycoplasmal pneumonia in swine up to 250 pounds body weight.</u>**

FDA File **200-345**
Firm: **Phoenix Scientific, Inc.**
Use: **Chickens: Water Soluble Powder**
Dosage: **2 Grams per gallon of drinking water for the first 5 to 7 days of life.**
Purpose: **<u>Control of airsacculitis and complicated respiratory disease.</u>**

FDA File **200-407**
Firm: **Agri-Laboratories, Ltd.**
Use: **Chickens: Water Soluble Powder**
Dosage: **2 Grams per gallon of drinking water for the first 5 to 7 days of life.**
Purpose: **<u>Control of airsacculitis and complicated respiratory disease.</u>**

MADURAMICIN (AMMONIUM)

FDA File **139-075**
Firm: **Alpharma, Inc.**
Use: **Chickens: Feed Additive**
Dosage: **5 to 6 parts per million in complete feed for broiler chickens.**
Purpose: **Prevention of coccidiosis.**

MARBOFLOXACIN

FDA File **141-151**
Firm: **Pfizer, Inc.**
Use: **Dogs, Cats:** Rx only **- Oral Tablet**
Dosage: **1.25 to 2.5 milligrams per pound of body weight once daily.**
Purpose: **Treatment of infections associated with bacteria susceptible to marbofloxacin.**

MERCAPTOBENZOTHIAZOLE

FDA File **005-236**
Firm: **Farnam Companies, Inc.**
Use: **Dogs: Topical Solution**
Dosage: **Apply freely to affected area.**
Purpose: **Treatment of hotspots (moist dermatitis) and first aid for scrapes and abrasions.**

MONENSIN (SODIUM)

FDA File **049-463**
Firm: **Elanco Animal Health, Div. Eli Lilly & Co.**
Use: **Chickens: Feed Additive**
Dosage: **90 to 110 grams per ton of feed.**
Purpose: **Prevention of coccidiosis.**

FDA File **049-464**
Firm: **Elanco Animal Health, Div. Eli Lilly & Co.**
Use: **Chickens: Feed Additive**
Dosage: **90 to 110 grams per ton of feed.**
Purpose: **Prevention of coccidiosis.**

FDA File **092-522**
Firm: **Pharmacia & Upjohn Co.**
Use: **Chickens: Feed Additive**

Dosage: **90 to 110 grams per ton of feed.**
Purpose: **Prevention of coccidiosis.**

FDA File **098-341**
Firm: **Intervet, Inc.**
Use: **Chickens: Feed Additive**
Dosage: **90 to 110 grams per ton of feed.**
Purpose: **Prevention of coccidiosis.**

FDA File **140-955**
Firm: **Elanco Animal Health, Div. Eli Lilly Co.**
Use: **Chickens: Feed Additive**
Dosage: **54 to 90 grams per ton of feed.**
Purpose: **Prevention of coccidiosis.**

FDA File **141-110**
Firm: **Elanco Animal Health, Div. Eli Lilly Co.**
Use: **Turkeys: Feed Additive**
Dosage: **54 to 90 grams per ton of feed.**
Purpose: **Prevention of coccidiosis.**

FDA File **141-138**
Firm: **Alpharma, Inc.**
Use: **Chickens: Feed Additive**
Dosage: **90 to 110 grams per ton of feed.**
Purpose: **Prevention of coccidiosis.**

FDA File **141-139**
Firm: **Alpharma, Inc.**
Use: **Chickens: Feed Additive**
Dosage: **90 to 110 grams per ton of feed.**
Purpose: **Prevention of coccidiosis.**

FDA File **141-140**
Firm: **Alpharma, Inc.**
Use: **Chickens: Feed Additive**

Dosage: **Chickens: 27.2 grams per ton of complete feed.** Purpose: **Prevention of coccidiosis.**
Use: **Chickens: Feed Additive**
Dosage: **90 to 110 grams per ton of feed.**
Purpose: **Prevention of coccidiosis.**

FDA File **141-149**
Firm: **Alpharma, Inc.**
Use: **Cattle: Feed Additive**
Dosage: **5 to 30 grams per ton of feed (50 to 360 milligrams per head per day). Only for cattle fed in confinement for slaughter.**
Purpose: **Prevention of coccidiosis.**

FDA File **141-164**
Firm: **Elanco Animal Health, Div. Eli Lilly & Co.**
Use: **Chickens: Feed Additive**
Dosage: **90 to 110 grams per ton of feed.**
Purpose: **Prevention of coccidiosis.**

FDA File **141-280**
Firm: **Intervet, Inc.**
Use: **Cattle: Feed Additive**
Dosage: **5 to 30 grams per ton of feed (50 to 360 milligrams per head per day). Only for cattle fed in confinement for slaughter.**
Purpose: **Prevention of coccidiosis.**

FDA File **141-282**
Firm: **Intervet, Inc.**
Use: **Cattle: Feed Additive**
Dosage: **5 to 30 grams per ton of feed (50 to 360 milligrams per head per day). Only for cattle fed in confinement for slaughter.**
Purpose: **Prevention of coccidiosis.**

FDA File **200-211**
Firm: **Alpharma, Inc.**
Use: **Chickens: Feed Additive**
Dosage: **90 to 110 grams per ton of feed.**
Purpose: **Prevention of coccidiosis.**

FDA File **038-878**
Firm: **Elanco Animal Health, Div. Eli Lilly & Co.**
Use: **Chickens, Quail: Feed Additive**
Dosage: **Chickens: 90 to 110 grams per ton of feed. Quail: 73 grams per ton of feed.**
Purpose: **Prevention of coccidiosis.**

FDA File **041-500**
Firm: **Elanco Animal Health, Div. Eli Lilly & Co.**
Use: **Chickens: Feed Additive**
Dosage: **90 to 110 grams per ton of feed.**
Purpose: **Prevention of coccidiosis.**

FDA File **047-933**
Firm: **Elanco Animal Health, Div. Eli Lilly & Co.**
Use: **Chickens: Feed Additive**
Dosage: **90 to 110 grams per ton of feed.**
Purpose: **Prevention of coccidiosis.**

FDA File **092-482**
Firm: **Pharmacia & Upjohn Co.**
Use: **Chickens: Feed Additive**
Dosage: **90 to 110 grams per ton of feed.**
Purpose: **Prevention of coccidiosis.**

FDA File **095-735**
Firm: **Elanco Animal Health, Div. Eli Lilly & Co.**
Use: **Cattle, Goats: Feed Additive**
Dosage: **Cattle: 0.14 to 360 milligrams per head per day. Goats: 20 grams per ton of feed.**
Purpose: **Beef and Dairy Cattle: Increased rate of weight gain, improved feed efficiency, and prevention and control of coccidiosis. Dairy Cattle: Increased milk production efficiency. Goats: Prevention of coccidiosis in goats maintained in confinement.**

FDA File **098-340**
Firm: **Intervet, Inc.**
Use: **Chickens: Feed Additive**
Dosage: **100 grams per ton of feed.**
Purpose: **Prevention of coccidiosis.**

FDA File **099-006**
Firm: **Phibro Animal Health, Inc.**
Use: **Chickens: Feed Additive**
Dosage: **90 to 110 grams per ton of feed.**
Purpose: **Prevention of coccidiosis.**

FDA File **104-646**
Firm: **Elanco Animal Health, Div. Eli Lilly & Co.**
Use: **Chickens: Feed Additive**
Dosage: **90 to 110 grams per ton of feed.**
Purpose: **Prevention of coccidiosis.**

FDA File **109-471**
Firm: **Ridley U.S. Holdings, Inc.**
Use: **Cattle: Feed Additive**
Dosage: **One 400 milligram per pound protein-mineral free choice feed block for each 5 head of dairy, beef, and beef replacement heifers on pasture.**
Purpose: **Increase rate of weight gain.**

FDA File **115-581**
Firm: **ADM Alliance Nutrition, Inc.**
Use: **Cattle: Feed Additive**
Dosage: **One 150 milligram per pound protein-mineral free choice feed block for each 10 to 12 head of cattle on pasture to provide 50 to 200 milligrams per head per day.**
Purpose: **Increase rate of weight gain.**

FDA File **116-088**
Firm: **Alpharma, Inc.**
Use: **Chickens: Feed Additive**
Dosage: **90 to 110 grams per ton of feed.**
Purpose: **Prevention of coccidiosis.**

FDA File **118-509**
Firm: **Farmland Industries**
Use: **Cattle: Feed Additive**
Dosage: **One 175 milligram per pound protein-mineral free choice feed block for each 4 head of cattle on pasture.**
Purpose: **Increase rate of weight gain.**

FDA File **119-253**
Firm: **Cooperative Res. Farms, Inc.**
Use: **Cattle: Feed Additive**
Dosage: **One 400 milligram per pound protein-mineral free choice feed block for each 5 head of cattle on pasture.**
Purpose: **Increase rate of weight gain.**

FDA File **120-724**
Firm: **Phibro Animal Health, Inc.**
Use: **Chickens: Feed Additive**
Dosage: **90 to 110 grams per ton of feed.**
Purpose: **Prevention of coccidiosis.**

FDA File **121-553**
Firm: **Alpharma, Inc.**
Use: **Chickens: Feed Additive**
Dosage: **90 to 110 grams per ton of feed.**
Purpose: **Prevention of coccidiosis.**

FDA File **122-481**
Firm: **Phibro Animal Health, Inc.**
Use: **Chickens: Feed Additive**
Dosage: **90 to 110 grams per ton of feed.**
Purpose: **Prevention of coccidiosis.**

FDA File **123-154**
Firm: **Alpharma, Inc.**
Use: **Chickens: Feed Additive**
Dosage: **90 to 110 grams per ton of feed.**
Purpose: **Prevention of coccidiosis.**

FDA File **124-309**
Firm: **Pharmacia & Upjohn Co.**
Use: **Cattle: Feed Additive**
Dosage: **5 to 30 grams per ton of feed (50 to 360 milligrams per head per day).**
Purpose: **Prevention and control of coccidiosis, increased rate of weight gain and improved feed efficiency in heifers being fed in confinement for slaughter.**

FDA File **125-476**
Firm: **Pharmacia & Upjohn Co.**
Use: **Cattle: Feed Additive**
Dosage: **5 to 30 grams per ton of feed (50 to 360 milligrams per head per day).**
Purpose: **Prevention and control of coccidiosis, increased rate of weight gain and improved feed efficiency in heifers being fed in confinement for slaughter.**

FDA File **130-736**
Firm: **Elanco Animal Health, Div. Eli Lilly & Co.**
Use: **Turkeys, Quail: Feed Additive**
Dosage: **Turkeys: 54 or 90 grams per ton of feed. Quail: 73 grams per ton of feed.**
Purpose: **Feed continuously for prevention of coccidiosis. Treat quail for 10 weeks.**

FDA File **134-830**
Firm: **Alpharma, Inc.**
Use: **Chickens: Feed Additive**
Dosage: **90 to 110 grams per ton of feed.**
Purpose: **Prevention of coccidiosis.**

FDA File **138-456**
Firm: **Alpharma, Inc.**
Use: **Chickens: Feed Additive**
Dosage: **90 to 110 grams per ton of feed.**
Purpose: **Prevention of coccidiosis.**

FDA File **138-703**
Firm: **Alpharma, Inc.**
Use: **Chickens: Feed Additive**
Dosage: **90 to 110 grams per ton of feed.**
Purpose: **Prevention of coccidiosis.**

FDA File **138-792**
Firm: **Pharmacia & Upjohn Co.**
Use: **Cattle: Feed Additive**
Dosage: **5 to 30 grams per ton of feed (50 to 360 milligrams per head per day).**
Purpose: **Prevention and control of coccidiosis, increased rate of weight gain and improved feed efficiency in heifers being fed in confinement for slaughter.**

FDA File **138-870**
Firm: **Pharmacia & Upjohn Co.**
Use: **Cattle: Feed Additive**
Dosage: **5 to 30 grams per ton of feed (50 to 360 milligrams per head per day).**
Purpose: **Prevention and control of coccidiosis, increased rate of weight gain and improved feed efficiency in heifers being fed in confinement for slaughter.**

FDA File **140-937**
Firm: **Elanco Animal Health, Div. Eli Lilly & Co.**
Use: **Turkeys: Feed Additive**
Dosage: **54 to 90 grams per ton of feed.**
Purpose: **Feed continuously for prevention of coccidiosis.**

FDA File **141-148**
Firm: **Alpharma, Inc.**
Use: **Chickens: Feed Additive**
Dosage: **90 to 110 grams per ton of feed up to 16 weeks of age.**
Purpose: **Feed continuously for prevention of coccidiosis.**

FDA File **141-224**
Firm: **Elanco Animal Health, Div. Eli Lilly & Co.**
Use: **Cattle: Feed Additive**
Dosage: **10 to 40 grams per ton of feed.**
Purpose: **Feed continuously for prevention and control of coccidiosis, increased rate of weight gain and improved feed efficiency.**

FDA File **141-225**
Firm: **Elanco Animal Health, Div. Eli Lilly & Co.**
Use: **Cattle: Feed Additive**

Dosage: **10 to 30 grams per ton of feed.**

Purpose: **Feed continuously for prevention and control of coccidiosis, increased rate of weight gain and improved feed efficiency.**

FDA File **141-233**
Firm: **Elanco Animal Health, Div. Eli Lilly & Co.**
Use: **Cattle: Feed Additive**
Dosage: **10 to 40 grams per ton of feed.**
Purpose: **Feed continuously for prevention and control of coccidiosis, increased rate of weight gain and improved feed efficiency.**

FDA File **141-234**
Firm: **Elanco Animal Health, Div. Eli Lilly & Co.**
Use: **Cattle: Feed Additive**
Dosage: **10 to 30 grams per ton of feed.**
Purpose: **Feed continuously for prevention and control of coccidiosis, increased rate of weight gain and improved feed efficiency.**

FDA File **141-276**
Firm: **Intervet, Inc.**
Use: **Cattle: Feed Additive**
Dosage: **10 to 40 grams per ton of feed.**
Purpose: **Feed during the last 20 to 40 days on feed for prevention and control of coccidiosis, increased rate of weight gain and improved feed efficiency.**

FDA File **141-278**
Firm: **Intervet, Inc.**
Use: **Cattle: Feed Additive**
Dosage: **10 to 40 grams per ton of feed.**

Purpose: **Feed during the last 20 to 40 days on feed for prevention and control of coccidiosis, increased rate of weight gain and improved feed efficiency.**

FDA File **200-263**
Firm: **Alpharma, Inc.**
Use: **Chickens: Feed Additive**
Dosage: **90 to 110 grams per ton of feed.**
Purpose: **Feed continuously for prevention of coccidiosis.**

FDA File **200-354**
Firm: **Pennfield Oil Co.**
Use: **Chickens: Feed Additive**
Dosage: **90 to 110 grams per ton of feed.**
Purpose: **Feed continuously for prevention of coccidiosis.**

FDA File **200-422**
Firm: **Ivy Laboratories, Div. of Ivy A.H., Inc.**
Use: **Cattle: Feed Additive**
Dosage: **50 to 360 milligrams per head per day.**
Purpose: **Feed continuously for increased rate of weight gain, improved feed efficiency, and prevention and control of coccidiosis in heifers being fed in confinement for slaughter.**

FDA File **200-424**
Firm: **Ivy Laboratories, Div. of Ivy A.H., Inc.**
Use: **Cattle: Feed Additive**
Dosage: **10 to 40 grams per ton of feed.**
Purpose: **Feed continuously for increased rate of weight gain, improved feed efficiency, and prevention and control of coccidiosis in**

heifers being fed in confinement for slaughter during the last 28 to 42 days on feed.

MUPIROCIN

FDA File **140-839**
Firm: **Pfizer, Inc.**
Use: **Dogs:** Rx only **- Topical Ointment**
Dosage: **Contains 20 milligrams per gram. Apply twice daily for not more than 30 days.**
Purpose: **Topical treatment of bacterial infections of the skin, including superficial pyoderma.**

FDA File **200-418**
Firm: **Altana, Inc.**
Use: **Dogs:** Rx only **- Topical Ointment**
Dosage: **Contains 20 milligrams per gram. Apply twice daily for not more than 30 days.**
Purpose: **Topical treatment of bacterial infections of the skin, including superficial pyoderma.**

MYRISTYL-GAMMA-PICOLINIUM CHLORIDE

FDA File **015-433**
Firm: **Pharmacia & Upjohn Co.**
Use: **Dogs, Cats, Horses:** Rx only **- Topical Powder**
Dosage: **Contains 0.2 milligrams per gram. Apply 1 to 3 times per day.**
Purpose: **Treatment of bacterial infections of the skin, including as a superficial dressing for minor cuts, wounds, lacerations, abrasions and for post surgical application.**

NARASIN

FDA File **118-980**
Firm: **Elanco Animal Health, Div. Eli Lilly & Co.**
Use: **Chickens: Feed Additive**
Dosage: **54 to 72 grams per ton of feed.**
Purpose: **Feed continuously for prevention of coccidiosis.**

FDA File **138-952**
Firm: **Elanco Animal Health, Div. Eli Lilly & Co.**
Use: **Chickens: Feed Additive**
Dosage: **27 to 45 grams per ton of feed.**
Purpose: **Feed continuously for prevention of coccidiosis.**

FDA File **140-445**
Firm: **Elanco Animal Health, Div. Eli Lilly & Co.**
Use: **Chickens: Feed Additive**
Dosage: **54 to 72 grams per ton of feed.**
Purpose: **Feed continuously for prevention of coccidiosis in broiler chickens.**

FDA File **140-843**
Firm: **Intervet, Inc.**
Use: **Chickens: Feed Additive**
Dosage: **54 to 72 grams per ton of feed.**
Purpose: **Feed continuously for prevention of coccidiosis in broiler chickens.**

FDA File **140-845**
Firm: **Intervet, Inc.**
Use: **Chickens: Feed Additive**
Dosage: **54 to 72 grams per ton of feed.**
Purpose: **Feed continuously for prevention of coccidiosis in broiler chickens.**

Thomas K. Shotwell

FDA File **140-852**
Firm: **Alpharma, Inc.**
Use: **Chickens: Feed Additive**
Dosage: **54 to 72 grams per ton of feed.**
Purpose: **Feed continuously for prevention of coccidiosis in broiler chickens.**

FDA File **140-853**
Firm: **Alpharma, Inc.**
Use: **Chickens: Feed Additive**
Dosage: **54 to 72 grams per ton of feed.**
Purpose: **Feed continuously for prevention of coccidiosis in broiler chickens.**

FDA File **140-865**
Firm: **Alpharma, Inc.**
Use: **Chickens: Feed Additive**
Dosage: **54 to 72 grams per ton of feed.**
Purpose: **Feed continuously for prevention of coccidiosis in broiler chickens.**

FDA File **140-926**
Firm: **Elanco Animal Health, Div. Eli Lilly & Co.**
Use: **Chickens: Feed Additive**
Dosage: **27 to 45 grams per ton of feed.**
Purpose: **Feed continuously for prevention of coccidiosis.**

FDA File **140-942**
Firm: **Elanco Animal Health, Div. Eli Lilly & Co.**
Use: **Chickens: Feed Additive**
Dosage: **27 to 45 grams per ton of feed.**
Purpose: **Feed continuously for prevention of coccidiosis.**

FDA File **140-947**
Firm: **Elanco Animal Health, Div. Eli Lilly & Co.**
Use: **Chickens: Feed Additive**
Dosage: **27 to 45 grams per ton of feed.**
Purpose: **Feed continuously for prevention of coccidiosis.**

FDA File **141-112**
Firm: **Alpharma, Inc.**
Use: **Chickens: Feed Additive**
Dosage: **27 to 45 grams per ton of feed.**
Purpose: **Feed continuously for prevention of coccidiosis.**

FDA File **141-113**
Firm: **Elanco Animal Health, Div. Eli Lilly & Co.**
Use: **Chickens: Feed Additive**
Dosage: **27 to 45 grams per ton of feed.**
Purpose: **Feed continuously for prevention of coccidiosis.**

FDA File **141-124**
Firm: **Alpharma, Inc.**
Use: **Chickens: Feed Additive**
Dosage: **27 to 45 grams per ton of feed.**
Purpose: **Feed continuously for prevention of coccidiosis.**

FDA File **141-170**
Firm: **Elanco Animal Health, Div. Eli Lilly & Co.**
Use: **Chickens: Feed Additive**
Dosage: **54 to 72 grams per ton of feed.**
Purpose: **Feed continuously for prevention of coccidiosis.**

NEOMYCIN (PALMITATE, SULFATE)

FDA File **010-524**
Firm: **Pharmacia & Upjohn Co.**
Use: **Dogs, Cats:** Rx only **- Otic Ointment**
Dosage: **Contains 5 milligrams (equivalent to 3.5 milligrams neomycin base) per gram of oint-**

ment. Fill ear canal 1 to 3 times per day.
Purpose: **Treatment of acute and chronic otitis externa.**

FDA File **011-315**
Firm: **Pharmacia & Upjohn Co.**
Use: **Cattle, Turkeys, Swine, Sheep, Goats: Soluble Powder**
Dosage: **10 milligrams neomycin sulfate per pound of body weight per day in divided doses for a maximum of 14 days (5 days in turkeys).**
Purpose: **Treatment and control of bacterial enteritis and for control of mortality associated with _E. coli._**

FDA File **011-347**
Firm: **Meriel Ltd.**
Use: **Dogs, Cats:** Rx only **- Ophthalmic Ointment**
Dosage: **Each gram of ointment contains 5 milligrams neomycin sulfate equivalent to 3.5 milligrams neomycin base. Apply a small amount to eye 4 times per day at 1 to 8 hour intervals. When favorable response occurs dosage may b reduced to twice daily until animal is asymptomatic.**
Purpose: **For treatment of superficial ocular inflammations or infections limited to the conjunctiva or anterior segment of the eye, such as those associated with allergic reactions or gross irritants.**

FDA File **011-703**
Firm: **Pharmacia & Upjohn Co.**
Use: **Dogs, Cats:** Rx only **- Otic Solution**
Dosage: **Contains 5 milligrams per milliliter neomycin: Administer**

1 to 2 drops in conjunctival sac 3 to 6 times per day, reducing with improvement. Otitis externa: 2 to 6 drops in ear 2 to 3 times daily. Limit treatment to period when local anesthetic action is essential to control self-inflicted trauma.
Purpose: **Treatment of infectious, allergic and traumatic keratitis and conjunctivitis, acute otitis externa, and to a lesser degree, chronic otitis externa.**

FDA File **094-975**
Firm: **Phibro Animal Health, Inc.**
Use: **Chickens, Swine, Turkeys: Feed Additive.**
Dosage: **10 to 500 grams per ton of feed depending on species and desired effect.**
Purpose: **Increased rate of weight gain and improved feed efficiency. For control of infectious synovitis, fowl cholera, chronic respiratory disease and airsacculitis in chickens and for hexamitiasis, infectious synovitis and bluecomb in turkeys. In swine, for treatment of bacterial enteritis, bacterial pneumonia, colibacillosis and for control and treatment of leptospirosis.**

FDA File **138-941**
Firm: **Pennfield Oil Co.**
Use: **Chickens, Swine, Turkeys: Feed Additive.**
Dosage: **10 to 500 grams per ton of feed depending on species and desired effect.**
Purpose: **Increased rate of weight gain and improved feed efficiency. For control of infectious synovitis, fowl cholera, chronic respiratory**

<u>disease and airsacculitis in chickens and for hexamitiasis, infectious synovitis and bluecomb in turkeys.</u> In swine, for treatment of bacterial enteritis, bacterial pneumonia, colibacillosis and <u>for control and</u> treatment of leptospirosis.

FDA File **140-810**
Firm: **Med-Pharmex, Inc.**
Use: **Dogs, Cats:** Rx only **- Otic Ointment**
Dosage: **Contains 5 milligrams per milliliter neomycin sulfate: Apply once daily to once a week. For severe conditions apply initially two to three times daily, decreasing frequency as improvement occurs.**
Purpose: **Treatment acute and chronic otitis of varied etiologies, interdigital cysts, anal gland infections in dogs, and for management of dermatologic disorders characterized by inflammation and dry or exudative dermatitis, particularly those caused, complicated, or threatened by bacterial or candidal infections. Also of value in eczematous dermatitis, contact dermatitis, and seborrheic dermatitis and as an adjunct in the treatment of dermatitis due to parasitic infections.**

FDA File **140-847**
Firm: **Altana, Inc.**
Use: **Dogs, Cats:** Rx only **- Otic Ointment**
Dosage: **Contains 5 milligrams per milliliter neomycin sulfate: Apply once daily to once a week. For severe conditions apply initially two to three times daily, decreasing frequency as improvement occurs.**

Purpose: **Treatment acute and chronic otitis of varied etiologies, interdigital cysts, anal gland infections in dogs, and for management of dermatologic disorders characterized by inflammation and dry or exudative dermatitis, particularly those caused, complicated, or threatened by bacterial or candidal infections. Also of value in eczematous dermatitis, contact dermatitis, and seborrheic dermatitis and as an adjunct in the treatment of dermatitis due to parasitic infections.**

FDA File **140-879**
Firm: **Pfizer, Inc.**
Use: **Dogs, Cats:** Rx only **- Otic Ointment**
Dosage: **Contains 5 milligrams per milliliter neomycin sulfate: Apply once daily to once a week. For severe conditions apply initially two to three times daily, decreasing frequency as improvement occurs.**
Purpose: **Treatment acute and chronic otitis of varied etiologies, interdigital cysts, anal gland infections in dogs, and for management of dermatologic disorders characterized by inflammation and dry or exudative dermatitis, particularly those caused, complicated, or threatened by bacterial or candidal infections. Also of value in eczematous dermatitis, contact dermatitis, and seborrheic dermatitis and as an adjunct in the treatment of dermatitis due to parasitic infections.**

FDA File **141-003**
Firm: **Fort Dodge Animal Health, Div. Of Wyeth**

Use: **Dogs, Cats:** Rx only **- Otic Ointment**

Dosage: **Contains 5 milligrams per milliliter neomycin sulfate: Apply once daily to once a week. For severe conditions apply initially two to three times daily, decreasing frequency as improvement occurs.**

Purpose: **Treatment acute and chronic otitis of varied etiologies, interdigital cysts, anal gland infections in dogs, and for management of dermatologic disorders characterized by inflammation and dry or exudative dermatitis, particularly those caused, complicated, or threatened by bacterial or candidal infections. Also of value in eczematous dermatitis, contact dermatitis, and seborrheic dermatitis and as an adjunct in the treatment of dermatitis due to parasitic infections.**

FDA File **200-245**
Firm: **Med-Pharmex, Inc.**
Use: **Dogs, Cats:** Rx only **- Topical Cream**

Dosage: **Each milliliter contains neomycin sulfate equivalent to 2.5 milligrams neomycin base. Apply once daily to once a week. For severe conditions apply initially two to three times daily, decreasing frequency as improvement occurs.**

Purpose: **Anti-inflammatory, antipruritic, antifungal agent for superficial bacterial infections and for dry or exudative dermatitis associated with candidal or bacterial infections.**

FDA File **200-330**
Firm: **Altana, Inc.**

Use: **Dogs, Cats:** Rx only **- Topical Cream**

Dosage: **Each milliliter contains neomycin sulfate equivalent to 2.5 milligrams neomycin base. Apply once daily to once a week. For severe conditions apply initially two to three times daily, decreasing frequency as improvement occurs.**

Purpose: **Anti-inflammatory, antipruritic, antifungal and antibacterial agent for treatment of superficial infections and for dry or exudative dermatitis associated with candidal or bacterial infections.**

FDA File **040-322**
Firm: **Schering-Plough Animal Health**
Use: **Dogs, Cats, Horses:** Rx only **- Topical Ointment**
Dosage: **Each milliliter contains neomycin sulfate equivalent to 2.5 milligrams neomycin base. Apply a thin coating of the ointment at least twice per day for 3 to 5 days.**
Purpose: **Treatment of skin wounds, superficial ulcers, and primary pyrogenic dermatitis in dogs and cats, and to minimize exuberant granulation tissue in traumatic wounds and promote healing of surgical or accidental wounds in horses.**

FDA File **010-542**
Firm: **Pharmacia & Upjohn Co.**
Use: **Dogs, Cats:** Rx only **- Otic Ointment**
Dosage: **Contains 3.5 milligrams neomycin base per gram of ointment. Apply to ear canal 1 to 3 times per day.**

Purpose: **Treatment of acute otitis externa and to a lesser degree chronic otitis externa. .**

FDA File **011-315**
Firm: **Pharmacia & Upjohn Co.**
Use: **Cattle, Turkeys, Swine, Sheep, Goats: Soluble Powder: Administer 10 milligrams neomycin sulfate per pound of body weight per day in divided doses for a maximum of 14 days. Add to drinking water or milk for use in liquid supplements. Continue for 2 to 3 days beyond remission of disease symptoms. In turkeys treatment to continue 24 to 48 hours beyond remission of symptoms but not to exceed a total of 5 consecutive days.**
Dosage: **Contains 20.3 grams neomycin sulfate, equivalent to 14.2 grams neomycin base per ounce.**
Purpose: **Treatment and** control of colibacillosis (bacterial enteritis). Also for control of mortality associated with *E. coli* in growing turkeys.

FDA File **011-437**
Firm: **Merial Ltd.**
Use: **Dogs, Cats:** Rx only **- Ophthalmic Ointment**
Dosage: **Contains 3.5 milligrams neomycin base per gram of ointment. Apply a small amount of ointment to eye 4 times per day at 1 to 8 hour intervals. When favorable response occurs, dosage may be reduced to twice per day until asymptomatic.**
Purpose: **Treatment of superficial ocular infections limited to the conjunctiva or anterior segment of the eye.**

FDA File **011-703**
Firm: **Pharmacia & Upjohn Co.**
Use: **Dogs, Cats:** Rx only **- Ophthalmic and Otic Solution**
Dosage: **Contains 3.5 milligrams neomycin base per milliliter. Apply 1 to 2 drops in conjunctival sac 3 to 6 times per day, reducing with improvement. For otitis externa: 2 to 6 drops in ear 2 to 3 times per day.**
Purpose: **Treatment of acute infections of the conjunctiva and acute otitis externa, and to a lesser degree, chronic otitis externa.**

FDA File **011-789**
Firm: **Pharmacia & Upjohn Co.**
Use: **Cattle, Swine, Horses:** Rx only **- Injection.**
Dosage: **Contains 3.5 milligrams neomycin base per milliliter. Inject deep intramuscularly for systemic effect, in joint cavity, tendon sheath, or bursa for local effect. Cattle: 10 to 20 milligrams may be repeated in 12 to 24 hours. Horse: 5 to 20 milligrams administered intramuscularly or IS. Swine: 5 milligrams per 300 pounds body weight.**
Purpose: **Treatment of overwhelming infection with severe toxicity and shock.**

FDA File **011-862**
Firm: **American Cyanamid, Division AHP Corp.**
Use: **Dogs:** Rx only **- Topical and Otic Solution**
Dosage: **Contains 3.5 milligrams neomycin base per milliliter. For chronic and deep seated lesions, apply 2 times per day; for less severe conditions apply once per day**

Purpose: **For treatment of bacterial conditions of the skin and ears, including acute and chronic otitis externa and acute moist dermatitis.**

FDA File **011-953**
Firm: **Pharmacia & Upjohn Co.**
Use: **Dogs, Cats:** Rx only **- Injectable Solution**
Dosage: **Contains 3.5 milligrams neomycin base per milliliter. Give 5 milligrams per pound of body weight per day by intramuscular or intravenous injection in divided doses every 6 to 8 hours for 3 to 5 days.**
Purpose: **Systemic treatment of bacterial infections.**

FDA File **012-258**
Firm: **Fort Dodge Animal Health, Div. Of Wyeth**
Use: **Dogs, Cats:** Rx only **- Topical and Otic Ointment**
Dosage: **Contains 3.5 milligrams neomycin base per gram of ointment. Apply as often as indicated, from once daily to weekly. For severe conditions apply initially 2 to 3 times per day, decreasing frequency as improvement occurs.**
Purpose: **Treatment of acute and chronic otitis externa of varied etiologies, interdigital cysts and in anal gland infections in dogs. Also for use in dermatologic disorders characterized by inflammation and dry or exudative dermatitis.**

FDA File **013-181**
Firm: **Schering-Plough Animal Health**
Use: **Dogs, Cats:** Rx only **- Oral Tablets**

Dosage: **Contains 50 milligrams neomycin base per tablet. Administer 1 to 2 tablets per 10 pounds of body weight.**
Purpose: <u>**Control of bacterial diarrhea.**</u>

FDA File **015-151**
Firm: **Medicis Dermatologics, Inc.**
Use: **Dogs, Cats:** Rx only **- Topical Cream**
Dosage: **Contains 3.5 milligrams neomycin base per milliliter of cream. Apply a small amount to the affected area 2 to 3 times per day.**
Purpose: **For treatment of wound infections.**

FDA File **015-433**
Firm: **Pharmacia & Upjohn Co.**
Use: **Dogs, Cats, Horses:** Rx only **- Dusting Powder**
Dosage: **Contains 3.5 milligrams neomycin base per gram of powder. Apply powder 1 to 3 times per day.**
Purpose: **Treatment of or as adjunctive therapy to certain ear and skin conditions and as a superficial dressing for minor cuts, wounds, lacerations, abrasions and for post-surgical application.**

FDA File **030-025**
Firm: **Pharmacia & Upjohn Co.**
Use: **Dogs, Cats, Horses:** Rx only **- Otic and Topical Ointment**
Dosage: **Contains 3.5 milligrams neomycin base per gram of ointment. For otic conditions, fill ear canal 1 to 3 times per day. For skin use, apply small amount of ointment 1 to 3 times per day.**

Purpose: **Treatment of acute otitis externa and to a lesser degree chronic otitis externa, anal gland infections and moist dermatitis in dogs and as a dressing for minor cuts, lacerations, abrasions and post-surgical therapy in dogs, cats and horses.**

FDA File **032-322**
Firm: **Evsco Pharmaceuticals**
Use: **Dogs, Cats:** Rx only **- Otic Solution**
Dosage: **Contains 3.5 milligrams neomycin base per milliliter of solution. Apply 2 to 3 times per day or as indicated. Severe infections should be supplemented with systemic therapy.**
Purpose: **For treatment of acute otitis externa.**

FDA File **034-872**
Firm: **Pharmacia & Upjohn Co.**
Use: **Dogs, Cats, Cattle, Horse:** Rx only **- Topical Ointment**
Dosage: **Contains 3.5 milligrams neomycin per milliliter of cream. For ophthalmic use, place a small amount into conjunctival sac 3 to 4 times per day. Otic: Fill the ear canal 1 to 3 times per day. For dermatological application, apply a small amount 1 to 3 times per day and rub or work in gently.**
Purpose: **For treatment or adjunctive therapy to certain eye, ear and skin conditions. As a superficial wound dressing for minor cuts, wounds, lacerations, and abrasions.**

FDA File **038-801**
Firm: **Fort Dodge Animal Health, Div. Of Wyeth**

Use: **Dogs, Cats:** Rx only **- Ophthalmic Solution**
Dosage: **Contains 3.5 milligrams neomycin base per milliliter of cream. Apply 2 to 3 drops per eye every 4 hours.**
Purpose: **For treatment of bacterial infections associated with topical conditions of the eye such as corneal injuries, keratoconjunctivitis and blepharitis.**

FDA File **042-633**
Firm: **Merial Ltd.**
Use: **Dogs, Cats:** Rx only **- Topical and Otic Solution**
Dosage: **Contains 3.5 milligrams neomycin base per milliliter of solution. Moisten lesion with 2 to 4 drops per square inch of surface to be treated. For otic conditions instill 5 to 15 drops in the ear twice per day for 7 days.**
Purpose: **Treatment of bacterial dermatoses and otitis externa.**

FDA File **044-655**
Firm: **Evsco Pharmaceuticals**
Use: **Dogs, Cats:** Rx only **- Ophthalmic Ointment**
Dosage: **Contains 3.5 milligrams neomycin base per milliliter of ointment. Apply to conjunctival sac 4 times per day. Severe infections should be supplemented by systemic therapy.**
Purpose: **For treatment superficial ocular bacterial infections limited to the conjunctiva or anterior segment of the eye.**

FDA File **045-288**
Firm: **Evsco Pharmaceuticals**
Use: **Dogs, Cats:** Rx only **- Ophthalmic**

Dosage: **Contains 3.5 milligrams neomycin base per milliliter. Apply 4 times per day for 7 days.**
Purpose: **Treatment of superficial ocular infections or inflammations limited to the conjunctiva or anterior segment of the eye.**

FDA File **049-725**
Firm: **Fort Dodge Animal Health. Div. Of Wyeth**
Use: **Dogs:** Rx only **- Ophthalmic Solution**
Dosage: **Contains 3.5 milligrams neomycin base per milliliter of solution. Apply 1 to 2 drops in eye every 6 hours.**
Purpose: **For treatment of secondary bacterial infections of the eye associated with conditions such as corneal injuries, conjunctivitis and blepharitis.**

FDA File **049-726**
Firm: **Fort Dodge Animal Health. Div. Of Wyeth**
Use: **Dogs:** Rx only **- Ophthalmic Solution**
Dosage: **Contains 3.5 milligrams neomycin base per milliliter of solution. Apply 1 to 2 drops in eye every 6 hours.**
Purpose: **For treatment of secondary bacterial infections of the eye associated with conditions such as corneal injuries, conjunctivitis and blepharitis.**

FDA File **065-015**
Firm: **Altana, Inc.**
Use: **Dogs, Cats:** Rx only **- Ophthalmic Ointment**

Dosage: **Contains 3.5 milligrams neomycin base per milliliter of ointment. Apply a thin film over the cornea 3 to 4 times per day.**
Purpose: **Treatment of acute or chronic conjunctivitis.**

FDA File **065-016**
Firm: **Altana, Inc.**
Use: **Dogs, Cats:** Rx only **- Ophthalmic Ointment**
Dosage: **Contains 3.5 milligrams neomycin base per milliliter of ointment. Apply a thin film over the cornea 3 to 4 times per day.**
Purpose: **Treatment of superficial bacterial infections of the eyelid and conjunctiva.**

FDA File **065-114**
Firm: **Pharmacia & Upjohn Co.**
Use: **Dogs, Cats:** Rx only **- Ophthalmic Ointment**
Dosage: **Contains 3.5 milligrams neomycin base per milliliter of ointment. Apply a thin film over the cornea 3 to 4 times per day.**
Purpose: **Treatment of superficial bacterial infections of the eyelid and conjuntiva.**

FDA File **065-119**
Firm: **Pharmacia & Upjohn Co.**
Use: **Dogs, Cats:** Rx only **- Ophthalmic and Topical Ointment**
Dosage: **Contains 17.5 milligrams neomycin base per milliliter of suspension. Apply to wound 1 to 3 times per day as necessary.**
Purpose: **Treatment of summer eczema, atopic dermatitis, interdigital eczema, and otitis externa caused by bacteria.**

FDA File **065-476**
Firm: **Schering-Plough Animal Health**
Use: **Dogs, Cats:** Rx only **- Ophthalmic Ointment**
Dosage: **Contains 3.5 milligrams neomycin base per milliliter of ointment. Apply a thin film over the cornea 3 to 4 times per day.**
Purpose: **Treatment of certain forms of conjunctivitis.**

FDA File **065-485**
Firm: **Schering-Plough Animal Health**
Use: **Dogs, Cats:** Rx only **- Ophthalmic Ointment**
Dosage: **Contains 3.5 milligrams neomycin base per gram of ointment. Apply a thin film over the cornea 3 to 4 times per day.**
Purpose: **Treatment of superficial bacterial infections of the eyelid and conjunctiva.**

FDA File **091-534**
Firm: **Pharmacia & Upjohn Co.**
Use: **Dogs, Cats:** Rx only **- Otic and Ophthalmic Suspension**
Dosage: **Contains 3.5 milligrams neomycin base per gram of ointment. Acute ocular inflammation: 1 to 2 drops in conjunctival sac 3 to 6 times per day. May be reduced to 1 drop 2 to 4 times per day. Otitis externa: 2 to 6 drops in external ear canal 2 to 3 times per day.**
Purpose: **Treatment of infectious traumatic keratitis and conjunctivitis, acute otitis externa and to a lesser degree, chronic otitis externa.**

FDA File **093-514**
Firm: **Pharmacia & Upjohn Co.**
Use: **Dogs, Cats:** Rx only **- Otic and Ophthalmic Ointment**
Dosage: **Contains 3.5 milligrams neomycin base per gram of ointment. Apply 3 to 4 times per day into the conjunctival sac. With improvement dosage may b reduced to 2 to 3 times per day. For otic conditions fill external ear canal 1 to 3 times per day.**
Purpose: **Treatment of infections, conjunctivitis, acute otitis externa and to a lesser extent chronic otitis externa.**

FDA File **096-676**
Firm: **Fort Dodge Animal Health, Div. Of Wyeth**
Use: **Dogs, Cats:** Rx only **- Topical Cream**
Dosage: **Contains 2.5 milligrams neomycin base per milliliter of cream. Apply a thin film. For mild conditions apply once per day for one week. In more severe conditions, apply 2 to 3 times per day, reducing dosage as conditions warrant.**
Purpose: **Treatment of superficial bacterial infections and for dry or exudative dermatitis associated with bacterial infections.**

FDA File **140-976**
Firm: **Pharmacia & Upjohn Co.**
Use: **Cattle, Turkeys, Swine, Sheep, Goats: Feed Additive**
Dosage: **Administer 250 to 2,250 grams per ton of dry complete feed to provide 10 milligrams neomycin sulfate per pound of body weight per day for a maximum of**

14 days. For milk replacers use 400 to 2,000 grams per ton of complete milk replacer to provide 10 milligrams neomycin sulfate per pound of body weight per day for a maximum of 14 days. Continue treatment 24 to 48 hours beyond remission of symptoms.

Purpose: **Treatment <u>and control</u> of colibacillosis (bacterial enteritis) caused by *E. coli.***

FDA File **200-046**
Firm: **Pfizer, Inc.**
Use: **Cattle, Swine, Sheep, Goats: Soluble Powder**
Dosage: **Contains 14.2 grams neomycin base per ounce. Administer 10 milligrams neomycin sulfate per pound of body weight per day in divided doses for a maximum of 14 days. Add to drinking water or milk. Continue treatment 24 to 48 hours beyond remission of symptoms, but not to exceed a total of 14 consecutive days.**
Purpose: **Treatment <u>and control</u> of colibacillosis (bacterial enteritis) caused by *E. coli.***

FDA File **200-050**
Firm: **Cross Vetpharm Group Ltd.**
Use: **Cattle, Swine, Sheep, Turkeys, Goats: Soluble Powder**
Dosage: **Contains 14.2 grams neomycin base per ounce. Administer 10 milligrams neomycin sulfate per pound of body weight per day in divided doses for a maximum of 14 days. Add to drinking water or milk. Continue treatment 24 to 48 hours beyond remission of symptoms, but not to exceed a total of 14 consecutive days. For turkeys administer 10 milligrams**

per pound of body weight per day in drinking water for 5 days. Treatment should continue for 2 or 3 days beyond remission of symptoms but not to exceed 5 consecutive days.

Purpose: **Treatment <u>and control</u> of colibacillosis (bacterial enteritis) caused by *E. coli.* <u>In turkeys for control of mortality associated with colibacillosis.</u>**

FDA File **200-113**
Firm: **Pharmacia & Upjohn Co.**
Use: **Cattle, Swine, Sheep, Goats: Water Additive Solution**
Dosage: **Contains 200 milligrams neomycin sulfate per milliliter. Administer 10 milligrams neomycin sulfate per pound of body weight per day in divided doses for a maximum of 14 days in drinking water. Continue treatment 24 to 48 hours beyond remission of symptoms, but not to exceed a total of 14 consecutive days.**
Purpose: **Treatment <u>and control</u> of colibacillosis (bacterial enteritis) caused by *E. coli.***

FDA File **200-118**
Firm: **Phoenix Scientific, Inc.**
Use: **Cattle, Swine, Sheep, Goats: Water Additive Solution**
Dosage: **Contains 200 milligrams neomycin sulfate per milliliter. Administer 10 milligrams neomycin sulfate per pound of body weight per day in divided doses for a maximum of 14 days in drinking water. Continue treatment 24 to 48 hours beyond remission of symptoms, but not to exceed a total of 14 consecutive days.**

Purpose: **Treatment and control of colibacillosis (bacterial enteritis) caused by** *E. coli.*

FDA File **200-130**
Firm: **Alpharma, Inc.**
Use: **Cattle, Swine, Turkeys, Sheep, Goats: Soluble Powder**
Dosage: **Contains 14.2 milligrams neomycin sulfate per ounce. Administer 10 milligrams neomycin sulfate per pound of body weight per day in divided doses for a maximum of 14 days in drinking water or milk. Continue treatment 2 to 3 days beyond remission of symptoms, but not to exceed a total of 14 consecutive days.**
Purpose: **Treatment and control of colibacillosis (bacterial enteritis) caused by** *E. coli.*

FDA File **200-153**
Firm: **Phoenix Scientific, Inc.**
Use: **Cattle, Swine, Sheep, Goats: Water Additive Solution**
Dosage: **Contains 200 milligrams neomycin sulfate per milliliter. Administer 10 milligrams neomycin sulfate per pound of body weight per day in divided doses for a maximum of 14 days in drinking water. Continue treatment 24 to 48 hours beyond remission of symptoms, but not to exceed a total of 14 consecutive days.**
Purpose: **Treatment and control of colibacillosis (bacterial enteritis) caused by** *E. coli.*

FDA File **200-235**
Firm: **Med-Pharmex, Inc.**
Use: **Cattle, Swine, Sheep, Goats: Soluble Powder**

Dosage: **Contains 14.2 milligrams neomycin sulfate per ounce. Administer 10 milligrams neomycin sulfate per pound of body weight per day in divided doses for a maximum of 14 days in drinking water or milk. Continue treatment 2 to 3 days beyond remission of symptoms, but not to exceed a total of 14 consecutive days.**
Purpose: **Treatment and control of colibacillosis (bacterial enteritis) caused by** *E. coli.*

FDA File **200-289**
Firm: **Med-Pharmex, Inc.**
Use: **Cattle, Swine, Sheep, Goats: Water Additive Solution**
Dosage: **Contains 200 milligrams neomycin sulfate per milliliter. Administer 10 milligrams neomycin sulfate per pound of body weight per day in divided doses for a maximum of 14 days in drinking water or milk. Continue treatment 2 to 3 days beyond remission of symptoms, but not to exceed a total of 14 consecutive days.**
Purpose: **Treatment and control of colibacillosis (bacterial enteritis) caused by** *E. coli.*

FDA File **200-378**
Firm: **Sparhawk Laboratories, Inc.**
Use: **Cattle, Swine, Sheep, Goats, Turkeys: Water Additive Powder**
Dosage: **Contains 20.3 grams neomycin sulfate per ounce. Cattle, Swine, Sheep, Goats: Administer 10 milligrams per pound of body weight per day in divided doses for a maximum of 14 days in drinking water. Turkeys: 10 milligrams per pound of body weight for 5 days. Continue treatment for 24 to 48**

hours beyond remission of disease symptoms.
Purpose: **Treatment and control** of colibacillosis in cattle, swine, sheep and goats, **and for control of mortality due to *E. coli* in growing turkeys.**

FDA File **200-379**
Firm: **Sparhawk Laboratories, Inc.**
Use: **Cattle, Swine, Sheep, Goats: Water Additive Solution**
Dosage: **Contains 200 milligrams neomycin sulfate per milliliter. Administer 10 milligrams per pound of body weight per day in divided doses for a maximum of 14 days in drinking water.**
Purpose: **Treatment and control** of colibacillosis.

NICARBAZIN

FDA File **009-476**
Firm: **Phibro Animal Health, Inc.**
Use: **Chickens: Feed Additive**
Dosage: **Administer 113.5 grams per ton of feed. Administer continuously from the time chicks are placed on litter until past the time when coccidiosis is ordinarily a hazard.**
Purpose: **Aid in preventing outbreaks of cecal and intestinal coccidiosis.**

FDA File **098-371**
Firm: **Phibro Animal Health, Inc.**
Use: **Chickens: Feed Additive**
Dosage: **Administer 90.8 to 181.6 grams per ton of feed. Administer continuously from the time chicks are placed on litter until past the time when coccidiosis is ordinarily a hazard.**

Purpose: **Aid in preventing outbreaks of cecal and intestinal coccidiosis.**

FDA File **098-374**
Firm: **Phibro Animal Health, Inc.**
Use: **Chickens: Feed Additive**
Dosage: **Administer 90.8 to 181.6 grams per ton of feed. Administer continuously from the time chicks are placed on litter until past the time when coccidiosis is ordinarily a hazard.**
Purpose: **Aid in preventing outbreaks of cecal and intestinal coccidiosis.**

FDA File **098-378**
Firm: **Phibro Animal Health, Inc.**
Use: **Chickens: Feed Additive**
Dosage: **Administer 113.5 grams per ton of feed. Administer continuously from the time chicks are placed on litter until past the time when coccidiosis is ordinarily a hazard.**
Purpose: **Aid in preventing outbreaks of cecal and intestinal coccidiosis.**

FDA File **100-853**
Firm: **Phibro Animal Health, Inc.**
Use: **Chickens: Feed Additive**
Dosage: **Administer 90.8 to 181.6 grams per ton of feed. Administer continuously from the time chicks are placed on litter until past the time when coccidiosis is ordinarily a hazard.**
Purpose: **Aid in preventing outbreaks of cecal and intestinal coccidiosis.**

FDA File **107-997**
Firm: **Phibro Animal Health, Inc.**

Use: **Chickens: Feed Additive**
Dosage: **Administer 113.5 grams
per ton of feed. Administer continuously from the time chicks are
placed on litter until past the time
when coccidiosis is ordinarily a
hazard.**
Purpose: **Aid in preventing outbreaks of cecal and intestinal
coccidiosis.**

FDA File **108-115**
Firm: **Phibro Animal Health, Inc.**
Use: **Chickens: Feed Additive**
Dosage: **Administer 113.5 grams
per ton of feed. Administer continuously from the time chicks are
placed on litter until past the time
when coccidiosis is ordinarily a
hazard.**
Purpose: **Aid in preventing outbreaks of cecal and intestinal
coccidiosis.**

FDA File **108-116**
Firm: **Phibro Animal Health, Inc.**
Use: **Chickens: Feed Additive**
Dosage: **Administer 113.5 grams
per ton of feed. Administer continuously from the time chicks are
placed on litter until past the time
when coccidiosis is ordinarily a
hazard.**
Purpose: **Aid in preventing outbreaks of cecal and intestinal
coccidiosis.**

FDA File **135-468**
Firm: **Elanco Animal Health, Div.
Eli Lilly & Co.**
Use: **Chickens: Feed Additive**
Dosage: **Administer 113.5 grams
per ton of feed. Administer con-
tinuously from the time chicks are
placed on litter until past the time**

when coccidiosis is ordinarily a
hazard.
Purpose: **Aid in preventing outbreaks of cecal and intestinal
coccidiosis.**

FDA File **138-952**
Firm: **Elanco Animal Health, Div.
Eli Lilly & Co.**
Use: **Chickens: Feed Additive**
Dosage: **Administer 27 to 45 grams
per ton of feed. Administer continuously from the time chicks are
placed on litter until past the time
when coccidiosis is ordinarily a
hazard.**
Purpose: **Prevention of cecal and
intestinal coccidiosis.**

FDA File **140-339**
Firm: **Intervet, Inc.**
Use: **Chickens: Feed Additive**
Dosage: **Administer 113.5 grams
per ton of feed. Administer continuously from the time chicks are
placed on litter until past the time
when coccidiosis is ordinarily a
hazard.**
Purpose: **Aid in preventing outbreaks of cecal and intestinal
coccidiosis.**

FDA File **140-926**
Firm: **Elanco Animal Health, Div.
Eli Lilly & Co.**
Use: **Chickens: Feed Additive**
Dosage: **Administer 27 to 45 grams
per ton of feed. Administer continuously from the time chicks are
placed on litter until past the time
when coccidiosis is ordinarily a
hazard.**
Purpose: **Prevention of cecal and
intestinal coccidiosis.**

FDA File **140-942**
Firm: **Elanco Animal Health, Div. Eli Lilly & Co.**
Use: **Chickens: Feed Additive**
Dosage: **Administer 45 grams per ton of feed. Administer continuously from the time chicks are placed on litter until past the time when coccidiosis is ordinarily a hazard.**
Purpose: **Prevention of cecal and intestinal coccidiosis.**

FDA File **140-947**
Firm: **Elanco Animal Health, Div. Eli Lilly & Co.**
Use: **Chickens: Feed Additive**
Dosage: **Administer 27 to 45 grams per ton of feed. Administer continuously from the time chicks are placed on litter until past the time when coccidiosis is ordinarily a hazard.**
Purpose: **Prevention of cecal and intestinal coccidiosis.**

FDA File **141-112**
Firm: **Alpharma, Inc.**
Use: **Chickens: Feed Additive**
Dosage: **Administer 27 to 45 grams per ton of feed. Administer continuously from the time chicks are placed on litter until past the time when coccidiosis is ordinarily a hazard.**
Purpose: **Prevention of cecal and intestinal coccidiosis.**

FDA File **141-113**
Firm: **Elanco Animal Health, Div. Eli Lilly & Co.**
Use: **Chickens: Feed Additive**
Dosage: **Administer 27 to 45 grams per ton of feed. Administer continuously from the time chicks are placed on litter until past the time when coccidiosis is ordinarily a hazard.**
Purpose: **Prevention of cecal and intestinal coccidiosis.**

FDA File **141-124**
Firm: **Alpharma, Inc.**
Use: **Chickens: Feed Additive**
Dosage: **Administer 27 to 45 grams per ton of feed. Administer continuously from the time chicks are placed on litter until past the time when coccidiosis is ordinarily a hazard.**
Purpose: **Prevention of cecal and intestinal coccidiosis.**

FDA File **141-146**
Firm: **Phibro Animal Health, Inc.**
Use: **Chickens: Feed Additive**
Dosage: **Administer 113.5 grams per ton of feed. Administer continuously from the time chicks are placed on litter until past the time when coccidiosis is ordinarily a hazard.**
Purpose: **Aid in preventing outbreaks of cecal and intestinal coccidiosis.**

FDA File **141-279**
Firm: **Alpharma, Inc.**
Use: **Chickens: Feed Additive**
Dosage: **Administer 113.5 grams per ton of feed. Administer continuously from the time chicks are placed on litter until past the time when coccidiosis is ordinarily a hazard.**
Purpose: **Aid in preventing outbreaks of cecal and intestinal coccidiosis.**

FDA File **200-027**
Firm: **Planalquimica Industrial Ltd.**
Use: **Chickens: Feed Additive**
Dosage: **Administer 113.5 grams per ton of feed. Administer continuously from the time chicks are placed on litter until past the time when coccidiosis is ordinarily a hazard.**
Purpose: **Aid in preventing outbreaks of cecal and intestinal coccidiosis.**

FDA File **200-164**
Firm: **Planalquimica Industrial Ltd.**
Use: **Chickens: Feed Additive**
Dosage: **Administer 113.5 grams per ton of feed. Administer continuously from the time chicks are placed on litter until past the time when coccidiosis is ordinarily a hazard.**
Purpose: **Aid in preventing outbreaks of cecal and intestinal coccidiosis.**

FDA File **200-170**
Firm: **Planalquimica Industrial Ltd.**
Use: **Chickens: Feed Additive**
Dosage: **Administer 113.5 grams per ton of feed. Administer continuously from the time chicks are placed on litter until past the time when coccidiosis is ordinarily a hazard.**
Purpose: **Aid in preventing outbreaks of cecal and intestinal coccidiosis.**

FDA File **200-171**
Firm: **Planalquimica Industrial Ltd.**
Use: **Chickens: Feed Additive**

Dosage: **Administer 113.5 grams per ton of feed. Administer continuously from the time chicks are placed on litter until past the time when coccidiosis is ordinarily a hazard.**
Purpose: **Aid in preventing outbreaks of cecal and intestinal coccidiosis.**

FDA File **200-172**
Firm: **Planalquimica Industrial Ltd.**
Use: **Chickens: Feed Additive**
Dosage: **Administer 113.5 grams per ton of feed. Administer continuously from the time chicks are placed on litter until past the time when coccidiosis is ordinarily a hazard.**
Purpose: **Aid in preventing outbreaks of cecal and intestinal coccidiosis.**

NITARSONE

FDA File **007-616**
Firm: **Alpharma Inc.**
Use: **Chickens, Turkeys: Feed Additive**
Dosage: **Administer 0.01875 percent in feed. Administer continuously when blackhead is ordinarily a hazard.**
Purpose: **Aid in prevention of blackhead (histomoniasis).**

FDA File **141-088**
Firm: **Alpharma Inc.**
Use: **Turkeys: Feed Additive**
Dosage: **Administer 0.01875 percent in complete feed of growing turkeys. Administer continuously when blackhead is ordinarily a hazard.**

Purpose: **Aid in prevention of black-head (histomoniasis).**

FDA File **141-132**
Firm: **Alpharma Inc.**
Use: **Turkeys: Feed Additive**
Dosage: **Administer 0.01875 per-cent in complete feed of growing turkeys. Administer continuously when blackhead is ordinarily a hazard.**
Purpose: **Aid in prevention of black-head (histomoniasis).**

NITAZOXANIDE

FDA File **141-178**
Firm: **Idexx Pharmaceuticals, Inc.**
Use: **Horses:** Rx only **- Oral Paste**
Dosage: **Each milligram of paste contains 0.72 milligrams ni-tazoxanide. Administer on days 1 through 5, 11.36 milligrams per pound of body weight. On days 6 through 28 administer 23.72 mil-ligrams per pound of body weight.**
Purpose: **Treatment of protozoal myeloencephalitis (EPM) caused by** *Sarcocystis neurona.*

NITROFURAZONE

FDA File **011-154**
Firm: **Hess & Clark, Inc.**
Use: **Cattle, Dogs, Cats, Sheep, Goats: Water Soluble Powder**
Dosage: **Powder contains 0.2 per-cent in a water soluble base. For pink eye in livestock and eye infec-tions in dogs and cats: remove cap and squeeze container to force a stream of powder directly into the eye. Repeat treatment daily. For ear infections insert nozzle** into ear canal and squeeze twice. Repeat daily until improvement is noted. For surface wounds, cuts, and abrasions apply daily until danger from infection is eliminat-ed or until healing occurs.**
Purpose: **In livestock species for the treatment of pink eye. In dogs and cats for treatment of eye and ear infections. In all species for treat-ment of surface wounds, cuts and abrasions.**

FDA File **100-854**
Firm: **Farnam Companies, Inc.**
Use: **Dogs, Horses: Ointment (0.2 percent)**
Dosage: **Apply directly on lesion with spatula or gauze. Keep in con-tact with lesion at least 24 hours and change as needed.**
Purpose: **Prevention and treatment of superficial bacterial infections of ears, wounds, burns and cuta-neous ulcers.**

FDA File **100-854**
Firm: **Cross Vetpharm Group, LTD**
Use: **Dogs, Cats, Horses: Ointment (0.2 percent)**
Dosage: **Apply directly on lesion with spatula or gauze. Keep in con-tact with lesion at least 24 hours and change as needed.**
Purpose: **Prevention and treatment of superficial bacterial infections of ears, wounds, burns and cuta-neous ulcers.**

FDA File **125-797**
Firm: **Boehringer Ingelheim Vet-medica, Inc.**
Use: **Dogs, Cats, Horses: Ointment (0.2 percent)**

Dosage: **Apply directly on lesion with spatula or gauze. Keep in contact with lesion at least 24 hours and change as needed.**
Purpose: **Prevention and treatment of superficial bacterial infections of ears, wounds, burns and cutaneous ulcers.**

FDA File **126-236**
Firm: **Boehringer Ingelheim Vetmedica, Inc.**
Use: **Dogs, Cats, Horses: Powder**
Dosage: **Apply several times per day. For deep or puncture wounds or serious burns use only as recommended by a veterinarian.**
Purpose: **Prevention and treatment of surface bacterial infections of wounds, burns, skin ulcers and abscesses after incision.**

FDA File **126-504**
Firm: **Cross Vetpharm Group, LTD**
Use: **Dogs, Cats, Horses: Ointment (0.2 percent)**
Dosage: **Apply directly on lesion with spatula or gauze. Keep in contact with lesion at least 24 hours and change as needed.**
Purpose: **Prevention and treatment of surface bacterial infections of wounds, burns and cutaneous ulcers.**

FDA File **130-872**
Firm: **Med-Pharmex, Inc.**
Use: **Dogs, Cats, Horses: Ointment (0.2 percent)**
Dosage: **Apply directly on lesion with spatula or gauze. Keep in contact with lesion at least 24 hours and change as needed.**
Purpose: **Prevention and treatment of surface bacterial infections of ears, wounds, burns and cutaneous ulcers.**

FDA File **132-427**
Firm: **Squire Laboratories, Inc.**
Use: **Horses: Ointment (0.2 percent)**
Dosage: **Apply directly on lesion with spatula or gauze. Keep in contact with lesion at least 24 hours and change as needed.**
Purpose: **Prevention and treatment of superficial bacterial infections of wounds, burns and cutaneous ulcers.**

FDA File **138-657**
Firm: **Sparhawk Laboratories, Inc.**
Use: **Dogs, Cats, Horses: Ointment (0.2 percent)**
Dosage: **Apply directly on lesion with spatula or gauze. Keep in contact with lesion at least 24 hours and change as needed.**
Purpose: **Prevention and treatment of superficial bacterial infections of wounds, burns and cutaneous ulcers.**

FDA File **140-851**
Firm: **Hess & Clark, Inc.**
Use: **Dogs, Cats, Horses: Ointment (0.2 percent)**
Dosage: **Apply directly on lesion with spatula or gauze. Keep in contact with lesion at least 24 hours and change as needed.**
Purpose: **Prevention and treatment of superficial bacterial infections of ears, wounds, burns and cutaneous ulcers.**

FDA File **140-881**
Firm: **Med-Pharmex, Inc.**

Use: **Dogs, Cats, Horses: Ointment (0.2 percent)**
Dosage: **Apply directly on lesion with spatula or gauze. Keep in contact with lesion at least 24 hours and change as needed.**
Purpose: **Prevention and treatment of superficial bacterial infections of ears, wounds, burns and cutaneous ulcers.**

FDA File **140-910**
Firm: **Hess & Clark, Inc.**
Use: **Dogs, Cats, Horses: Powder**
Dosage: **Apply several times per day. For deep or puncture wounds or serious burns use only as recommended by a veterinarian.**
Purpose: **Prevention and treatment of surface bacterial infections of wounds, burns, skin ulcers and abscesses after incision.**

NITROMIDE

FDA File **011-141**
Firm: **Fort Dodge Animal Health, Div. Of Wyeth**
Use: **Chickens: Feed Additive**
Dosage: **Finished feed to contain 227 grams per ton. Feed continuously.**
Purpose: **Prevention of coccidiosis.**

FDA File **039-666**
Firm: **Fort Dodge Animal Health, Div. Of Wyeth**
Use: **Chickens: Feed Additive**
Dosage: **Premix contains 25 percent active. Finished feed to contain 227 grams per ton. Feed continuously.**
Purpose: **Prevention of coccidiosis.**

NOVOBIOCIN (BASE, SODIUM)

FDA File **012-375**
Firm: **Pharmacia & Upjohn Co.**
Use: **Chickens, Turkeys, Mink, Ducks: Feed Additive**
Dosage: **Type B medicate feed contains 17.5 grams per ton and is intend for use in preparing finished feed contain 200 to 350 grams per ton. Feed continuously for 5 to 7 or 14 days.**
Purpose: **Chickens and Turkeys: Treatment of staph synovitis and generalized staph infections; treating breast blisters. Turkeys: Treating acute outbreaks of fowl cholera, <u>control of recurring fowl cholera</u>. Mink: Treatment of infections, abscesses, urinary infections. Ducks: <u>Control of infectious serositis and fowl cholera.</u>**

FDA File **055-072**
Firm: **Pharmacia & Upjohn Co.**
Use: **Cattle: Intramammary Infusion.**
Dosage: **Each 10 milliliter dose contains 150 milligrams. Infuse 10 milliliters into each infected quarter and massage into udder.**
Purpose: **Treatment of mastitis in lactating cows.**

FDA File **055-076**
Firm: **Pharmacia & Upjohn Co.**
Use: **Dogs:** Rx only **- Oral Tablets**
Dosage: **Administer 60 milligrams per 6 pounds of body weight every 12 hours for at least 48 hours after signs of infection have disappeared, but not to exceed 10 days.**
Purpose: **Treatment of acute or chronic upper respiratory infections such as tonsillitis, bronchitis, and tracheobronchitis.**

FDA File **100-808**
Firm: **Pharmacia & Upjohn Co.**
Use: **Cattle:** Rx only **- Intramammary Infusion.**
Dosage: **Each 10 milliliter dose contains 150 milligrams. Infuse 10 milliliters into each infected quarter and massage into udder.**
Purpose: **Treatment of mastitis in lactating cows.**

FDA File **102-511**
Firm: **Pharmacia & Upjohn Co.**
Use: **Cattle: Intramammary Infusion.**
Dosage: **Each 10 milliliter dose contains 400 milligrams. Infuse 10 milliliters into each quarter at drying off but not less than 30 days before calving.**
Purpose: **Treatment of mastitis in non-lactating cows.**

FDA File **055-098**
Firm: **Pharmacia & Upjohn Co.**
Use: **Cattle: Intramammary Infusion.**
Dosage: **Each 10 milliliter dose contains 400 milligrams. Infuse 10 milliliters into each quarter at the time of drying off but not less than 30 days before calving.**
Purpose: **Treatment of subclinical mastitis in non-lactating cows.**

FDA File **065-090**
Firm: **Pharmacia & Upjohn Co.**
Use: **Dogs:** Rx only **- Oral Tablets**
Dosage: **Administer 60 milligrams per 6 pounds of body weight. Continue treatment for an additional 3 days or every 12 hours for 48 hours.**
Purpose: **Treatment of acute or chronic upper respiratory infec-**

tions such as tonsillitis, bronchitis, and tracheobronchitis.

FDA File **065-099**
Firm: **Pharmacia & Upjohn Co.**
Use: **Dogs, Cats:** Rx only **- Oral Capsules**
Dosage: **Dogs: Administer 60 to 120 milligrams per 5 to 15 pounds of body weight daily for at least 48 hours after animal is asymptomatic. Mature Cats: 60 milligrams every 12 hours. Daily dose should be divided and equally spaced. Continue for 48 hours after animal is asymptomatic.**
Purpose: **Treatment of infections such as respiratory, urinary or gastrointestinal tract infections and other infections.**

OLEANDOMYCIN

FDA File **011-545**
Firm: **Pfizer, Inc.**
Use: **Chickens, Turkeys: Feed Additive.**
Dosage: **Premix contains 5 grams per pound. Feeds to contain 1 to 2 grams per ton.**
Purpose: **Increased rate of weight gain and improved feed efficiency in floor raised broilers and growing turkeys.**

FDA File **035-287**
Firm: **Phibro Animal Health, Inc.**
Use: **Swine: Feed Additive.**
Dosage: **Premix contains 5 grams per pound. Feeds to contain 5 to 11.25 grams per ton.**
Purpose: **Increased rate of weight gain and improved feed efficiency**

in floor raised broilers and grow-ing turkeys.

ORBIFLOXACIN

FDA File **141-081**
Firm: **Schering-Plough Animal Health**
Use: **Dogs, Cats:** Rx only **- Oral Tablets**
Dosage: **Administer 2.5 milligrams per kilogram of body weight once daily for 2 to 3 days beyond ces-sation of clinical signs for up to a maximum of 30 days. May be increased to 7.5 milligrams per kilogram of body weight for skin and associated soft tissue infec-tions. For treatment of urinary tract infections, use for at least 10 consecutive days.**
Purpose: **Treatment of diseases as-sociated with bacteria susceptible to orbifloxacin.**

ORMETOPRIM

FDA File **040-209**
Firm: **Alpharma, Inc.**
Use: **Chickens, Turkeys, Ducks: Feed Additive.**
Dosage: **Chickens: Administer 68.1 grams per ton of feed. Turkeys: Administer 34.05 grams per ton of feed. Chukar partridges: 68.2 grams per ton. Ducks: 136.2 to 272.4 grams per ton.**
Purpose: **Chickens: Prevention of infectious coryza, colibacillosis, fowl cholera, and an aid in im-proving growth and feed efficiency and improved pigmentation. Tur-keys: prevention of fowl cholera. Ducks: Control of infections due to** P. multocida**, and in the control**

of bacterial infections due to *E. coli, Riemerella anatipestifer*, and severe challenge of *P. multocida*.

FDA File **041-984**
Firm: **Alpharma, Inc.**
Use: **Chickens: Feed Additive.**
Dosage: **Administer 68.1 grams per ton of feed.**
Purpose: Prevention of infectious coryza, colibacillosis, and an aid in improving growth and feed ef-ficiency.

FDA File **100-929**
Firm: **Pfizer, Inc.**
Use: **Dogs:** Rx only **- Oral Tablets**
Dosage: **Each 120, 240, 600 or 1200 milligram tablet contains sulfadi-methoxine/ormetoprim in a 5 to 1 ratio. On the first day administer 25 milligrams per pound of body weight then follow with a daily dosage of 12.5 milligrams per pound of body weight. Continue treatment until dog is asymptom-atic for 48 hours, but not to exceed a total of 21 consecutive days.**
Purpose: **Treatment of skin and soft tissue infections (wounds and abscesses) caused by strains of** Staphylococcus aureus **and** E. coli **and urinary tract infections caused by** E. coli, Staphylococcus spp.**, and** Proetus mirabilis.

FDA File **125-933**
Firm: **Pharmaq AS**
Use: **Fish, Catfish: Feed Additive.**
Dosage: **Premix contains 113.5 grams sulfadimethoxine and 27.2 grams ormetoprim per pound. Fish and Catfish: Use premix to provide a feed containing 50 mil-ligrams total drug ingredients per**

kilogram of body weight of live fish per day. Administer for 5 consecutive days.
Purpose: **Fish: Control of furunculosis in salmonids. Catfish: Control of enteric septicemia.**

OXYTETRACYCLINE (BASE, DIHYDRATE BASE, HYDROCHLORIDE, QUATERNARY SALT

FDA File **032-946**
Firm: **Pfizer, Inc.**
Use: **Chickens: Soluble Powder**
Dosage: **Incorporate into drinking water at a rate of 1.0 gram per gallon for up to 5 days.**
Purpose: **Prevention and** treatment of complicated respiratory disease, and to prevent and treat secondary infections due to *E. coli.*

FDA File **038-439**
Firm: **Phibro Animal Health, Inc.**
Use: **Fish (Rainbow Trout and Salmonids), Lobster: Feed Additive**
Dosage: **Fish: 3.75 g per 100 pounds of fish per day in mixed ration for 10 days in salmonids and rainbow trout. Incorporate 113.5 grams into 100 pounds of feed for skeletal marking and 2.5 to 3.75 grams per 100 pounds for other indications. Lobster: Administer as the sole ration for 5 consecutive days in feed containing monoalkyl (C8-C18) trimethyl ammonium oxytetracycline.**
Purpose: **Fish: Control of mortality due to coldwater disease associated with *Flavobacterium psychrophilum* and control of columnaris disease associated with *Flavobacterium columnare* in rainbow**

trout, control of bacterial hemorrhagic septicemia, and pseudomonas disease; for marking of skeletal tissue, and for control of ulcer disease and furunculosis. Lobster: Control of gaffkemia (red tail) caused by *Aerococcus viridans.*

FDA File **046-719**
Firm: **Pharmacia & Upjohn Co.**
Use: **Cattle: Feed Additive**
Dosage: **Administer in feed at the rate of 75 milligrams per head per day.**
Purpose: **Increased rate of weight gain, improved feed efficiency, and reduction of liver condemnations due to liver abscesses.**

FDA File **094-975**
Firm: **Phibro Animal Health, Inc.**
Use: **Chickens, Swine, Turkey: Feed Additive**
Dosage: **Add to feed to provide 10 to 500 grams per ton of complete feed for chickens; 10 to 50 grams per ton or 0.05 to 0.1 milligrams per pound of body weight for swine; and 10 to 100 grams oxytetracycline per ton of finished feed for turkeys.**
Purpose: **Increased rate of weight gain and improved feed efficiency. Also for control of infectious synovitis, fowl cholera, chronic respiratory disease, and air sacculitis in chickens, and for hexamitiasis, infectious synovitis, and bluecomb in turkeys.** For treatment of bacterial enteritis, bacterial pneumonia, colibacillosis and for the control and treatment of leptospirosis in swine.

FDA File **099-006**
Firm: **Phibro Animal Health, Inc.**
Use: **Chickens: Feed Additive**
Dosage: **Add to feed to provide 500 grams oxytetracycline per ton of finished feed.**
Purpose: **Control of chronic respiratory disease.**

FDA File **101-666**
Firm: **Phibro Animal Health, Inc.**
Use: **Chickens: Feed Additive**
Dosage: **Add to feed to provide 200 grams oxytetracycline per ton of finished feed.**
Purpose: **Control of complicated chronic respiratory disease.**

FDA File **113-232**
Firm: **Pfizer, Inc.**
Use: **Cattle, Swine: Injection**
Dosage: **Cattle: Administer 3 to 5 milligrams per pound of body weight per day, not to exceed 4 days or 9 milligrams in a single dose where retreatment is impractical. Swine: Administer 3 milligrams per pound of body weight 8 hours before farrowing or immediately after farrowing for infectious enteritis. For other claims give 3 to 5 milligrams per pound of body weight per day.**
Purpose: **Cattle: Treatment of anaplasmosis, anthrax, pneumonia and shipping fever complex, foot rot, diphtheria, bacterial enteritis, wooden tongue, leptospirosis, acute metritis and wound infections, and infectious bovine keratoconjunctivitis (pinkeye). Swine: Control of infectious enteritis in suckling pigs and treatment of bacterial enteritis, pneumonia, and leptospirosis.**

FDA File **138-939**
Firm: **Penfield Oil Co.**
Use: **Chickens, Swine, Turkey: Feed Additive**
Dosage: **Add to feed to provide 10 to 500 grams per ton of complete feed for chickens; 10 to 50 grams per ton or 0.05 to 0.1 milligrams per pound of body weight for swine; and 10 to 100 grams oxytetracycline per ton of finished feed for turkeys.**
Purpose: **Increased rate of weight gain and improved feed efficiency. Also for control of infectious synovitis, fowl cholera, chronic respiratory disease, and air sacculitis in chickens, and for hexamitiasis, infectious synovitis, and bluecomb in turkeys. For treatment of bacterial enteritis, bacterial pneumonia, colibacillosis and for the control and treatment of leptospirosis in swine.**

FDA File **140-579**
Firm: **Alpharma, Inc.**
Use: **Cattle: Feed Additive**
Dosage: **Add to feed to provide 7.5 grams oxytetracycline per ton of finished feed.**
Purpose: **Increased rate of weight gain and improved feed efficiency. Reduction of the incidence and severity of liver abscesses in beef cattle fed in confinement for slaughter. Feed continuously as the sole ration.**

FDA File **141-143**
Firm: **Norbrook Laboratories**
Use: **Cattle, Swine: Injection**
Dosage: **Cattle: R/O - Administer 3 to 5 milligrams per pound of**

body weight per day, not to exceed 4 days or 9 milligrams in a single dose where retreatment is impractical. For control of respiratory disease in cattle at high risk administer 13.6 milligrams per pound. Swine: Administer 3 milligrams per pound of body weight 8 hours before farrowing or immediately after farrowing for infectious enteritis. For other claims give 3 to 5 milligrams per pound of body weight per day.

Purpose: **Cattle:** Rx only − for treatment of anaplasmosis, anthrax; OTC for pneumonia and shipping fever complex, foot rot, diphtheria, bacterial enteritis, wooden tongue, leptospirosis, acute metritis and wound infections, and infectious bovine keratoconjunctivitis (pinkeye). Swine: Control of infectious enteritis in suckling pigs and treatment of bacterial enteritis, pneumonia, and leptospirosis.

FDA File **141-211**
Firm: **Phibro Animal Health, Inc.**
Use: **Swine: Feed Additive**
Dosage: **Add to feed to provide 10 milligrams oxytetracycline per pound of body weight. Feed continuously for 7 to 14 days.**
Purpose: **Treatment of bacterial enteritis and bacterial pneumonia and for increased rate of weight gain and improved feed efficiency.**

FDA File **200-008**
Firm: **Boehringer Ingelheim Vetmedica, Inc.**
Use: **Cattle, Swine: Injection**

Dosage: **Cattle: Administer 3 to 5 milligrams per pound of body weight per day, not to exceed 4 days or 9 milligrams in a single dose where retreatment is impractical. Swine: Administer 3 milligrams per pound of body weight 8 hours before farrowing or immediately after farrowing for infectious enteritis. For other claims give 3 to 5 milligrams per pound of body weight per day.**
Purpose: **Cattle:** Rx only - Treatment of anaplasmosis, anthrax, OTC for pneumonia and shipping fever complex, foot rot, diphtheria, bacterial enteritis, wooden tongue, leptospirosis, acute metritis and wound infections, and infectious bovine keratoconjunctivitis (pinkeye). Swine: OTC for control of infectious enteritis in suckling pigs and treatment of bacterial enteritis, pneumonia, and leptospirosis.

FDA File **200-117**
Firm: **Cross Vetpharm Group Ltd.**
Use: **Cattle,** Rx only **for treatment of anaplasmosis, anthrax, Swine: Injection**
Dosage: **Cattle: Administer 3 to 5 milligrams per pound of body weight per day, not to exceed 4 days or 9 milligrams in a single dose where retreatment is impractical. Swine: Administer 3 milligrams per pound of body weight 8 hours before farrowing or immediately after farrowing for infectious enteritis. For other claims give 3 to 5 milligrams per pound of body weight per day.**

Purpose: **Cattle: Treatment of ana-plasmosis, anthrax, pneumonia and shipping fever complex, foot rot, diphtheria, bacterial enteritis, wooden tongue, leptospirosis, acute metritis and wound infections, and infectious bovine keratoconjunctivitis (pinkeye). Swine:** <u>Control of infectious enteritis in suckling pigs and</u> **treatment of bacterial enteritis, pneumonia, and leptospirosis.**

FDA File **200-123**
Firm: **Phoenix Scientific, Inc.**
Use: **Cattle, Swine:** R/O - **Injection**
Dosage: **Cattle: Administer 3 to 5 milligrams per pound of body weight per day, not to exceed 4 days or 9 milligrams in a single dose where retreatment is impractical. Swine: Administer 3 milligrams per pound of body weight 8 hours before farrowing or immediately after farrowing for infectious enteritis. For other claims give 3 to 5 milligrams per pound of body weight per day.**
Purpose: **Cattle:** Rx only – **For treatment of anaplasmosis, anthrax,** OTC - **for treatment of pneumonia and shipping fever complex, foot rot, diphtheria, bacterial enteritis, wooden tongue, leptospirosis, acute metritis and wound infections, and infectious bovine keratoconjunctivitis (pinkeye). Swine:** <u>Control of infectious enteritis in suckling pigs and treatment of bacterial enteritis, pneumonia, and leptospirosis.</u>

FDA File **200-128**
Firm: **Agri-Laboratories, Ltd.**

Use: **Cattle:** R/O, **Swine: Injection**
Dosage: **Cattle: Administer 3 to 5 milligrams per pound of body weight per day, not to exceed 4 days or 9 milligrams in a single dose where retreatment is impractical. Swine: Administer 3 milligrams per pound of body weight 8 hours before farrowing or immediately after farrowing for infectious enteritis. For other claims give 3 to 5 milligrams per pound of body weight per day.**
Purpose: **Cattle:** Rx only – **for treatment of anaplasmosis, anthrax,** OTC **for pneumonia and shipping fever complex, foot rot, diphtheria, bacterial enteritis, wooden tongue, leptospirosis, acute metritis and wound infections, and infectious bovine keratoconjunctivitis (pinkeye). Swine:** <u>Control of infectious enteritis in suckling pigs and</u> **treatment of bacterial enteritis, pneumonia, and leptospirosis.**

FDA File **200-154**
Firm: **Penfield Oil Co.**
Use: **Cattle** Rx only **-, Swine: Injection**
Dosage: **Cattle: Administer 3 to 5 milligrams per pound of body weight per day, not to exceed 4 days or 9 milligrams in a single dose where retreatment is impractical. Swine: Administer 3 milligrams per pound of body weight 8 hours before farrowing or immediately after farrowing for infectious enteritis. For other claims give 3 to 5 milligrams per pound of body weight per day.**
Purpose: **Cattle:** Rx only – **For treatment of anaplasmosis, anthrax,**

OTC for pneumonia and shipping fever complex, foot rot, diphtheria, bacterial enteritis, wooden tongue, leptospirosis, acute metritis and wound infections, and infectious bovine keratoconjunctivitis (pinkeye). Swine: Control of infectious enteritis in suckling pigs and treatment of bacterial enteritis, pneumonia, and leptospirosis.

FDA File **130-435**
Firm: **Vetoquinol N.-A., Inc.**
Use: **Chickens, Turkeys, Swine, Fish**
Dosage: **Turkeys: 200 to 400 milligrams per gallon of drinking water for 7 to 14 days. Chickens: 400 to 800 milligrams per gallon of drinking water for 7 to 14 days. Swine: 10 milligrams per pound of body weight for up to 14 days. Finfish: Immerse fish in a solution of water containing 200 to 700 milligrams per liter of water for 2 to 6 hours.**
Purpose: **For control of infectious synovitis, chronic respiratory disease, air sac disease, and fowl cholera in chickens. Control of hexamitiasis, bluecomb, and infectious synovitis in turkeys. Control and treatment of bacterial enteritis, leptospirosis, and bacterial pneumonia in swine. For skeletal marking in finfish fry and fingerlings.**

FDA File **200-306**
Firm: **Norbrook Laboratories**
Use: **Cattle, Swine: Injection**
Dosage: **Cattle: Administer 3 to 5 milligrams per pound of body weight per day, not to exceed 4 days or 9 milligrams in a single dose where retreatment is impractical. For control of respiratory disease in cattle at high risk administer 13.6 milligrams per pound. Swine: Administer 3 milligrams per pound of body weight 8 hours before farrowing or immediately after farrowing for infectious enteritis. For other claims give 3 to 5 milligrams per pound of body weight per day.**
Purpose: **Cattle:** Rx only − **For treatment of anaplasmosis, anthrax,** OTC **for pneumonia and shipping fever complex, foot rot, diphtheria, bacterial enteritis, wooden tongue, leptospirosis, acute metritis and wound infections, and infectious bovine keratoconjunctivitis (pinkeye). Swine: Control of infectious enteritis in suckling pigs and treatment of bacterial enteritis, pneumonia, and leptospirosis.**

FDA File **095-143**
Firm: **Phibro Animal Health, Inc.**
Use: **Cattle, Bees, Chickens, Sheep, Swine, Turkeys: Feed Additive**
Dosage: **Cattle: Administer 10 to 500 grams per ton of feed.**
Purpose: **Calves, Sheep, Chickens, Swine: Increased rate of weight gain and improved feed efficiency. Turkeys: Control of hexamitiasis and infectious synovitis. Chickens: Control of infectious synovitis and fowl cholera; reduction of mortality due to airsacculitis. Sheep: Treatment of bacterial enteritis and bacterial pneumonia. Bees: Control of American and European foulbrood.**

FDA File **007-879**
Firm: **Pfizer, Inc.**

Use: **Dogs, Cats:** Rx only **- Oral Capsule**
Dosage: **Administer 25 to 50 milligrams per pound of body weight per day in divided doses at 12 hour intervals. Continue for 48 hours after symptoms subside.**
Purpose: **Treatment of bacterial pneumonia, tonsillitis, bacterial enteritis, urinary tract infections and wound infections.**

FDA File **008-622**
Firm: **Pfizer, Inc.**
Use: **Cattle, Bees, Chickens, Sheep, Swine, Fish, Turkeys: Soluble Powder**
Dosage: **Cattle, swine and sheep: Add to drinking water at the rate of 200 to 400 milligrams per gallon or 10 milligrams per pound of body weight. Finfish fry: Immerse fish in a solution containing 200 to 700 milligrams per liter of water for 2 to 6 hours.**
Purpose: **Cattle, Sheep, Swine: Prevention and/or treatment of bacterial enteritis. Chickens, Turkeys: Control of hexamitiasis and infectious synovitis. Chickens: Control of infectious synovitis and fowl cholera; reduction of mortality due to airsacculitis. Sheep: Treatment of bacterial enteritis and bacterial pneumonia. Bees: Control of American and European foulbrood. Fish: Finfish fry: For skeletal marking.**

FDA File **008-763**
Firm: **Pfizer, Inc.**

Use: **Dogs, Cats:** Rx only **- Cattle, Sheep, Horse:** OTC **- Topical-Ophthalmic Ointment**
Dosage: **Contains 5 milligrams per gram. Administer topically to eyes 2 to 4 times per day.**
Purpose: **Prophylaxis and treatment of superficial ocular infections.**

FDA File **008-769**
Firm: **Pfizer, Inc.**
Use: **Cattle, Swine, Chickens, Turkeys: Injection**
Dosage: **Administer 3 to 5 milligrams per pound of body weight per day for up to 4 days for cattle; 6.25 to 100 milligrams per bird.**
Purpose: **Prophylaxis and treatment of diseases caused by organisms sensitive to oxytetracycline. Rx only – in cattle for treatment of anaplasmosis or anthrax.**

FDA File **011-060**
Firm: **Pfizer, Inc.**
Use: **Cattle: Oral Tablet**
Dosage: **For control administer 250 milligrams and for treatment administer 500 milligrams per 100 pounds of body weight per day in two doses and continue for 24 to 48 hours after animal is asymptomatic.**
Purpose: **Control and treatment of bacterial enteritis and bacterial pneumonia (shipping fever complex).**

FDA File **013-146**
Firm: **Pfizer, Inc.**
Use: **Dogs:** Rx only **- Injection**
Dosage: **Administer 5 milligrams per pound of body weight per day**

in divided doses at 6 to 12 hour intervals. Continue treatment for 24 hours after dog is asymptomatic.
Purpose: **Treatment of infectious diseases of the urinary tract, bacterial pulmonary infections and secondary infections.**

FDA File **013-293**
Firm: **Pfizer, Inc.**
Use: **Dogs, Cats: Topical Spray**
Dosage: **Contains 300 milligrams per three ounces of spray. Hold container 6 inches from area to be treated and spray for 1 to 2 seconds. Repeat frequently.**
Purpose: **Relief of discomfort associated with allergic, infectious and traumatic skin conditions.**

FDA File **038-200**
Firm: **Boehringer Ingelheim Vetmedica, Inc.**
Use: **Chickens, Turkeys: Water Additive**
Dosage: **Dissolve in water to provide 3 to 5 milligrams per pound of body weight per day based on normal water consumption.**
Purpose: **Chickens: <u>Control of infectious synovitis caused by Mycoplasma synoviae, chronic respiratory disease and air sac infections caused by M. gallisepticum and E. coli, and control of fowl cholera. In growing turkeys for control of complicating bacterial organisms associated with bluecomb disease and for control of hexamitiasis.</u>**

FDA File **045-143**
Firm: **Boehringer Ingelheim Vetmedica, Inc.**

Use: **Cattle: Injection**
Dosage: **Administer 3 to 5 milligrams per pound of body weight per day. Continue treatment for 24 to 48 hours after animal is asymptomatic but not to exceed a total of 4 consecutive days.**
Purpose: **Cattle: Treatment of pneumonia and shipping fever complex, foot rot, diphtheria, bacterial enteritis, wooden tongue, leptospirosis, acute metritis, wound infections and acute metritis.**

FDA File **047-278**
Firm: **Boehringer Ingelheim Vetmedica, Inc.**
Use: **Cattle,** Rx only **– for anaplasmosis or anthrax: Swine:** OTC **- Injection**
Dosage: **Cattle: Administer 3 to 5 milligrams per pound of body weight per day, not to exceed 4 days or 9 milligrams in a single dose where retreatment is impractical. Swine: Administer 3 to 5 milligrams per pound of body weight per day. For sows administer 3 milligrams per pound of body weight 8 hours before farrowing or immediately after farrowing for infectious enteritis. For other claims give 3 to 5 milligrams per pound of body weight per day. Continue treatment for 24 to 48 hours after animal is asymptomatic but not to exceed a total of 4 days therapy.**
Purpose: **Cattle: Treatment of anaplasmosis, anthrax, pneumonia and shipping fever complex, foot rot, diphtheria, bacterial enteritis, wooden tongue, leptospirosis, acute metritis and wound infec-**

tions, and infectious bovine keratoconjunctivitis (pinkeye). Swine: Control of infectious enteritis in suckling pigs and treatment of bacterial enteritis, pneumonia, and leptospirosis.

FDA File **048-287**
Firm: **Phoenix Scientific, Inc.**
Use: **Cattle: Injection**
Dosage: **Administer 3 to 5 milligrams per pound of body weight per day, not to exceed consecutive 4 days.**
Purpose: **Cattle: Treatment of pneumonia and shipping fever complex, foot rot, diphtheria, bacterial enteritis, wooden tongue, leptospirosis, acute metritis and wound infections.**

FDA File **049-948**
Firm: **Pfizer, Inc.**
Use: **Dogs:** Rx only **- Injection**
Dosage: **Administer 5 milligrams per pound of body weight per day in divided doses at 6 to 12 hour intervals. Continue treatment for at least 24 hours after dog is asymptomatic.**
Purpose: **Treatment of infectious diseases of the urinary tract, bacterial pulmonary infections and secondary infections.**

FDA File **091-127**
Firm: **Pfizer, Inc.**
Use: **Cattle: Injection**
Dosage: **Administer 3 to 5 milligrams per pound of body weight per day, not to exceed consecutive 4 days. Continue treatment for 24 to 48 hours after animal is asymptomatic.**

Purpose: **Cattle: Treatment of pneumonia and shipping fever complex, foot rot, diphtheria, bacterial enteritis, wooden tongue, leptospirosis, acute metritis and wound infections.**

FDA File **094-114**
Firm: **Pfizer, Inc.**
Use: **Cattle, Swine: Injection**
Dosage: **Administer 3 to 5 milligrams per pound of body weight per day, not to exceed consecutive 4 days. Continue treatment for 24 to 48 hours after animal is asymptomatic. Swine: Inject 3 to 5 milligrams per pound of body weight per day. For sows inject 3 milligrams per pound of body weight once approximately 8 hours before farrowing or immediately afterwards.**
Purpose: **Cattle: Treatment of pneumonia and shipping fever complex, foot rot, diphtheria, bacterial enteritis, wooden tongue, leptospirosis, acute metritis and wound infections. Swine: Treatment of bacterial enteritis, pneumonia and leptospirosis. Sows: Aid in the control of infectious enteritis in suckling pigs.**

FDA File **095-642**
Firm: **Boehringer Ingelheim Vetmedica, Inc.**
Use: **Cattle,** Rx only – **for anaplasmosis or anthrax: Swine:** OTC **- Injection**
Dosage: **Administer 3 to 5 milligrams per pound of body weight per day, not to exceed consecutive 4 days. Continue treatment for 24 to 48 hours after animal is asymptomatic. Swine: Inject 3 to**

5 milligrams per pound of body weight per day. For sows inject 3 milligrams per pound of body weight once approximately 8 hours before farrowing or immediately afterwards.
Purpose: **Cattle: Treatment of anaplasmosis, pneumonia and shipping fever complex, foot rot, diphtheria, bacterial enteritis, wooden tongue, leptospirosis, acute metritis and wound infections. Swine: Treatment of bacterial enteritis, pneumonia and leptospirosis. Sows: Aid in the control of infectious enteritis in suckling pigs.**

FDA File **097-452**
Firm: **Boehringer Ingelheim Vetmedica, Inc.**
Use: **Cattle:** Rx only **–for anaplasmosis or anthrax, Swine:** OTC **- Injection**
Dosage: **Administer 3 to 5 milligrams per pound of body weight per day, not to exceed consecutive 4 days. Continue treatment for 24 to 48 hours after animal is asymptomatic. Swine: Inject 3 to 5 milligrams per pound of body weight per day. For sows inject 3 milligrams per pound of body weight once approximately 8 hours before farrowing or immediately afterwards.**
Purpose: **Cattle: Treatment of anaplasmosis, pneumonia and shipping fever complex, foot rot, diphtheria, bacterial enteritis, wooden tongue, leptospirosis, acute metritis and wound infections. Swine: Treatment of bacterial enteritis, pneumonia and leptospirosis. Sows: Aid in the control of infectious enteritis in suckling pigs.**

FDA File **099-402**
Firm: **Pfizer, Inc.**
Use: **Cattle:** Rx only **for treatment of anaplasmosis.** OTC **for other uses - Injection**
Dosage: **Administer 3 to 5 milligrams per pound of body weight per day, not to exceed consecutive 4 days. Continue treatment for 24 to 48 hours after animal is asymptomatic.**
Purpose: **Cattle: Treatment of anaplasmosis, pneumonia and shipping fever complex, foot rot, diphtheria, bacterial enteritis, wooden tongue, leptospirosis, acute metritis and wound infections.**

FDA File **108-963**
Firm: **Boehinger Ingelheim, Inc.**
Use: **Cattle:** Rx only **if labeled for anaplasmosis:** OTC **- other uses - Injection**
Dosage: **Administer 3 to 5 milligrams per pound of body weight per day, not to exceed consecutive 4 days. Continue treatment for 24 to 48 hours after animal is asymptomatic.**
Purpose: **Treatment of anaplasmosis, pneumonia and shipping fever complex, foot rot, diphtheria, bacterial enteritis, wooden tongue, leptospirosis, acute metritis and wound infections.**

FDA File **130-435**
Firm: **Alpharma, Inc.**
Use: **Chickens, Turkeys, Swine, Fish**
Dosage: **Turkeys: 200 to 400 milligrams per gallon of drinking water for 7 to 14 days. Chickens: 400 to 800 milligrams per gallon of drinking water for 7 to 14 days.**

Swine: 10 milligrams per pound of body weight for up to 14 days. Finfish: Immerse fish in a solution of water containing 200 to 700 milligrams per liter of water for 2 to 6 hours.
Purpose: **For control of infectious synovitis, chronic respiratory disease, air sac disease, and fowl cholera in chickens. Control of hexamitiasis, bluecomb, and infectious synovitis in turkeys. Control and treatment of bacterial enteritis, leptospirosis, and bacterial pneumonia in swine. For skeletal marking in finfish fry and fingerlings.**

FDA File **140-582**
Firm: **Cross Vetpharm Group LTD.**
Use: **Cattle:** Rx only **if labeled for anaplasmosis;** OTC **other uses- Injection**
Dosage: **Administer 3 to 5 milligrams per pound of body weight per day, not to exceed consecutive 4 days. Continue treatment for 24 to 48 hours after animal is asymptomatic.**
Purpose: **Treatment of anaplasmosis, pneumonia and shipping fever complex, foot rot, diphtheria, bacterial enteritis, wooden tongue, leptospirosis, acute metritis and wound infections.**

FDA File **141-002**
Firm: **Boehinger Ingelheim, Inc.**
Use: **Cattle: Oral bolus**
Dosage: **Administer 500 milligrams per 100 pounds of body weight every 12 hours until animal is normal bit not to exceed 4 consecutive days. Continue treatment for 24**

to 48 hours after animal is asymptomatic.
Purpose: **Control of bacterial enteritis, bacterial pneumonia, and pasteurellosis.**

FDA File **200-026**
Firm: **Pennfield Oil Co.**
Use: **Cattle, Chickens, Sheep, Swine, Turkeys: Soluble Powder Water Additive**
Dosage: **Cattle, swine and sheep: Add to drinking water at the rate of 10 milligrams per pound of body weight for up to 14 days.**
Purpose: **Cattle, Sheep, Swine: Prevention and/or treatment of bacterial enteritis. Chickens, Turkeys: Control of hexamitiasis and infectious synovitis. Chickens: Control of infectious synovitis and fowl cholera; reduction of mortality due to airsacculitis. Sheep: Treatment of bacterial enteritis and bacterial pneumonia.**

FDA File **200-066**
Firm: **Agri-Laboratories, LTD.**
Use: **Chickens, Swine, Turkeys: Soluble Powder Water Additive**
Dosage: **Cattle, swine and sheep: Add to drinking water at the rate of 200, 400 or 800 milligrams per gallon for 7 to 14 days.**
Purpose: **Cattle, Sheep, Swine: Prevention and/or treatment of bacterial enteritis. Chickens, Turkeys: Control of hexamitiasis and infectious synovitis. Turkeys: Control of bluecomb. Chickens: Control of infectious synovitis and fowl cholera; reduction of mortality due to airsacculitis. Swine: Control and treatment of bacterial pneumonia and leptospirosis.**

FDA File **200-068**
Firm: **Phoenix Scientific, Inc.**
Use: **Cattle: Injection**
Dosage: **Administer 3 to 5 milligrams per pound of body weight per day, not to exceed consecutive 4 days. Continue treatment for 24 to 48 hours after animal is asymptomatic.**
Purpose: **Treatment of pneumonia and shipping fever complex, foot rot, diphtheria, bacterial enteritis, wooden tongue, leptospirosis, acute metritis and wound infections.**

FDA File **200-144**
Firm: **Cross Vetpharm Group LTD.**
Use: **Chickens, Swine, Turkeys: Soluble Powder Water Additive**
Dosage: **Add to drinking water at the rate of 200, 400 or 800 milligrams per gallon for 7 to 14 days.**
Purpose: **Swine: Prevention and/or treatment of bacterial enteritis, Chickens, Turkeys: Control of hexamitiasis and infectious synovitis. Turkeys: Control of bluecomb. Chickens: Control of infectious synovitis and fowl cholera; reduction of mortality due to airsacculitis. Swine: Control and treatment of bacterial pneumonia and leptospirosis.**

FDA File **200-146**
Firm: **Phoenix Scientific, Inc.**
Use: **Beef, Chickens, Swine, Turkeys, Sheep: Soluble Powder Water Additive**
Dosage: **Cattle, swine and sheep: Add to drinking water at the rate of 200, 400 or 800 milligrams per gallon for 7 to 14 days.**
Purpose: **Cattle, Sheep, Swine: Prevention and/or treatment of bacterial enteritis. Chickens, Turkeys: Control of hexamitiasis and infectious synovitis. Turkeys: Control of bluecomb. Chickens: Control of infectious synovitis and fowl cholera; reduction of mortality due to airsacculitis. Swine: Control and treatment of bacterial pneumonia and leptospirosis. Prevention or treatment of shipping fever complex in cattle and sheep.**

FDA File **200-247**
Firm: **Phoenix Scientific, Inc.**
Use: **Cattle, Bees, Chickens, Sheep, Swine, Fish, Turkeys: Soluble Powder**
Dosage: **Cattle, swine and sheep: Add to drinking water at the rate of 200, 400 or 800 milligrams per gallon. Finfish fry: Immerse fish in a solution containing 200 to 700 milligrams per liter of water for 2 to 6 hours.**
Purpose: **Cattle, Sheep, Swine: Prevention and/or treatment of bacterial enteritis. Chickens, Turkeys: Control of hexamitiasis and infectious synovitis. Turkeys: Control of bluecomb. Chickens: Control of infectious synovitis and fowl cholera; reduction of mortality due to airsacculitis. Sheep: Treatment of bacterial enteritis and bacterial pneumonia. Bees: Control of American and European foulbrood. Fish: Finfish fry: For skeletal marking.**

FDA File **008-804**
Firm: **Phibro Animal Health, Inc.**
Use: **Cattle, Bees, Catfish, Chickens, Sheep, Swine, Lobster, Salmon, Turkeys: Feed Additive**

241

Dosage: **10 to 500 grams per ton. For fish 250 mg per kilogram of body weight per day. For lobsters 1 gram per pound of complete feed.**
Purpose: **Increased rate of weight gain and improved feed efficiency in calves, sheep, chickens, and swine. Control of hexamitiasis and infectious synovitis in turkeys and control of infectious synovitis and fowl cholera in chickens. Reduction of mortality due to air sacculitis in chickens.** Treatment of bacterial enteritis and bacterial pneumonia in sheep. **Control of American and European foulbrood in honey bees. Marking of skeletal tissue in Pacific salmon and control of ulcer disease and pseudomonas disease in salmonids. Control of bacterial hemorrhagic septicemia and pseudomonas in catfish. Control of gaffkernia in lobsters.**

FDA File **138-939**
Firm: **Pennfield Oil Co.**
Use: **Cattle, Bees, Chickens, Sheep, Swine, Turkeys: Feed Additive**
Dosage: **10 to 500 grams per ton of feed.**
Purpose: **Increased rate of weight gain and improved feed efficiency in calves, sheep, chickens, and swine. Control of hexamitiasis and infectious synovitis in turkeys and control of infectious synovitis and fowl cholera in chickens. Reduction of mortality due to air sacculitis in chickens.** Treatment of bacterial enteritis and bacterial pneumonia in sheep. **Control of**

American and European foulbrood in honey bees.

FDA File **130-435**
Firm: **Cross Vetpharm Group LTD**
Use: **Fish**
Dosage: **Finfish: Immerse fish in a solution of water containing 200 to 700 milligrams per liter of water for 2 to 6 hours.**
Purpose: **For skeletal marking in finfish fry and fingerlings.**

PENICILLIN (BENZATHINE, POTASSIUM, PROCAINE, POTASSIUM PHENOXYMETHYL)

FDA File **035-207**
Firm: **Merial LTD.**
Use: **Chickens: Feed Additive**
Dosage: **2.4 to 50 grams per ton of finished feed.**
Purpose: **Growth promotion and improved feed efficiency.**

FDA File **035-688**
Firm: **Alpharma, Inc.**
Use: **Swine: Feed Additive**
Dosage: **50 Grams per ton of finished feed.**
Purpose: **Reduction of the incidence of cervical abscesses,** treatment of bacterial enteritis, **maintenance of weight gains in the presence of atrophic rhinitis. Increased rate of weight gain and improved feed efficiency in swine up to 75 pounds body weight.**

FDA File **039-077**
Firm: **Alpharma, Inc.**
Use: **Swine: Feed Additive**

Dosage: **50 Grams per ton of finished feed.**
Purpose: <u>**Reduction of the incidence of cervical abscesses,** treatment of bacterial enteritis, **maintenance of weight gains in the presence of atrophic rhinitis. Increased rate of weight gain and improved feed efficiency in swine 10 pounds to 6 weeks post weaning. Swine 6 to 16 weeks post weaning above claims except improved feed efficiency.**</u>

FDA File **046-666**
Firm: **Alpharma, Inc.**
Use: **Chickens, Turkeys, Swine Pheasant, Quail: Feed Additive**
Dosage: **2.4 to 50 Grams per ton of finished feed.**
Purpose: <u>**Increased rate of weight gain and improved feed efficiency.**</u>

FDA File **046-668**
Firm: **Phibro Animal Health, Inc.**
Use: **Chickens, Turkeys, Swine Pheasant, Quail: Feed Additive**
Dosage: **2.4 to 50 Grams per ton of finished feed.**
Purpose: <u>**Increased rate of weight gain and improved feed efficiency.**</u>

FDA File **055-028**
Firm: **West Chemical Products, Inc.**
Use: **Dairy Cattle:** Rx only **- Intramammary**
Dosage: **1 Million units per quarter at last milking before drying off.**
Purpose: <u>**Reduce the frequency of existing infections and to prevent new infections of *Staphylococcus aureus* in dry cows.**</u>

FDA File **055-060**
Firm: **Fort Dodge Animal Health, Div. Of Wyeth**

Use: **Turkeys: Water Additive**
Dosage: **Administer 1,500,000 units per gallon of drinking water at first sign of erysipelas.**
Purpose: **Treatment of erysipelas caused by *Erysipelothrix rhustopathiae*.**

FDA File **055-072**
Firm: **Pharmacia & Upjohn Co.**
Use: **Dairy Cattle: Intramammary**
Dosage: **100,000 units per quarter.**
Purpose: **Treatment of mastitis caused by *Staphylococcus aureus, Streptococcus agalactiae, S. dysgalactiae,* and *S. uberis* in lactating cows.**

FDA File **055-097**
Firm: **Boehringer Ingelheim Vetmedica, Inc.**
Use: **Dairy Cattle: Intramammary**
Dosage: **200,000 units per quarter.**
Purpose: <u>**Treatment of subclinical mastitis caused by *Staphylococcus aureus* and *Streptococcus agaluctia* at the time of drying off.**</u>

FDA File **055-098**
Firm: **Pharmacia & Upjohn Co.**
Use: **Dairy Cattle: Intramammary**
Dosage: **200,000 units per quarter.**
Purpose: <u>**Treatment of subclinical mastitis caused by *Staphylococcus aureus* and *Streptococcus agalactia* at the time of drying off.**</u>

FDA File **065-010**
Firm: **Norbrook Laboratories**
Use: **Cattle, Swine, Sheep, Horses: Injection**
Dosage: **3000 Units per pound of body weight per day for not more than 4 days. Continue for 24 hours after animal is asymptomatic.**

Purpose: **Treatment of bacterial pneumonia in cattle and sheep, erysipelas in swine and strangles in horses.**

FDA File **065-081**
Firm: **G.C. Handford Mfg. Co.**
Use: **Dairy Cattle: Intramammary**
Dosage: **100,000 units per quarter in dry or lactating cattle. In lactating cattle repeat up to 3 times at 12 hour intervals.**
Purpose: **Treatment of mastitis.**

FDA File **065-119**
Firm: **Pharmacia & Upjohn Co.**
Use: **Dogs, Cats:** Rx only **- Topical Ointment**
Dosage: **Each milliliter contains 10,000 units. Apply 1 to 3 times per day.**
Purpose: **Treatment of summer eczema, atopic dermatitis, interdigital eczema and otitis externa.**

FDA File **065-087**
Firm: **Fort Dodge Animal Health, Div. Of Wyeth**
Use: **Dogs, Cattle, Horses:** Rx only **- Injection**
Dosage: **Dogs: Inject subcutaneously or intramuscularly 1 milliliter per 10 to 25 pounds body weight and repeat in 48 hours; Cattle: Inject subcutaneously 2 milliliters per 150 pounds body weight and repeat in 48 hours; Horses: Inject intramuscularly 2 milliliters per 150 pounds body weight and repeat in 48 hours. Each milliliter contains 150,000 IU benzathine penicillin G.**

Purpose: **Treatment of bacterial infections susceptible to the drug, such as pneumonia, respiratory tract infections, equine strangles, blackleg, anthrax, and shipping fever.**

FDA File **065-130**
Firm: **Fort Dodge Animal Health, Div. Wyeth**
Use: **Cattle, Dogs, Horses:** Rx only **- Injection**
Dosage: **Dogs, Cats: 10,000 units per pound of body weight per day and continue for 24 to 36 hours after animal is asymptomatic. Horses: 3,000 units per pound of body weight per day continued until 24 to 36 hours after animal is asymptomatic.**
Purpose: **Treatment of bacterial infections.**

FDA File **065-169**
Firm: **Fort Dodge Animal Health, Div. Of Wyeth**
Use: **Dogs** Rx only **- Cattle, Horses:** OTC**: Injection**
Dosage: **Dogs: Inject subcutaneously or intramuscularly 1 milliliter per 10 to 25 pounds body weight and repeat in 48 hours; Cattle: Inject subcutaneously 2 milliliters per 150 pounds body weight and repeat in 48 hours; Horses: Inject intramuscularly 2 milliliters per 150 pounds body weight and repeat in 48 hours. Each milliliter contains 150,000 IU benzathine penicillin G.**
Purpose: **Treatment of bacterial infections susceptible to the drug, such as pneumonia, respiratory**

tract infections, equine strangles, blackleg, anthrax, and shipping fever.

FDA File **065-174**
Firm: **Fort Dodge Animal Health, Div. Of Wyeth**
Use: **Dogs** Rx only**, Cattle, Swine, Sheep, Horses:** OTC**: Injection**
Dosage: **Dogs: 100,000 units per pound of body weight per day and continue at least 48 hours after animal is asymptomatic; Cattle, Swine, Horses and Sheep: 3000 units per pound of body weight per day and continue for 48 hours after animal is asymptomatic.**
Purpose: **Dogs and Cats: Treatment of diseases caused by penicillin-sensitive diseases. Cattle and Sheep: Treatment of bacterial pneumonia. Swine: Treatment of erysipelas. Horses: Treatment of strangles.**

FDA File **065-383**
Firm: **Merial LTD.**
Use: **Dairy Cattle: Intramammary**
Dosage: **100,000 units per quarter in dry or lactating cattle. In dry cows inject each quarter at the time of drying off. In lactating cattle repeat up to 3 times at 12-hour intervals.**
Purpose: **Treatment of mastitis.**

FDA File **065-488**
Firm: **Walco International, Inc.**
Use: **Dogs:** Rx only**, Cattle, Horses:** OTC**: Injection**
Dosage: **Dogs: Inject 1 milliliter per 10 to 25 pounds body weight and repeat in 48 hours; Cattle: Inject subcutaneously 2 milliliters per 150 pounds body weight and**

repeat in 48 hours; Horses: Inject intramuscularly 2 milliliters per 150 pounds body weight and repeat in 48 hours. Each milliliter contains 150,000 IU benzathine penicillin G.
Purpose: **Treatment of bacterial infections susceptible to the drug, such as pneumonia, respiratory tract infections, equine strangles, blackleg, anthrax, and shipping fever.**

FDA File **065-493**
Firm: **G.C. Hanford Mfg. Co.**
Use: **Cattle, Swine, Sheep, Horses: Injection**
Dosage: **Inject 3000 units per pound body weight. Continue until 24 hours after animal is asymptomatic but not to exceed 4 consecutive days.**
Purpose: **Treatment of bacterial pneumonia in all species and erysipelas in swine and horses. Treatment of strangles in horses.**

FDA File **065-498**
Firm: **Phoenix Scientific, Inc.**
Use: **Cattle: Injection**
Dosage: **Inject 2 milliliters per 150 pounds body weight and repeat in 48 hours; each milliliter contains 150,000 IU benzathine penicillin G.**
Purpose: **Treatment of bacterial pneumonia, (shipping fever complex), upper respiratory infections, and blackleg.**

FDA File **065-500**
Firm: **G.C. Hanford Mfg. Co.**
Use: **Dogs:** Rx only**; Cattle, Horses:** OTC **Injection**

Dosage: **Dogs: Inject 1 milliliter per 10 to 25 pounds body weight and repeat in 48 hours; Cattle: Inject subcutaneously 2 milliliters per 150 pounds body weight and repeat in 48 hours; Horses: Inject intramuscularly 2 milliliters per 150 pounds body weight and repeat in 48 hours. Each milliliter contains 150,000 IU benzathine penicillin G.**
Purpose: **Treatment of bacterial infections susceptible to the drug, such as rhinitis or pharyngitis, pneumonia, respiratory tract infections, equine strangles, blackleg, anthrax, and shipping fever.**

FDA File **065-505**
Firm: **Cross Vetpharm Group LTD.**
Use: **Cattle, Swine, Sheep, Horses: Injection**
Dosage: **Inject subcutaneously 3000 units per pound body weight.**
Purpose: **Treatment of bacterial pneumonia in all species and erysipelas in horses. Treatment of strangles.**

FDA File **065-506**
Firm: **Cross Vetpharm Group Ltd.**
Use: **Dogs:** Rx only**, Cattle, Horses: OTC - Injection**
Dosage: **Dogs: Inject subcutaneously or intramuscularly 1 milliliter per 10 to 25 pounds body weight and repeat in 48 hours; Cattle: Inject subcutaneously 2 milliliters per 150 pounds body weight and repeat in 48 hours; Horses: Inject intramuscularly 2 milliliters per 150 pounds body weight and repeat in 48 hours. Each milliliter contains 150,000 IU benzathine penicillin G.**

Purpose: **Treatment of bacterial infections such as pneumonia, respiratory tract infections, equine strangles, blackleg, anthrax, and shipping fever.**

FDA File **200-103**
Firm: **Cross Vetpharm Group LTD.**
Use: **Turkeys: Water Additive**
Dosage: **Administer 1,500,000 units per gallon of drinking water at first sign of erysipelas.**
Purpose: **Treatment of erysipelas caused by *Erysipelothrix rhustopathiae*.**

FDA File **200-106**
Firm: **Alpharma, Inc.**
Use: **Turkeys: Water Additive**
Dosage: **Administer 1,500,000 units per gallon of drinking water at first sign of erysipelas.**
Purpose: **Treatment of erysipelas caused by *Erysipelothrix rhustopathiae*.**

FDA File **200-122**
Firm: **Alpharma, Inc.**
Use: **Turkeys: Water Additive**
Dosage: **Administer 1,500,000 units per gallon of drinking water at first sign of erysipelas.**
Purpose: **Treatment of erysipelas caused by *Erysipelothrix rhustopathiae*.**

FDA File **200-347**
Firm: **Phoenix Scientific, Inc.**
Use: **Turkeys: Water Additive**
Dosage: **Administer 1,500,000 units per gallon of drinking water at first sign of erysipelas.**
Purpose: **Treatment of erysipelas caused by *Erysipelothrix rhustopathiae*.**

FDA File **200-372**
Firm: **G.C. Hanford Mfg. Co.**
Use: **Turkeys: Water Additive**
Dosage: **Administer 1,500,000 units per gallon of drinking water at first sign of erysipelas.**
Purpose: **Treatment of erysipelas caused by** *Erysipelothrix rhustopathiae.*

FDA File **065-110**
Firm: **Phoenix Scientific, Inc.**
Use: **Dogs, Cats:** Rx only **-, Cattle, Horses, Swine, Sheep:** OTC: **Injectable Suspension**
Dosage: **Dogs, Cats: 10,000 units per pound of body weight daily at 24 hour intervals by intramuscular injection. Continue treatment for 48 hours after symptoms disappear. Cattle, Sheep, Swine, Horses: Inject subcutaneously 2 milliliters (300,000 units) per 150 pounds body weight and repeat in 48 hours; Horses: Inject intramuscularly 2 milliliters per pound of body weight and continue treatment for in 48 hours after symptoms disappear. Not to exceed 7 days of treatment. Each milliliter contains 150,000 IU procaine penicillin G.**
Purpose: **Cattle and Sheep: Treatment of bacterial pneumonia. Swine: For treatment of erysipelas. Horses: Treatment of strangles caused by** *Streptococcus equi.* **Dogs and Cats: For treatment of infections caused by penicillin sensitive organisms.**

FDA File **091-668**
Firm: **Alpharma, Inc.**
Use: **Swine: Feed Additive**
Dosage: **50 grams per ton of feed.**

Purpose: **Reduction in the incidence of cervical abscesses, treatment of bacterial enteritis or necrotic enteritis and prevention of enteritis during stress. Maintenance of weight gains in the presence of atrophic rhinitis, improved rate of weight gain and improved feed efficiency in swine weighing up to 75 pounds.**

FDA File **094-295**
Firm: **ADM Animal Health & Nutrition Div.**
Use: **Chickens: Feed Additive**
Dosage: **2.4 to 50 grams per ton of feed.**
Purpose: **Growth promotion and feed efficiency.**

FDA File **098-371**
Firm: **Phibro Animal Health, Inc.**
Use: **Chickens: Feed Additive**
Dosage: **2.4 to 50 grams per ton of feed.**
Purpose: **Growth promotion and feed efficiency.**

FDA File **098-374**
Firm: **Phibro Animal Health, Inc.**
Use: **Chickens: Feed Additive**
Dosage: **2.4 to 50 grams per ton of feed.**
Purpose: **Increased rate of weight gain and improved feed efficiency.**

FDA File **138-934**
Firm: **Pennfield Oil Co.**
Use: **Swine: Feed Additive**
Dosage: **50 grams per ton of feed.**
Purpose: **Reduce the incidence of cervical abscesses; treatment of bacterial swine enteritis and vibrionic dysentery, and for the preven-**

tion of these diseases during times of stress; maintenance of weight gains in the presence of atrophic rhinitis; and for growth promotion and increased feed efficiency in swine up to 75 pounds.

FDA File **200-140**
Firm: **Alpharma, Inc.**
Use: **Swine: Feed Additive**
Dosage: **50 grams per ton of feed.**
Purpose: **Reduction in the incidence of cervical abscesses,** treatment of bacterial enteritis or necrotic enteritis and vibrionic dysentery, **maintenance of weight gains in the presence of atrophic rhinitis, improved rate of weight gain and improved feed efficiency in swine 10 pounds body weight to 6 weeks after weaning. For swine in confinement (dry-lot) or on limited pasture up to 16 weeks after weaning.**

FDA File **200-167**
Firm: **Alpharma, Inc.**
Use: **Swine: Feed Additive**
Dosage: **50 grams per ton of feed.**
Purpose: **Reduction in the incidence of cervical abscesses,** treatment of bacterial enteritis or necrotic enteritis and vibrionic dysentery, **maintenance of weight gains in the presence of atrophic rhinitis, improved rate of weight gain and improved feed efficiency in swine 10 pounds body weight to 6 weeks after weaning. For swine in confinement (dry-lot) or on limited pasture up to 16 weeks after weaning.**

FDA File **200-307**
Firm: **Vetoquinol N.-A., Inc.**
Use: **Turkeys: Water Additive**
Dosage: **Administer 1,500,000 units per gallon of drinking water at first sign of erysipelas.**
Purpose: **Treatment of erysipelas caused by** *Erysipelothrix rhustopathiae.*

FDA File **065-275**
Firm: **Merial LTD.**
Use: **Dogs, Cats:** Rx only **- Oral Tablet**
Dosage: **10 to 15 milligrams per pound of body weight every 6 to 8 hours, 1 to 2 hours before feeding.**
Purpose: **Treatment of respiratory, urogenital, skin, and soft tissue infections and septicsemia.**

FDA File **065-276**
Firm: **Merial LTD.**
Use: **Dogs, Cats:** Rx only **- Oral Granules**
Dosage: **10 to 15 milligrams per pound of body weight every 6 to 8 hours, 1 to 2 hours before feeding.**
Purpose: **Treatment of respiratory, urogenital, skin, and soft tissue infections and septicsemia.**

PIRLIMYCIN (HYDROCHLORIDE)

FDA File **141-036**
Firm: **Pharmacia & Upjohn Co.**
Use: **Dairy Cattle: Intramammary Infusion**
Dosage: **50 milligrams per quarter repeated at 24 hour intervals for up to 8 treatments.**
Purpose: **Treatment of clinical and subclinical mastitis.**

POLYMYXIN B (SULFATE)

FDA File **008-763**
Firm: **Pfizer, Inc.**
Use: **Dogs, Cats:** Rx only **- Cattle, Sheep, Horse:** OTC **Ophthalmic**
Dosage: **Contains 10,000 units polymyxin B per gram. Administer topically to eyes 2 to 4 times per day.**
Purpose: **Prophylaxis and treatment of superficial ocular infections.**

FDA File **038-801**
Firm: **Fort Dodge Animal Health, Div. Of Wyeth**
Use: **Dogs, Cats:** Rx only **- Ophthalmic Solution**
Dosage: **Contains 10,000 units polymyxin B per milliliter. Apply 2 to 3 drops per eye every 4 hours.**
Purpose: **For treatment of bacterial infections associated with topical conditions of the eye such as corneal injuries, keratoconjunctivitis and blepharitis.**

FDA File **049-725**
Firm: **Fort Dodge Animal Health. Div. Of Wyeth**
Use: **Dogs:** Rx only **- Ophthalmic Solution**
Dosage: **Contains 10,000 units polymyxin B per milliliter. Apply 1 to 2 drops in eye every 6 hours.**
Purpose: **For treatment of secondary bacterial infections of the eye associated with conditions such as corneal injuries, conjunctivitis and blepharitis.**

FDA File **049-726**
Firm: **Fort Dodge Animal Health. Div. Of Wyeth**

Use: **Dogs:** Rx only **- Ophthalmic Solution**
Dosage: **Contains 10,000 units polymyxin B per milliliter. Apply 1 to 2 drops in eye every 6 hours.**
Purpose: **For treatment of secondary bacterial infections of the eye associated with conditions such as corneal injuries, conjunctivitis and blepharitis.**

FDA File **065-015**
Firm: **Altana, Inc.**
Use: **Dogs, Cats:** Rx only **- Ophthalmic Ointment**
Dosage: **Contains 10,000 units polymyxin B per gram. Apply a thin film over cornea 3 to 4 times per day.**
Purpose: **For treatment of acute or chronic conjunctivitis.**

FDA File **065-016**
Firm: **Altana, Inc.**
Use: **Dogs, Cats:** Rx only **- Ophthalmic Ointment**
Dosage: **Contains 10,000 units polymyxin B per gram. Apply a thin film over cornea 3 to 4 times per day.**
Purpose: **For treatment of superficial bacterial infections of the eyelid and conjunctiva.**

FDA File **065-114**
Firm: **Pharmacia & Upjohn Co.**
Use: **Dogs, Cats:** Rx only **- Ophthalmic Ointment**
Dosage: **Contains 10,000 units polymyxin B per gram. Apply a thin film over cornea 3 to 4 times per day.**
Purpose: **For treatment of superficial bacterial infections of the eyelid and conjunctiva.**

FDA File **065-119**
Firm: **Pharmacia & Upjohn Co.**
Use: **Dogs, Cats:** Rx only **- Ophthal-mic Suspension**
Dosage: **Contains 5,000 units poly-myxin B per milliliter. Apply a thin film over cornea 3 to 4 times per day.**
Purpose: **For treatment of summer eczema, atopic dermatitis, inter-digital eczema, and otitis externa.**

FDA File **065-476**
Firm: **Schering-Plough Animal Health.**
Use: **Dogs, Cats:** Rx only **- Ophthal-mic Ointment**
Dosage: **Contains 10,000 units polymyxin B per gram. Apply a thin film over cornea 3 to 4 times per day.**
Purpose: **For treatment of superfi-cial bacterial infections of con-junctivitis.**

FDA File **065-485**
Firm: **Schering-Plough Animal Health.**
Use: **Dogs, Cats:** Rx only **- Ophthal-mic Ointment**
Dosage: **Contains 10,000 units polymyxin B per gram. Apply a thin film over cornea 3 to 4 times per day.**
Purpose: **For treatment of super-ficial bacterial infections of the eyelid and conjunctivitis.**

ROBENIDINE (HYDROCHLO-RIDE)

FDA File **048-486**
Firm: **Alpharma, Inc.**
Use: **Chickens: Feed Additive**
Dosage: **30 grams per ton of feed.**
Purpose: **Prevention of coccidiosis.**

FDA File **092-507**
Firm: **Alpharma, Inc.**
Use: **Chickens: Feed Additive**
Dosage: **30 grams per ton of feed.**
Purpose: **Prevention of coccidiosis.**

FDA File **093-106**
Firm: **Pharmacia & Upjohn Co.**
Use: **Chickens: Feed Additive**
Dosage: **30 grams per ton of feed.**
Purpose: **Prevention of coccidiosis.**

FDA File **095-546**
Firm: **Alpharma, Inc.**
Use: **Chickens: Feed Additive**
Dosage: **30 grams per ton of feed.**
Purpose: **Prevention of coccidiosis.**

FDA File **096-933**
Firm: **Alpharma, Inc.**
Use: **Chickens: Feed Additive**
Dosage: **30 grams per ton of feed.**
Purpose: **Prevention of coccidiosis.**

FDA File **097-085**
Firm: **Alpharma, Inc.**
Use: **Chickens: Feed Additive**
Dosage: **30 grams per ton of feed.**
Purpose: **Prevention of coccidiosis.**

FDA File **101-666**
Firm: **Phibro Animal Health, Inc.**
Use: **Chickens: Feed Additive**
Dosage: **30 grams per ton of feed.**
Purpose: **Prevention of coccidiosis.**

FDA File **141-154**
Firm: **Alpharma, Inc.**
Use: **Chickens: Feed Additive**
Dosage: **30 grams per ton of feed.**
Purpose: **Prevention of coccidiosis.**

FDA File **141-155**
Firm: **Alpharma, Inc.**
Use: **Chickens: Feed Additive**
Dosage: **30 grams per ton of feed.**
Purpose: **Prevention of coccidiosis.**

FDA File **200-212**
Firm: **Alpharma, Inc.**
Use: **Chickens: Feed Additive**
Dosage: **30 grams per ton of feed.**
Purpose: **Prevention of coccidiosis.**

ROXARSONE

FDA File **005-414**
Firm: **Alpharma, Inc.**
Use: **Chickens, Turkeys, Swine: Water Soluble Tablets**
Dosage: **Chickens and Turkeys: 0.002 to 0.008 percent in water. Swine: 400 milligrams per gallon of drinking water or 400 milligrams in 2 fluid ounces of water per 50 pounds body weight as a drench.**
Purpose: **Chickens and Turkeys: Prevention of coccidiosis, increased rate of weight gain and improved feed efficiency. Swine: Treatment of swine dysentery.**

FDA File **006-419**
Firm: **Alpharma, Inc.**
Use: **Chickens, Turkeys: Water Soluble Tablets**
Dosage: **0.002 percent in drinking water continuously throughout the growing period.**
Purpose: **Increased rate of weight gain, improved feed efficiency and improved pigmentation.**

FDA File **006-081**
Firm: **Alpharma, Inc.**

Use: **Chickens, Turkeys: Water Soluble Solution**
Dosage: **0.002 percent in drinking water continuously throughout the growing period.**
Purpose: **Increased rate of weight gain, improved feed efficiency and improved pigmentation.**

FDA File **007-891**
Firm: **Alpharma, Inc.**
Use: **Chickens, Turkeys, Swine: Feed Additive**
Dosage: **22.7 to 45.4 grams per ton of complete feed throughout the growing period. For treatment of dysentery in swine use 181.5 grams per ton.**
Purpose: **Increased rate of weight gain, improved feed efficiency and improved pigmentation. Swine: Increased rate of weight gain, improved feed efficiency use 22.7 to 45.4 grams per ton; and for treatment of swine dysentery use 181.5 grams per ton for not more than 6 days. For increased rate of weight gain and improved feed efficiency in swine.**

FDA File **008-274**
Firm: **Alpharma, Inc.**
Use: **Swine: Water Soluble Tablets**
Dosage: **400 milligrams per gallon of drinking water for not more than 6 days or 400 milligrams in 2 ounces of water for 1 to 2 days administered by drench. Repeat treatment after 5 days if needed.**
Purpose: **Treatment of swine dysentery.**

FDA File **013-461**
Firm: **Merial LTD.**
Use: **Chickens: Feed Additive**

Dosage: **45.4 Grams per ton of complete feed throughout the growing period.**
Purpose: **Growth promotion.**

FDA File **034-537**
Firm: **Fort Dodge Animal Health, Div. Wyeth**
Use: **Chickens: Feed Additive**
Dosage: **22.7 to 45.4 Grams per ton of complete feed throughout the growing period.**
Purpose: **Growth promotion, improved feed efficiency, and improved pigmentation.**

FDA File **039-284**
Firm: **Swisher Feed Division**
Use: **Chickens: Feed Additive**
Dosage: **34 Grams per ton of complete feed throughout the growing period.**
Purpose: **Increased rate of weight gain.**

FDA File **039-366**
Firm: **Fort Dodge Animal Health, Div. Wyeth**
Use: **Chickens: Feed Additive**
Dosage: **45.4 Grams per ton of complete feed throughout the growing period.**
Purpose: **Growth promotion, improved feed efficiency and improved pigmentation.**

FDA File **040-264**
Firm: **Merial LTD.**
Use: **Chickens: Feed Additive**
Dosage: **45.4 Grams per ton of complete feed throughout the growing period.**
Purpose: **Growth promotion, improved feed efficiency, and improved pigmentation.**

FDA File **040-435**
Firm: **Alpharma, Inc.**
Use: **Chickens: Feed Additive**
Dosage: **45.4 Grams per ton of complete feed throughout the growing period.**
Purpose: **Growth promotion, improved feed efficiency, and improved pigmentation.**

FDA File **041-177**
Firm: **Merial LTD.**
Use: **Chickens: Feed Additive**
Dosage: **45.4 Grams per ton of complete feed throughout the growing period.**
Purpose: **Increased rate of weight gain.**

FDA File **041-178**
Firm: **Pharmacia & Upjohn Co.**
Use: **Chickens: Feed Additive**
Dosage: **45.4 Grams per ton of complete feed throughout the growing period.**
Purpose: **Growth promotion, improved feed efficiency, and improved pigmentation.**

FDA File **041-500**
Firm: **Elanco Animal Health, Div. Eli Lilly & Co.**
Use: **Chickens: Feed Additive**
Dosage: **45.4 Grams per ton of complete feed throughout the growing period.**
Purpose: **Growth promotion, improved feed efficiency, and improved pigmentation.**

FDA File **041-541**
Firm: **Merial LTD.**
Use: **Chickens: Feed Additive**

Dosage: **45.4 Grams per ton of complete feed throughout the growing period.**
Purpose: **Growth promotion, improved feed efficiency, and improved pigmentation.**

FDA File **041-984**
Firm: **Alpharma, Inc.**
Use: **Chickens: Feed Additive**
Dosage: **22.7 Grams per ton of complete feed throughout the growing period.**
Purpose: **Growth promotion, improved feed efficiency, and improved pigmentation.**

FDA File **044-016**
Firm: **Merial LTD.**
Use: **Chickens: Feed Additive**
Dosage: **45.4 Grams per ton of complete feed throughout the growing period.**
Purpose: **Growth promotion, improved feed efficiency, and improved pigmentation.**

FDA File **049-179**
Firm: **Merial LTD.**
Use: **Chickens: Feed Additive**
Dosage: **22. 7 to 45.4 grams per ton of complete feed throughout the growing period.**
Purpose: **Growth promotion, improved feed efficiency, and improved pigmentation.**

FDA File **049-180**
Firm: **Merial LTD.**
Use: **Chickens: Feed Additive**
Dosage: **34 Grams per ton of complete feed throughout the growing period.**

Purpose: **Growth promotion, improved feed efficiency, and improved pigmentation.**

FDA File **049-464**
Firm: **Elanco Animal Health, Div. Eli Lilly & Co.**
Use: **Chickens: Feed Additive**
Dosage: **11.3 to 22.7 grams per ton of complete feed throughout the growing period.**
Purpose: **Growth promotion, improved feed efficiency.**

FDA File **091-326**
Firm: **Alpharma, Inc.**
Use: **Chickens: Feed Additive**
Dosage: **11 to 45 grams per ton of complete feed throughout the growing period.**
Purpose: **Increased rate of weight gain, improved feed efficiency.**

FDA File **092-522**
Firm: **Pharmacia & Upjohn Co.**
Use: **Chickens: Feed Additive**
Dosage: **15 to 45 grams per ton of complete feed throughout the growing period.**
Purpose: **Increased rate of weight gain, improved feed efficiency, and improved pigmentation.**

FDA File **092-953**
Firm: **Alpharma, Inc.**
Use: **Chickens: Feed Additive**
Dosage: **22.7 to 45.4 grams per ton of complete feed throughout the growing period.**
Purpose: **Increased rate of weight gain, improved feed efficiency, and improved pigmentation.**

FDA File **093-025**
Firm: **Alpharma, Inc.**

Use: **Chickens, Turkeys, Swine: Soluble Powder**
Dosage: **Chickens and Turkeys: 0.002 percent in drinking water. Swine: 0.01 percent in drinking water. As a drench in swine administer 30 milliliters of a 1.55 percent solution for 1 to 2 days. Treatment may be repeated in 5 days.**
Purpose: **Increased rate of weight gain, improved feed efficiency and improved pigmentation. Swine: For treatment of swine dysentery.**

FDA File **095-546**
Firm: **Alpharma, Inc.**
Use: **Chickens: Feed Additive**
Dosage: **22.5 to 45.4 grams per ton of complete feed throughout the growing period.**
Purpose: **Increased rate of weight gain.**

FDA File **095-547**
Firm: **Intervet, Inc.**
Use: **Chickens: Feed Additive**
Dosage: **22.8 to 34.1 grams per ton of complete feed throughout the growing period.**
Purpose: **Increased rate of weight gain, improved feed efficiency, and improved pigmentation.**

FDA File **095-548**
Firm: **Intervet, Inc.**
Use: **Chickens: Feed Additive**
Dosage: **22.8 to 34.1 grams per ton of complete feed throughout the growing period.**
Purpose: **Increased rate of weight gain, improved feed efficiency, and improved pigmentation.**

FDA File **095-549**
Firm: **Intervet, Inc.**
Use: **Chickens: Feed Additive**
Dosage: **22.8 to 34.1 grams per ton of complete feed throughout the growing period.**
Purpose: **Increased rate of weight gain, improved feed efficiency, and improved pigmentation.**

FDA File **098-341**
Firm: **Intervet, Inc.**
Use: **Chickens: Feed Additive**
Dosage: **22.7 to 45.4 grams per ton of complete feed throughout the growing period.**
Purpose: **Increased rate of weight gain, improved feed efficiency.**

FDA File **098-371**
Firm: **Phibro Animal Health, Inc.**
Use: **Chickens: Feed Additive**
Dosage: **22.7 to 45.4 grams per ton of complete feed throughout the growing period.**
Purpose: **Increased rate of weight gain, improved feed efficiency, and improved pigmentation.**

FDA File **100-853**
Firm: **Phibro Animal Health, Inc.**
Use: **Chickens: Feed Additive**
Dosage: **22.7 to 45.4 grams per ton of complete feed throughout the growing period.**
Purpose: **Increased rate of weight gain, improved feed efficiency, and improved pigmentation.**

FDA File **101-628**
Firm: **Intervet, Inc.**
Use: **Chickens: Feed Additive**
Dosage: **22.7 grams per ton of complete feed throughout the growing period.**

Purpose: **Increased rate of weight gain, improved feed efficiency.**

FDA File **102-485**
Firm: **Alpharma, Inc.**
Use: **Chickens: Feed Additive**
Dosage: **45.4 grams per ton of complete feed throughout the growing period.**
Purpose: **Increased rate of weight gain, improved feed efficiency, and improved pigmentation.**

FDA File **105-758**
Firm: **Alpharma, Inc.**
Use: **Chickens: Feed Additive**
Dosage: **15.4 grams per ton of complete feed throughout the growing period.**
Purpose: **Increased rate of weight gain, improved feed efficiency, and improved pigmentation.**

FDA File **107-997**
Firm: **Phibro Animal Health, Inc.**
Use: **Chickens: Feed Additive**
Dosage: **22.7 grams per ton of complete feed throughout the growing period.**
Purpose: **Increased rate of weight gain.**

FDA File **108-115**
Firm: **Phibro Animal Health, Inc.**
Use: **Chickens: Feed Additive**
Dosage: **22.7 grams per ton of complete feed throughout the growing period.**
Purpose: **Increased rate of weight gain.**

FDA File **112-661**
Firm: **Alpharma, Inc.**
Use: **Chickens: Feed Additive**

Dosage: **45.4 grams per ton of complete feed throughout the growing period.**
Purpose: **Increased rate of weight gain, improved feed efficiency.**

FDA File **112-687**
Firm: **Alpharma, Inc.**
Use: **Chickens: Feed Additive**
Dosage: **45.4 grams per ton of complete feed throughout the growing period.**
Purpose: **Increased rate of weight gain, improved feed efficiency.**

FDA File **116-082**
Firm: **Alpharma, Inc.**
Use: **Chickens: Feed Additive**
Dosage: **45.4 grams per ton of complete feed throughout the growing period.**
Purpose: **Increased rate of weight gain, improved feed efficiency.**

FDA File **116-088**
Firm: **Alpharma, Inc.**
Use: **Chickens: Feed Additive**
Dosage: **22.7 to 45.4 grams per ton of complete feed throughout the growing period.**
Purpose: **Increased rate of weight gain, improved feed efficiency.**

FDA File **120-724**
Firm: **Phibro Animal Health, Inc.**
Use: **Chickens: Feed Additive**
Dosage: **22.7 grams per ton of complete feed throughout the growing period.**
Purpose: **Increased rate of weight gain.**

FDA File **123-154**
Firm: **Alpharma, Inc.**
Use: **Chickens: Feed Additive**

Dosage: **15 to 45.4 grams per ton of complete feed throughout the growing period.**
Purpose: **Increased rate of weight gain, improved feed efficiency.**

FDA File **126-052**
Firm: **Alpharma, Inc.**
Use: **Chickens: Feed Additive**
Dosage: **22.7 to 45.4 grams per ton of complete feed throughout the growing period.**
Purpose: **Increased rate of weight gain, improved feed efficiency.**

FDA File **131-894**
Firm: **Alpharma, Inc.**
Use: **Chickens: Feed Additive**
Dosage: **45.4 grams per ton of complete feed throughout the growing period.**
Purpose: **Increased rate of weight gain.**

FDA File **132-447**
Firm: **Alpharma, Inc.**
Use: **Chickens: Feed Additive**
Dosage: **22.7 to 45.4 grams per ton of complete feed throughout the growing period.**
Purpose: **Improved feed efficiency.**

FDA File **134-185**
Firm: **Alpharma, Inc.**
Use: **Chickens: Feed Additive**
Dosage: **45.4 grams per ton of complete feed throughout the growing period.**
Purpose: **Improved feed efficiency and control of coccidiosis.**

FDA File **135-321**
Firm: **Alpharma, Inc.**
Use: **Chickens: Feed Additive**

Dosage: **34.1 or 45.4 grams per ton of complete feed throughout the growing period.**
Purpose: **Increased rate of weight gain and control of coccidiosis.**

FDA File **137-536**
Firm: **Alpharma, Inc.**
Use: **Chickens: Feed Additive**
Dosage: **45.4 grams per ton of complete feed throughout the growing period.**
Purpose: **Increased rate of weight gain, improved feed efficiency.**

FDA File **138-703**
Firm: **Alpharma, Inc.**
Use: **Chickens: Feed Additive**
Dosage: **22.7 to 45.4 grams per ton of complete feed throughout the growing period.**
Purpose: **Improved feed efficiency.**

FDA File **138-953**
Firm: **Phibro Animal Health, Inc.**
Use: **Chickens: Feed Additive**
Dosage: **45.4 grams per ton of complete feed throughout the growing period.**
Purpose: **Improved feed efficiency and control of coccidiosis.**

FDA File **139-190**
Firm: **Alpharma, Inc.**
Use: **Chickens: Feed Additive**
Dosage: **34.1 grams per ton of complete feed throughout the growing period.**
Purpose: **Increased rate of weight gain and improved feed efficiency.**

FDA File **140-445**
Firm: **Elanco Animal Health, Div. Eli Lilly Co.**
Use: **Chickens: Feed Additive**

Dosage: **45.4 grams per ton of complete feed throughout the growing period.**
Purpose: **Control of coccidiosis.**

FDA File **140-533**
Firm: **Intervet, Inc.**
Use: **Chickens: Feed Additive**
Dosage: **22.7 to 45.4 grams per ton of complete feed throughout the growing period.**
Purpose: **Increased rate of weight gains and improved feed efficiency.**

FDA File **140-581**
Firm: **Alpharma, Inc.**
Use: **Chickens: Feed Additive**
Dosage: **45.4 grams per ton of complete feed throughout the growing period.**
Purpose: **Improved feed efficiency and control of coccidiosis.**

FDA File **140-821**
Firm: **American Cyanamid, Div. AHP Corp.**
Use: **Chickens: Feed Additive**
Dosage: **22.7 to 45.4 grams per ton of complete feed throughout the growing period.**
Purpose: **Increased rate of weight gains and improved feed efficiency.**

FDA File **140-843**
Firm: **Intervet, Inc.**
Use: **Chickens: Feed Additive**
Dosage: **22.8 to 34.1 grams per ton of complete feed throughout the growing period.**
Purpose: **Increased rate of weight gain, improved feed efficiency, and improved pigmentation.**

FDA File **140-852**
Firm: **Alpharma, Inc.**
Use: **Chickens: Feed Additive**
Dosage: **22.7 to 45.4 grams per ton of complete feed throughout the growing period.**
Purpose: **Increased rate of weight gain, improved feed efficiency, and improved pigmentation.**

FDA File **140-867**
Firm: **Alpharma, Inc.**
Use: **Chickens: Feed Additive**
Dosage: **45 grams per ton of complete feed for up to 5 days.**
Purpose: **Prevention of coccidiosis.**

FDA File **141-058**
Firm: **Phibro Animal Health, Inc.**
Use: **Chickens: Feed Additive**
Dosage: **45.4 grams per ton of complete feed throughout the growing period.**
Purpose: **Improved feed efficiency and control of coccidiosis.**

FDA File **141-066**
Firm: **Phibro Animal Health, Inc.**
Use: **Chickens: Feed Additive**
Dosage: **45.4 grams per ton of complete feed throughout the growing period.**
Purpose: **Control of coccidiosis.**

FDA File **141-100**
Firm: **Alpharma, Inc.**
Use: **Chickens: Feed Additive**
Dosage: **22.7 to 45.4 grams per ton of complete feed throughout the growing period.**
Purpose: **Increased rate of weight gain, improved feed efficiency, and improved pigmentation.**

FDA File **141-112**
Firm: **Alpharma, Inc.**
Use: **Chickens: Feed Additive**
Dosage: **22.7 to 45.4 grams per ton
of complete feed throughout the
growing period.**
Purpose: **Increased rate of weight
gain, improved feed efficiency, and
improved pigmentation.**

FDA File **141-113**
Firm: **Elanco Animal Health, Div.
Eli Lilly & Co.**
Use: **Chickens: Feed Additive**
Dosage: **45.4 Grams per ton of com-
plete feed throughout the growing
period.**
Purpose: **Increased rate of weight
gain, improved feed efficiency, and
improved pigmentation.**

FDA File **141-121**
Firm: **Alpharma, Inc.**
Use: **Chickens: Feed Additive**
Dosage: **22.7 to 45.4 grams per ton
of complete feed throughout the
growing period.**
Purpose: **Increased rate of weight
gain, improved feed efficiency, and
improved pigmentation.**

FDA File **141-131**
Firm: **Alpharma, Inc.**
Use: **Chickens: Feed Additive**
Dosage: **22.7 to 45.4 grams per ton
of complete feed throughout the
growing period.**
Purpose: **Increased rate of weight
gain, improved feed efficiency, and
improved pigmentation.**

FDA File **141-135**
Firm: **Alpharma, Inc.**
Use: **Chickens: Feed Additive**

Dosage: **22.7 to 45.4 grams per ton
of complete feed throughout the
growing period.**
Purpose: **Increased rate of weight
gain, improved feed efficiency, and
improved pigmentation.**

FDA File **141-138**
Firm: **Alpharma, Inc.**
Use: **Chickens: Feed Additive**
Dosage: **22.7 to 45.4 grams per ton
of complete feed throughout the
growing period.**
Purpose: **Increased rate of weight
gain, improved feed efficiency, and
improved pigmentation.**

FDA File **141-139**
Firm: **Alpharma, Inc.**
Use: **Chickens: Feed Additive**
Dosage: **22.7 to 45.4 grams per ton
of complete feed throughout the
growing period.**
Purpose: **Increased rate of weight
gain, improved feed efficiency, and
improved pigmentation.**

FDA File **141-142**
Firm: **Alpharma, Inc.**
Use: **Chickens: Feed Additive**
Dosage: **22.7 to 45.4 grams per ton
of complete feed throughout the
growing period.**
Purpose: **Increased rate of weight
gain, improved feed efficiency, and
improved pigmentation.**

FDA File **141-155**
Firm: **Alpharma, Inc.**
Use: **Chickens: Feed Additive**
Dosage: **22.7 to 45.4 grams per ton
of complete feed throughout the
growing period.**

Purpose: **Increased rate of weight gain, improved feed efficiency, and improved pigmentation.**

FDA File **141-157**
Firm: **Alpharma, Inc.**
Use: **Chickens: Feed Additive**
Dosage: **22.7 to 45.4 grams per ton of complete feed throughout the growing period.**
Purpose: **Increased rate of weight gain, improved feed efficiency, and improved pigmentation.**

FDA File **141-190**
Firm: **Schering-Plough Animal Health**
Use: **Chickens: Feed Additive**
Dosage: **22.7 to 45.4 grams per ton of complete feed throughout the growing period.**
Purpose: **Increased rate of weight gain, improved feed efficiency, and improved pigmentation.**

FDA File **141-223**
Firm: **Alpharma, Inc.**
Use: **Chickens: Feed Additive**
Dosage: **22.7 to 45.4 grams per ton of complete feed throughout the growing period.**
Purpose: **Increased rate of weight gain, improved feed efficiency, and improved pigmentation.**

FDA File **141-226**
Firm: **Phibro Animal Health, Inc.**
Use: **Chickens: Feed Additive**
Dosage: **22.7 grams per ton of complete feed throughout the growing period.**
Purpose: **Increased rate of weight gain, improved feed efficiency, and improved pigmentation.**

FDA File **200-080**
Firm: **Intervet, Inc.**
Use: **Chickens: Feed Additive**
Dosage: **45.4 grams per ton of complete feed throughout the growing season.**
Purpose: **Prevention of coccidiosis and improved feed efficiency.**

FDA File **200-081**
Firm: **Intervet, Inc.**
Use: **Chickens: Feed Additive**
Dosage: **45.4 grams per ton of complete feed throughout the growing season.**
Purpose: **Prevention of coccidiosis and increased rate of weight gain.**

FDA File **200-086**
Firm: **Intervet, Inc.**
Use: **Chickens: Feed Additive**
Dosage: **45.4 grams per ton of complete feed throughout the growing season.**
Purpose: **Increased rate of weight gain and improved feed efficiency.**

FDA File **200-090**
Firm: **Intervet, Inc.**
Use: **Chickens: Feed Additive**
Dosage: **45.4 grams per ton of complete feed throughout the growing season.**
Purpose: **Improved feed efficiency.**

FDA File **200-091**
Firm: **Intervet, Inc.**
Use: **Chickens: Feed Additive**
Dosage: **45 grams per ton of complete feed throughout the growing season.**
Purpose: **Prevention of coccidiosis.**

FDA File **200-094**
Firm: **Intervet, Inc.**
Use: **Chickens: Feed Additive**
Dosage: **45.4 grams per ton of complete feed throughout the growing season.**
Purpose: **Prevention of coccidiosis and improved feed efficiency.**

FDA File **200-097**
Firm: **Intervet, Inc.**
Use: **Chickens: Feed Additive**
Dosage: **22.7 to 45.4 grams per ton of complete feed throughout the growing season.**
Purpose: **Improved feed efficiency.**

FDA File **200-143**
Firm: **Intervet, Inc.**
Use: **Chickens: Feed Additive**
Dosage: **34.1 grams per ton of complete feed throughout the growing season.**
Purpose: **Increased rate of weight gain and improved feed efficiency.**

FDA File **200-170**
Firm: **Planalquimica Industrial LTDA.**
Use: **Chickens: Feed Additive**
Dosage: **22.7 grams per ton of complete feed throughout the growing season.**
Purpose: **Increased rate of weight gain.**

FDA File **200-172**
Firm: **Planalquimica Industrial LTDA.**
Use: **Chickens: Feed Additive**
Dosage: **22.7 grams per ton of complete feed throughout the growing season.**
Purpose: **Increased rate of weight gain.**

FDA File **200-206**
Firm: **Alpharma, Inc.**
Use: **Chickens: Feed Additive**
Dosage: **11 to 45 grams per ton of complete feed throughout the growing period.**
Purpose: **Increased rate of weight gain and improved feed efficiency.**

FDA File **200-207**
Firm: **Alpharma, Inc.**
Use: **Chickens: Feed Additive**
Dosage: **45.4 grams per ton of complete feed throughout the growing period.**
Purpose: **Increased rate of weight gain, improved feed efficiency, and improved pigmentation.**

FDA File **200-208**
Firm: **Alpharma, Inc.**
Use: **Chickens: Feed Additive**
Dosage: **34.1 grams per ton of complete feed throughout the growing period.**
Purpose: **Increased rate of weight gain or improved feed efficiency.**

FDA File **200-209**
Firm: **Alpharma, Inc.**
Use: **Chickens: Feed Additive**
Dosage: **34.1 grams per ton of complete feed throughout the growing period.**
Purpose: **Increased rate of weight gain and improved feed efficiency.**

FDA File **200-211**
Firm: **Alpharma, Inc.**
Use: **Chickens: Feed Additive**
Dosage: **15 to 45.4 grams per ton of complete feed throughout the growing period.**

Purpose: **Increased rate of weight gain and/or improving pigmentation, depending on dosage.**

FDA File **200-214**
Firm: **Alpharma, Inc.**
Use: **Chickens: Feed Additive**
Dosage: **45.4 grams per ton of complete feed throughout the growing period.**
Purpose: **Increased rate of weight gain and improved feed efficiency, and improved pigmentation.**

FDA File **200-215**
Firm: **Alpharma, Inc.**
Use: **Chickens: Feed Additive**
Dosage: **34.1 grams per ton of complete feed throughout the growing period.**
Purpose: **Increased rate of weight gain and improved feed efficiency.**

FDA File **200-217**
Firm: **Alpharma, Inc.**
Use: **Chickens: Feed Additive**
Dosage: **34 grams per ton of complete feed throughout the growing period.**
Purpose: **Increased rate of weight gain.**

FDA File **200-259**
Firm: **Alpharma, Inc.**
Use: **Chickens: Feed Additive**
Dosage: **45 grams per ton of complete feed for not more than 5 days.**
Purpose: **Prevention of coccidiosis.**

FDA File **200-260**
Firm: **Alpharma, Inc.**
Use: **Chickens: Feed Additive**

Dosage: **45 grams per ton of complete feed for not more than 5 days.**
Purpose: **Prevention of coccidiosis.**

FDA File **200-355**
Firm: **Pennfield Oil Co.**
Use: **Chickens: Feed Additive**
Dosage: **45 grams per ton of complete feed for not more than 5 days.**
Purpose: **Prevention of coccidiosis.**

SALINOMYCIN (SODIUM)

FDA File **128-686**
Firm: **Roche Vitamins, Inc.**
Use: **Chickens, Quail: Feed Additive**
Dosage: **Chickens: 40 to 60 grams per ton of complete feed throughout the growing period. Quail: 50 grams per ton throughout the growing period.**
Purpose: **Prevention of coccidiosis.**

FDA File **134-284**
Firm: **Roche Vitamins, Inc.**
Use: **Chickens: Feed Additive**
Dosage: **40 to 60 grams per ton of complete feed throughout the growing period.**
Purpose: **Prevention of coccidiosis.**

FDA File **135-321**
Firm: **Alpharma, Inc.**
Use: **Chickens: Feed Additive**
Dosage: **40 to 60 grams per ton of complete feed throughout the growing period.**
Purpose: **Prevention of coccidiosis.**

FDA File **135-746**
Firm: **Alpharma, Inc.**
Use: **Chickens: Feed Additive**

Dosage: **40 to 60 grams per ton of complete feed throughout the growing period.**
Purpose: **Prevention of coccidiosis.**

FDA File **138-828**
Firm: **Phibro Animal Health, Inc.**
Use: **Chickens: Feed Additive**
Dosage: **40 to 60 grams per ton of complete feed throughout the growing period.**
Purpose: **Prevention of coccidiosis.**

FDA File **139-235**
Firm: **Alpharma, Inc.**
Use: **Chickens: Feed Additive**
Dosage: **40 to 60 grams per ton of complete feed throughout the growing period.**
Purpose: **Prevention of coccidiosis.**

FDA File **141-121**
Firm: **Alpharma, Inc.**
Use: **Chickens: Feed Additive**
Dosage: **40 to 60 grams per ton of complete feed throughout the growing period.**
Purpose: **Prevention of coccidiosis.**

FDA File **141-135**
Firm: **Alpharma, Inc.**
Use: **Chickens: Feed Additive**
Dosage: **40 to 60 grams per ton of complete feed throughout the growing period.**
Purpose: **Prevention of coccidiosis.**

FDA File **131-136**
Firm: **Alpharma, Inc.**
Use: **Chickens: Feed Additive**
Dosage: **40 to 60 grams per ton of complete feed throughout the growing period.**
Purpose: **Prevention of coccidiosis.**

FDA File **132-447**
Firm: **Alpharma, Inc.**
Use: **Chickens: Feed Additive**
Dosage: **40 to 60 grams per ton of complete feed throughout the growing period.**
Purpose: **Prevention of coccidiosis.**

FDA File **134-185**
Firm: **Alpharma, Inc.**
Use: **Chickens: Feed Additive**
Dosage: **40 to 60 grams per ton of complete feed throughout the growing period.**
Purpose: **Prevention of coccidiosis.**

FDA File **137-536**
Firm: **Alpharma, Inc.**
Use: **Chickens: Feed Additive**
Dosage: **40 to 60 grams per ton of complete feed throughout the growing period.**
Purpose: **Prevention of coccidiosis.**

FDA File **134-185**
Firm: **Roche Vitamins, Inc.**
Use: **Chickens: Feed Additive**
Dosage: **40 to 60 grams per ton of complete feed throughout the growing period.**
Purpose: **Prevention of coccidiosis.**

FDA File **138-053**
Firm: **Phibro Animal Health, Inc.**
Use: **Chickens: Feed Additive**
Dosage: **40 to 60 grams per ton of complete feed throughout the growing period.**
Purpose: **Prevention of coccidiosis.**

FDA File **139-190**
Firm: **Alpharma, Inc.**
Use: **Chickens: Feed Additive**

Dosage: **40 to 60 grams per ton of complete feed throughout the growing period.**
Purpose: **Prevention of coccidiosis.**

FDA File **140-448**
Firm: **Phibro Animal Health, Inc.**
Use: **Chickens: Feed Additive**
Dosage: **40 to 60 grams per ton of complete feed for up to 5 days.**
Purpose: **Prevention of coccidiosis.**

FDA File **140-581**
Firm: **Alpharma, Inc.**
Use: **Chickens: Feed Additive**
Dosage: **40 to 60 grams per ton of complete feed throughout the growing period.**
Purpose: **Prevention of coccidiosis.**

FDA File **140-859**
Firm: **Alpharma, Inc.**
Use: **Chickens: Feed Additive**
Dosage: **40 to 60 grams per ton of complete feed for up to 5 days.**
Purpose: **Prevention of coccidiosis.**

FDA File **140-867**
Firm: **Alpharma, Inc.**
Use: **Chickens: Feed Additive**
Dosage: **40 to 60 grams per ton of complete feed for up to 5 days.**
Purpose: **Prevention of coccidiosis.**

FDA File **141-198**
Firm: **Elanco Animal Health, Div. Eli Lilly & Co.**
Use: **Chickens: Feed Additive**
Dosage: **40 to 60 grams per ton of complete feed throughout the growing period.**
Purpose: **Prevention of coccidiosis.**

FDA File **200-075**
Firm: **Intervet, Inc.**

Use: **Chickens, Quail: Feed Additive**
Dosage: **Chickens, Quail: 40 to 60 grams per ton of complete feed throughout the growing period.**
Purpose: **Prevention of coccidiosis.**

FDA File **200-080**
Firm: **Intervet, Inc.**
Use: **Chickens: Feed Additive**
Dosage: **40 to 60 grams per ton of complete feed throughout the growing period.**
Purpose: **Prevention of coccidiosis.**

FDA File **200-081**
Firm: **Intervet, Inc.**
Use: **Chickens: Feed Additive**
Dosage: **40 to 60 grams per ton of complete feed throughout the growing period.**
Purpose: **Prevention of coccidiosis.**

FDA File **200-082**
Firm: **Intervet, Inc.**
Use: **Chickens: Feed Additive**
Dosage: **40 to 60 grams per ton of complete feed throughout the growing period.**
Purpose: **Prevention of coccidiosis.**

FDA File **200-083**
Firm: **Intervet, Inc.**
Use: **Chickens: Feed Additive**
Dosage: **40 to 60 grams per ton of complete feed throughout the growing period.**
Purpose: **Prevention of coccidiosis.**

FDA File **200-086**
Firm: **Intervet, Inc.**
Use: **Chickens: Feed Additive**
Dosage: **40 to 60 grams per ton of complete feed throughout the growing period.**
Purpose: **Prevention of coccidiosis.**

FDA File **200-089**
Firm: **Intervet, Inc.**
Use: **Chickens: Feed Additive**
Dosage: **40 to 60 grams per ton
of complete feed throughout the
growing period.**
Purpose: **Prevention of coccidiosis.**

FDA File **200-090**
Firm: **Intervet, Inc.**
Use: **Chickens: Feed Additive**
Dosage: **40 to 60 grams per ton
of complete feed throughout the
growing period.**
Purpose: **Prevention of coccidiosis.**

FDA File **200-091**
Firm: **Intervet, Inc.**
Use: **Chickens: Feed Additive**
Dosage: **Chickens: 40 to 60 grams
per ton of complete feed for up to
5 days.**
Purpose: **Prevention of coccidiosis.**

FDA File **200-092**
Firm: **Intervet, Inc.**
Use: **Chickens: Feed Additive**
Dosage: **40 to 60 grams per ton
of complete feed throughout the
growing period.**
Purpose: **Prevention**

FDA File **200-093**
Firm: **Intervet, Inc.**
Use: **Chickens: Feed Additive**
Dosage: **40 to 60 grams per ton
of complete feed throughout the
growing period.**
Purpose: **Prevention of coccidiosis.**

FDA File **200-094**
Firm: **Intervet, Inc.**
Use: **Chickens: Feed Additive**
Dosage: **40 to 60 grams per ton
of complete feed throughout the
growing period.**
Purpose: **Prevention of coccidiosis.**

FDA File **200-095**
Firm: **Intervet, Inc.**
Use: **Chickens: Feed Additive**
Dosage: **40 to 60 grams per ton of
complete feed for up to 5 days.**
Purpose: **Prevention of coccidiosis.**

FDA File **200-096**
Firm: **Intervet, Inc.**
Use: **Chickens: Feed Additive**
Dosage: **40 to 60 grams per ton of
complete feed for up to 5 days.**
Purpose: **Prevention of coccidiosis.**

FDA File **200-097**
Firm: **Intervet, Inc.**
Use: **Chickens: Feed Additive**
Dosage: **40 to 60 grams per ton
of complete feed throughout the
growing period.**
Purpose: **Prevention of coccidiosis.**

FDA File **200-143**
Firm: **Intervet, Inc.**
Use: **Chickens: Feed Additive**
Dosage: **40 to 60 grams per ton
of complete feed throughout the
growing period.**
Purpose: **Prevention of coccidiosis.**

FDA File **200-204**
Firm: **Alpharma, Inc.**
Use: **Chickens: Feed Additive**
Dosage: **40 to 60 grams per ton
of complete feed throughout the
growing period.**
Purpose: **Prevention of coccidiosis.**

FDA File **200-209**
Firm: **Alpharma, Inc.**
Use: **Chickens: Feed Additive**
Dosage: **40 to 60 grams per ton**
of complete feed throughout the
growing period.
Purpose: **Prevention of coccidiosis.**

FDA File **200-210**
Firm: **Alpharma, Inc.**
Use: **Chickens: Feed Additive**
Dosage: **40 to 60 grams per ton**
of complete feed throughout the
growing period.
Purpose: **Prevention of coccidiosis.**

FDA File **200-215**
Firm: **Alpharma, Inc.**
Use: **Chickens: Feed Additive**
Dosage: **40 to 60 grams per ton**
of complete feed throughout the
growing period.
Purpose: **Prevention of coccidiosis.**

FDA File **200-259**
Firm: **Alpharma, Inc.**
Use: **Chickens: Feed Additive**
Dosage: **40 to 60 grams per ton of**
complete feed for up to 5 days.
Purpose: **Prevention of coccidiosis.**

FDA File **200-260**
Firm: **Alpharma, Inc.**
Use: **Chickens: Feed Additive**
Dosage: **40 to 60 grams per ton of**
complete feed for up to 5 days.
Purpose: **Prevention of coccidiosis.**

FDA File **200-261**
Firm: **Alpharma, Inc.**
Use: **Chickens: Feed Additive**
Dosage: **40 to 60 grams per ton of**
complete feed for up to 5 days.
Purpose: **Prevention of coccidiosis.**

FDA File **200-262**
Firm: **Alpharma, Inc.**
Use: **Chickens: Feed Additive**
Dosage: **40 to 60 grams per ton of**
complete feed for up to 5 days.
Purpose: **Prevention of coccidiosis.**

FDA File **200-355**
Firm: **Pennfield Oil Co.**
Use: **Chickens: Feed Additive**
Dosage: **40 to 60 grams per ton of**
complete feed for not more than 5
days.
Purpose: **Prevention of coccidiosis.**

FDA File **200-357**
Firm: **Pennfield Oil Co.**
Use: **Chickens: Feed Additive**
Dosage: **40 to 60 grams per ton of**
complete feed for not more than 5
days.
Purpose: **Prevention of coccidiosis.**

FDA File **200-091**
Firm: **Alpharma, Inc.**
Use: **Chickens: Feed Additive**
Dosage: **40 to 60 grams per ton of**
complete feed for up to 5 days.
Purpose: **Prevention of coccidiosis.**

SEMDURAMICIN (SODIUM)

FDA File **140-940**
Firm: **Phibro Animal Health, Inc.**
Use: **Chickens: Feed Additive**
Dosage: **25 parts per million in**
complete feed.
Purpose: **Prevention of coccidiosis.**

FDA File **141-058**
Firm: **Phibro Animal Health, Inc.**
Use: **Chickens: Feed Additive**
Dosage: **22.7 grams per ton of com-**
plete feed.

Purpose: **Prevention of coccidiosis.**

FDA File **141-065**
Firm: **Phibro Animal Health, Inc.**
Use: **Chickens: Feed Additive**
Dosage: **22.7 grams per ton of complete feed.**
Purpose: **Prevention of coccidiosis.**

FDA File **141-066**
Firm: **Phibro Animal Health, Inc.**
Use: **Chickens: Feed Additive**
Dosage: **22.7 grams per ton of complete feed.**
Purpose: **Prevention of coccidiosis.**

FDA File **141-114**
Firm: **Phibro Animal Health, Inc.**
Use: **Chickens: Feed Additive**
Dosage: **22.7 grams per ton of complete feed.**
Purpose: **Prevention of coccidiosis.**

FDA File **141-226**
Firm: **Phibro Animal Health, Inc.**
Use: **Chickens: Feed Additive**
Dosage: **22.7 grams per ton of complete feed.**
Purpose: **Prevention of coccidiosis.**

FDA File **141-281**
Firm: **Phibro Animal Health, Inc.**
Use: **Chickens: Feed Additive**
Dosage: **22.7 grams per ton of complete feed.**
Purpose: **Prevention of coccidiosis.**

SPECTINOMYCIN (DIHYDRO-CHLORIDE PENTAHYDRATE, SULFATE TETRAHYDRATE)

FDA File **015-126**
Firm: **Fort Dodge Animal Health, Div. Of Wyeth**

Use: **Dogs:** Rx only **- Oral Tablets or Injection**
Dosage: **10 milligrams per pound of body weight twice per day for 4 days.**
Purpose: **Treatment of diarrhea and gastroenteritis.**

FDA File **033-157**
Firm: **IVX Animal Health**
Use: **Swine: Oral Doser**
Dosage: **Swine: 30 to 45 milligrams per 10 pounds of body weight twice per day for 3 to 5 days.**
Purpose: **Treatment and control of enteric colibacillosis in pigs less than 4 weeks of age and under 15 pounds body weight.**

FDA File **038-661**
Firm: **Cross Vetpharm Group LTD.**
Use: **Chickens: Water Additive**
Dosage: **For prevention or control of losses due to chronic respiratory disease administer 2 grams per gallon. For increased rate of weight gain and improved feed efficiency administer 0.5 grams per gallon. For control of infectious synovitis administer 1 gram per gallon.**
Purpose: **Prevention or control of losses due to chronic respiratory disease, increased rate of weight gain, and control of infectious synovitis.**

FDA File **040-040**
Firm: **Phoenix Scientific, Inc.**
Use: **Dogs:** Rx only **- Chickens, Turkeys:** OTC: **Injection**
Dosage: **Dogs: 2.5 to 5 milligrams per pound of body weight twice per day for up to 4 days. Chickens and Turkeys: Injec4t 1.5 to 5 mil-**

266

ligrams per chick; inject turkey poults at 1 to 2 milligrams per poult. For chronic respiratory disease inject 5 milligrams per poult.
Purpose: **Dogs: Treatment of infections caused by gram-negative and gram positive organisms. Chickens and Turkeys: <u>Reduction of mortality associated with Arizona group infection and control of chronic respiratory disease.</u>**

FDA File **041-629**
Firm: **Fort Dodge Animal Health, Div. Wyeth**
Use: **Swine: Oral Solution**
Dosage: **Swine: 50 milligrams per 10 pounds of body weight twice per day for 3 to 5 days.**
Purpose: **Treatment <u>and control</u> of enteric colibacillosis in pigs under 4 weeks of age and under 15 pounds body weight.**

FDA File **016-109**
Firm: **Pharmacia & Upjohn Co.**
Use: **Chickens: Water Additive Powder**
Dosage: **For prevention or control of losses due to chronic respiratory disease administer 2 grams per gallon. For increased rate of weight gain and improved feed efficiency administer 0.5 grams per gallon. For control of infectious synovitis administer 1 gram per gallon.**
Purpose: **<u>For increased rate of weight gain and improved feed efficiency. For prevention or control of airsacculitis and complicated chronic respiratory disease.</u>**

FDA File **093-483**
Firm: **Phoenix Scientific, Inc.**

Use: **Dogs:** Rx only **- Injection**
Dosage: **Inject 2.5 to 5.0 milligrams per pound of body weight twice per day. May be continued for 4 days. .**
Purpose: **Treatment of susceptible gram positive and negative bacterial infections.**

FDA File **093-515**
Firm: **Cross Vetpharm Group LTD.**
Use: **Dogs:** Rx only **- Oral Tablets or Injection**
Dosage: **10 milligrams per pound of body weight twice per day for 4 days.**
Purpose: **Treatment of infectious diarrhea and gastroenteritis.**

FDA File **141-077**
Firm: **Pharmacia & Upjohn Co.**
Use: **Cattle:** Rx only **- Injection**
Dosage: **10 to 15 milligrams per kilogram of body weight at 24-hour intervals for 3 to 5 days.**
Purpose: **For treatment of bovine respiratory disease.**

FDA File **200-127**
Firm: **Pharmacia & Upjohn Co.**
Use: **Dogs:** Rx only, **Chickens, Turkeys: OTC: Injection**
Dosage: **Dogs: 2.5 to 5 milligrams per pound of body weight twice per day for up to 4 days. Chickens and Turkeys: Inject 1.5 to 5 milligrams per chick; inject turkey poults at 1 to 2 milligrams per poult. For chronic respiratory disease inject 5 milligrams per poult.**
Purpose: **Dogs: Treatment of infections caused by gram-negative and gram positive organisms. Chick-**

ens and Turkeys: <u>Reduction of mortality associated with Arizona group infection and control of chronic respiratory disease.</u>

FDA File **200-345**
Firm: **Phoenix Scientific, Inc.**
Use: **Chickens: Water Additive Powder**
Dosage: **For prevention or control of losses due to chronic respiratory disease administer 2 grams per gallon. For increased rate of weight gain and improved feed efficiency administer 0.5 grams per gallon. For control of infectious synovitis administer 1 gram per gallon.**
Purpose: <u>**For increased rate of weight gain and improved feed efficiency. For control of infectious synovitis and for control of airsacculitis and complicated chronic respiratory disease.**</u>

FDA File **200-364**
Firm: **Cross Vetpharm Group LTD.**
Use: **Swine: Oral Doser**
Dosage: **Swine: 5 milligrams per pound of body weight twice per day for 3 to 5 days.**
Purpose: **Treatment <u>and control</u> of enteric colibacillosis in pigs under 4 weeks of age and under 15 pounds body weight.**

FDA File **200-380**
Firm: **Cross Vetpharm Group LTD.**
Use: **Chickens: Water Soluble Powder**

Dosage: **Control of airsacculitis and complicated chronic respiratory disease administer 2 grams per gallon.**
Purpose: <u>**Control of airsacculitis and complicated chronic respiratory disease.**</u>

STREPTOMYCIN (SULFATE)

FDA File **065-107**
Firm: **Veterinary Specialties, Inc.**
Use: **Dogs:** Rx only **- Oral Powder**
Dosage: **Each gram contains 20 milligrams streptomycin. Administer one level teaspoon per 10 pounds of body weight three times daily.**
Purpose: **For treatment of bacterial enteritis and the relief of associated diarrhea.**

FDA File **065-252**
Firm: **Veterinary Service, Inc.**
Use: **Cattle, Swine, Chickens: Oral Solution**
Dosage: **0.5 to 1.5 grams per gallon of drinking water. In calves and chickens dose for up to 5 days; in swine for up to 4 days.**
Purpose: **For treatment of bacterial enteritis.**

FDA File **200-197**
Firm: **Contemporary Products, Inc.**
Use: **Cattle, Swine, Chickens: Oral Solution**
Dosage: **0.5 to 1.5 grams per gallon of drinking water. In calves and chickens dose for up to 5 days; in swine for up to 4 days.**
Purpose: **For treatment of bacterial enteritis.**

SULFABROMOMETHAZINE (SODIUM)

FDA File **011-532**
Firm: **Merial Ltd.**
Use: **Cattle: Oral Bolus**
Dosage: **90 milligrams per pound of body weight and repeat in 48 hours if necessary.**
Purpose: **Treatment of necrotic pododermatitis (foot rot), colibacillosis (scours), bacterial pneumonia, bovine respiratory disease complex, acute metritis, and acute mastitis.**

SULFACHLOROPYRAZINE (SODIUM, MONOHYDRATE)

FDA File **015-160**
Firm: **Fort Dodge Animal Health, Div. Of Wyeth**
Use: **Chickens: Water Additive**
Dosage: **0.03% in drinking water.**
Purpose: **Treatment of coccidiosis.**

FDA File **031-553**
Firm: **American Cyanamid, Division AHP Corp.**
Use: **Chickens: Water Additive**
Dosage: **0.03% in drinking water.**
Purpose: **Treatment of coccidiosis.**

SULFACHLORPYRIDAZINE (SODIUM)

FDA File **033-127**
Firm: **Fort Dodge Animal Health, Div. Of Wyeth**
Use: **Cattle: Oral Bolus**
Dosage: **Calves: 30 to 45 milligrams per pound of body weight per day** in divided doses twice per day for 1 to 5 days.
Purpose: **Treatment of diarrhea.**

FDA File **033-318**
Firm: **Fort Dodge Animal Health, Div. Of Wyeth**
Use: **Cattle: Injection**
Dosage: **Calves: 30 to 45 milligrams per pound of body weight per day in divided doses twice per day for 1 to 5 days.**
Purpose: **Treatment of diarrhea.**

FDA File **033-319**
Firm: **Fort Dodge Animal Health, Div. Of Wyeth**
Use: **Dogs:** Rx only **- Oral Tablets**
Dosage: **500 milligrams per 10 to 15 pounds of body weight per day in 2 to 3 divided doses for up to 7 days.**
Purpose: **Treatment of infectious tracheobronchitis and treatment of infections susceptible to the drug.**

FDA File **033-373**
Firm: **Fort Dodge Animal Health, Div. Of Wyeth**
Use: **Cattle, Swine: Soluble Powder**
Dosage: **Calves: 30 to 45 milligrams per pound of body weight in milk or milk replacer per day in divided doses twice per day for 1 to 5 days. Swine: 20 to 35 milligrams per pound of body weight per day in divided doses for 1 to 5 days.**
Purpose: **Treatment of diarrhea.**

FDA File **040-181**
Firm: **Fort Dodge Animal Health, Div. Of Wyeth**
Use: **Swine: Oral Suspension**

Dosage:. **Swine: 20 to 35 milligrams per pound of body weight per day in two divided doses for 1 to 5 days.**

Purpose: **Treatment of diarrhea.**

SULFADIAZINE (SILVER)

FDA File **095-614**
Firm: **Schering-Plough Animal Health**
Use: **Dogs:** Rx only **- Oral Tablet**
Dosage: **30 milligrams per kilogram of body weight per day until 2 to 3 days after animal is asymptomatic but not to exceed 14 consecutive days.**
Purpose: **Treatment of bacterial infections where potent systemic antibacterial is required, either alone or as an adjunct to surgery or debridement with associated infection; also in acute infections and for acute infections of the urinary, respiratory, or alimentary tracts, abscesses, or acute bacterial complications of distemper.**

FDA File **105-093**
Firm: **Schering-Plough Animal Health**
Use: **Dogs:** Rx only **- Injection**
Dosage: **Each milliliter contains 200 milligrams sulfadiazine. Inject one milliliter per 20 pounds of body weight per day for 3 to 5 days. May be used alone or in conjunction with oral dosing. Not to exceed 14 consecutive days.**
Purpose: **Treatment of acute urinary tract infections, bacterial complications of distemper, respiratory tract or alimentary tract infections, wounds and abscesses, and acute septicemia.**

FDA File **106-965**
Firm: **Schering-Plough Animal Health**
Use: **Horses:** Rx only **- Injection**
Dosage: **800 milligrams per 100 pounds of body weight as a single daily dose for 5 to 7 days. Daily dose may be halved and given morning and evening. Continue until 2 to 3 days after clinical signs have subsided.**
Purpose: **For use where systemic antibacterial action against sensitive organisms is required during treatment of acute strangles, respiratory tract infections, acute urogenital infections, wound infections and abscesses.**

FDA File **095-614**
Firm: **Schering-Plough Animal Health**
Use: **Dogs:** Rx only **- Oral Tablet**
Dosage: **30 milligrams per kilogram of body weight per day until 2 to 3 days after animal is asymptomatic but not to exceed 14 consecutive days.**
Purpose: **Treatment of bacterial infections where potent systemic antibacterial is required, either alone or as an adjunct to surgery or debridement with associated infection; also in acute infections and for acute infections of the urinary, respiratory, or alimentary tracts, abscesses, or acute bacterial complications of distemper.**

FDA File **115-578**
Firm: **Fort Dodge Animal Health, Div. Of Wyeth**
Use: **Dogs:** Rx only **- Oral Tablets**

Dosage: **14 milligrams per pound of body weight per day and continue for 2-3 days after clinical signs have subsided but not more than 14 consecutive days.**

Purpose: **For control of acute bacterial infections of the urinary, respiratory and alimentary tracts, of wounds and abscesses, and of complications of distemper.**

FDA File **131-918**
Firm: **Schering-Plough Animal Health**
Use: **Horses:** Rx only **- Oral Paste**
Dosage: **25 milligrams per kilogram of body weight as a single daily dose for 5 to 7 days. Daily dose may be halved and given morning and evening. Continue until 2 to 3 days after clinical signs have subsided.**

Purpose: **For use where systemic antibacterial action against sensitive organisms is required during treatment of acute strangles, respiratory tract infections, acute urogenital infections, wound infections and abscesses.**

FDA File **132-486**
Firm: **Fort Dodge Animal Health, Div. Wyeth**
Use: **Dogs:** Rx only **- Injection**
Dosage: **Each milliliter contains 200 milligrams. Administer 1 milliliter per 20 pounds of body weight. For severe infections, after the initial dose subsequent doses may be halved and given every 12 hours. Continue until 2 to 3 days after clinical signs have subsided.**

Purpose: **For treatment of acute urinary tract infections, acute bacterial complications of distemper, acute respiratory tract infections, acute alimentary tract infections and acute septicemia due to *Streptococcus zooepidemicus*.**

FDA File **134-778**
Firm: **Fort Dodge Animal Health, Div. Wyeth**
Use: **Horses:** Rx only **- Injection**
Dosage: **Each milliliter contains 400 milligrams sulfadiazine. Administer 2 milliliters per 100 pounds of body weight per day for 5 to 7 days. Daily dose may be halved and given morning and evening. Continue acute infection therapy for 2 to 3 days after clinical signs have subsided.**

Purpose: **For control of bacterial infections during treatment of strangles, respiratory tract infections, and acute urogenital tract infections, and wound infections and abscesses.**

FDA File **136-342**
Firm: **Fort Dodge Animal Health, Div. Wyeth**
Use: **Horses: Oral Paste**
Dosage: **1665 milligrams per 500 pounds of body weight per day as a single dose for 5 to 7 days. Daily dosage may be halved and given morning and evening. For acute infections therapy, continue for 2 to 3 days after clinical signs have subsided.**

Purpose: **Control of bacterial infections when required during treatment of acute strangles, respiratory and acute urogenital infections, wound infections and abscesses.**

SUPERBUGS

FDA File **136-741**
Firm: **Schering-Plough Animal Health**
Use: **Dogs:** Rx only **- Oral Suspension**
Dosage: **50 milligrams per 5 pounds of body weight per day or one-half daily dose every 12 hours. Administer until 2 to 3 days after animal is asymptomatic but not to exceed 14 consecutive days.**
Purpose: **Control of bacterial infection during the treatment of acute urinary, respiratory or alimentary tract infections, acute bacterial complications of distemper and for wound infections and abscesses.**

FDA File **141-240**
Firm: **Animal Health Pharmaceuticals, LLC.**
Use: **Horses:** Rx only **- Oral Suspension**
Dosage: **Each milliliter contains 250 milligrams sulfadiazine. Administer orally 20 milligrams per kilogram of body weight per day.**
Purpose: **Treatment of equine protozoal myeloencephalitis caused by *Sarcocystis neurona*.**

FDA File **200-033**
Firm: **Macleod Pharmaceuticals**
Use: **Horses:** Rx only **- Oral Powder**
Dosage: **Each gram of powder contains 333 milligrams sulfadiazine. Administer 3.75 grams per 110 pounds of body weight per day. Administer orally in a small amount of feed, as a single daily dose for 5 to 7 days. Continue until 2 to 3 days after clinical signs have subsided.**

Purpose: **For use in feed for control of bacterial infections during the treatment of acute strangles, respiratory tract infections, acute urogenital infections, wound infections and abscesses.**

FDA File **200-244**
Firm: **Pharmacia & Upjohn Co.**
Use: **Horses:** Rx only **- Oral Powder**
Dosage: **Each gram of powder contains 333 milligrams sulfadiazine. Administer 3.75 grams per 110 pounds of body weight per day. Administer orally in a small amount of feed, as a single daily dose for 5 to 7 days. Continue until 2 to 3 days after clinical signs have subsided.**
Purpose: **For use in feed for control of bacterial infections during the treatment of acute strangles, respiratory tract infections, acute urogenital infections, wound infections and abscesses.**

SULFADIMETHOXINE

FDA File **012-087**
Firm: **Schering-Plough Animal Health**
Use: **Dogs:** Rx only **- Oral Tablets**
Dosage: **25 milligrams per pound of body weight first day followed by 12.5 milligrams per pound until 48 hours after symptoms have subsided.**
Purpose: **Treatment of respiratory and genitourinary tract infections, enteritis and soft tissue infections.**

FDA File **015-102**
Firm: **Pfizer, Inc.**

Use: **Dogs:** Rx only **- Oral Tablets**
Dosage: **25 milligrams per pound of body weight first day followed by 12.5 milligrams per pound until 48 hours after symptoms have subsided.**
Purpose: **Treatment of infections caused by organisms susceptible to sulfadimethoxine.**

FDA File **031-205**
Firm: **Pfizer, Inc.**
Use: **Cattle, Chickens, Turkey: Water Soluble**
Dosage: **Cattle: 2.5 grams per 100 pounds of body weight first day followed by 1.25 grams per 100 pounds for the next 4 days in drinking water or as a drench. Chickens: 1.875 grams per gallon for 6 days. Turkeys: Add to drinking water at 0.938 grams per gallon for 6 days.**
Purpose: **Cattle: Treatment of shipping fever complex, calf diphtheria, bacterial pneumonia and foot rot. Chickens, Turkeys: Treatment of coccidiosis, fowl cholera, and in chickens for treatment of infectious coryza.**

FDA File **031-715**
Firm: **Pfizer, Inc.**
Use: **Cattle: Water Soluble**
Dosage: **25 milligrams per pound of body weight first day followed by 12.5 milligrams per pound until 48 hours after symptoms have subsided.**
Purpose: **Treatment of outbreaks of shipping fever complex, diphtheria, bacterial pneumonia and foot rot. .**

FDA File **037-700**
Firm: **Schering-Plough Animal Health**
Use: **Dogs:** Rx only **- Oral Suspension**
Dosage: **25 milligrams per pound of body weight first day followed by 12.5 milligrams per pound until 48 hours after symptoms have subsided.**
Purpose: **Treatment of infections caused by organisms susceptible to sulfadimethoxine.**

FDA File **040-209**
Firm: **Schering-Plough Animal Health**
Use: **Chickens, Turkeys, Chukar Partridges, Ducks: Feed Additive**
Dosage: **Chickens: 113.5 grams per ton. Turkeys: 56.75 grams per ton. Chukar partridges: 113.5 grams per ton. Ducks: 227 to 454 grams per ton.**
Purpose: **Prevention of coccidiosis, infectious coryza, coilbacillosis, fowl cholera and growth promotion, feed efficiency and improved pigmentation in chickens. Prevention of coccidiosis and fowl cholera in turkeys. For prevention of coccidiosis in Chukar partridges. Control of infections in ducks.**

FDA File **041-245**
Firm: **Pfizer, Inc.**
Use: **Dogs, Cats:** Rx only**, Horse, Cattle: OTC - Injection**
Dosage: **Dogs, Cats: 55 milligrams per kilogram of body weight first day followed by 27.5 milligrams per kilogram. Horse, Cattle: 55 milligrams per kilogram of body weight followed by 27.5 milligrams per kilogram per day until**

48 hours after animal is asymptomatic.
Purpose: **Dog, Cat: Treatment of infections caused by organisms susceptible to sulfadimethoxine. Horses: Treatment of respiratory disease caused by** *Streptococcus equi* **(strangles). Cattle: Treatment of shipping fever complex, diphtheria, bacterial pneumonia and foot rot.**

FDA File **041-984**
Firm: **Alpharma, Inc.**
Use: **Chickens: Feed Additive**
Dosage: **113.5 grams per ton of complete feed.**
Purpose: **Prevention of coccidiosis, infectious coryza, and colibacillosis.**

FDA File **046-285**
Firm: **Pfizer, Inc.**
Use: **Cattle, Chickens, Turkey: Water Soluble Powder**
Dosage: **Cattle: 2.5 grams per 100 pounds of body weight first day followed by 1.25 grams per 100 pounds for the next 4 days in drinking water or as a drench. Chickens: 1.875 grams per gallon for 6 days. Turkeys: Add to drinking water at 0.938 grams per gallon for 6 days.**
Purpose: **Cattle: Treatment of shipping fever complex, calf diphtheria, bacterial pneumonia and foot rot. Chickens, Turkeys: Treatment of coccidiosis, fowl cholera, and in chickens for treatment of infectious coryza.**

FDA File **093-107**
Firm: **Pfizer, Inc.**
Use: **Cattle: Oral Bolus**

Dosage: **12.5 milligrams per 200 pounds of body weight. Do not retreat for 7 days.**
Purpose: **Treatment of outbreaks of shipping fever complex, diphtheria, bacterial pneumonia, calf diphtheria, and foot rot.**

FDA File **100-929**
Firm: **Pfizer, Inc.**
Use: **Dogs:** Rx only **- Oral Tablets**
Dosage: **25 milligrams per pound of body weight followed by 12.5 milligrams per pound of body weight. Continue treatment until patient is asymptomatic for 4 8 hours but not to exceed a total of 21 consecutive days.**
Purpose: **Treatment of skin and soft tissue infections and urinary tract infections.**

FDA File **125-033**
Firm: **Pharmaq AS**
Use: **Fish, Catfish: Feed Additive**
Dosage: **40 Milligrams per kilogram of body weight of live fish per day for 5 consecutive days.**
Purpose: **Control of furunculosis in salmonids. Control of enteric septicemia in catfish.**

FDA File **200-030**
Firm: **Agri-Laboratories, LTD.**
Use: **Cattle, Chickens, Turkey: Water Soluble Solution**
Dosage: **Cattle: 2.5 grams per 100 pounds of body weight first day followed by 1.25 grams per 100 pounds for the next 4 days in drinking water or as a drench. Chickens: 1.875 grams per gallon for 6 days. Turkeys: Add to drink-**

ing water at 0.938 grams per gallon for 6 days.

Purpose: **Cattle: Treatment of shipping fever complex, calf diphtheria, bacterial pneumonia and foot rot. Chickens, Turkeys: Treatment of coccidiosis, fowl cholera, and in chickens for treatment of infectious coryza.**

FDA File **200-031**
Firm: **Agri-Laboratories, LTD.**
Use: **Cattle, Chickens, Turkey: Water Soluble Powder**
Dosage: **Cattle: 2.5 grams per 100 pounds of body weight first day followed by 1.25 grams per 100 pounds for the next 4 days in drinking water or as a drench. Chickens: 1.875 grams per gallon for 6 days. Turkeys: Add to drinking water at 0.938 grams per gallon for 6 days.**
Purpose: **Cattle: Treatment of shipping fever complex, calf diphtheria, bacterial pneumonia and foot rot. Chickens, Turkeys: Treatment of coccidiosis, fowl cholera, and in chickens for treatment of infectious coryza.**

FDA File **200-038**
Firm: **Agri-Laboratories, LTD.**
Use: **Cattle: Injection**
Dosage: **25 milligrams per pound of body weight followed by 12.5 milligrams per pound per day until 48 hours after animal is asymptomatic.**
Purpose: **Cattle: Treatment of bovine respiratory disease (shipping fever complex), diphtheria, bacterial pneumonia and foot rot.**

FDA File **200-165**
Firm: **Boehringer Ingelheim Vetmedica, Inc.**
Use: **Cattle, Chickens, Turkey: Water Soluble Powder**
Dosage: **Cattle: 2.5 grams per 100 pounds of body weight first day followed by 1.25 grams per 100 pounds for the next 4 days in drinking water or as a drench. Chickens: 1.875 grams per gallon for 6 days. Turkeys: Add to drinking water at 0.938 grams per gallon for 6 days.**
Purpose: **Cattle: Treatment of shipping fever complex, calf diphtheria, bacterial pneumonia and foot rot. Chickens, Turkeys: Treatment of coccidiosis, fowl cholera, and in chickens for treatment of infectious coryza.**

FDA File **200-177**
Firm: **Phoenix Scientific, Inc.**
Use: **Cattle: Injection**
Dosage: **55 milligrams per kilogram of body weight followed by 27.5 milligrams per kilogram per day until 48 hours after animal is asymptomatic.**
Purpose: **Cattle: Treatment of bovine respiratory disease (shipping fever complex), diphtheria, bacterial pneumonia and foot rot.**

FDA File **200-192**
Firm: **Phoenix Scientific, Inc.**
Use: **Cattle, Chickens, Turkey: Water Soluble Solution**
Dosage: **Cattle: 2.5 grams per 100 pounds of body weight first day followed by 1.25 grams per 100 pounds for the next 4 days in drinking water or as a drench.**

Chickens: 1.875 grams per gallon for 6 days. Turkeys: Add to drinking water at 0.938 grams per gallon for 6 days.

Purpose: **Cattle: Treatment of shipping fever complex, calf diphtheria, bacterial pneumonia and foot rot. Chickens, Turkeys: Treatment of coccidiosis, fowl cholera, and in chickens for treatment of infectious coryza.**

FDA File **200-238**
Firm: **Med-Pharmex, Inc.**
Use: **Cattle, Chickens, Turkey: Water Soluble Powder**
Dosage: **Cattle: 2.5 grams per 100 pounds of body weight first day followed by 1.25 grams per 100 pounds for the next 4 days in drinking water or as a drench. Chickens: 1.875 grams per gallon for 6 days. Turkeys: Add to drinking water at 0.938 grams per gallon for 6 days.**
Purpose: **Cattle: Treatment of shipping fever complex, calf diphtheria, bacterial pneumonia and foot rot. Chickens, Turkeys: Treatment of coccidiosis, fowl cholera, and in chickens for treatment of infectious coryza.**

FDA File **200-251**
Firm: **Med-Pharmex, Inc.**
Use: **Cattle, Chickens, Turkey: Water Soluble Solution**
Dosage: **Cattle: 2.5 grams per 100 pounds of body weight first day followed by 1.25 grams per 100 pounds for the next 4 days in drinking water or as a drench. Chickens: 1.875 grams per gallon for 6 days. Turkeys: Add to drink-**

ing water at 0.938 grams per gallon for 6 days.

Purpose: **Cattle: Treatment of shipping fever complex, calf diphtheria, bacterial pneumonia and foot rot. Chickens, Turkeys: Treatment of coccidiosis, fowl cholera, and in chickens for treatment of infectious coryza.**

FDA File **200-258**
Firm: **Phoenix Scientific, Inc.**
Use: **Cattle, Chickens, Turkey: Water Soluble Powder**
Dosage: **Cattle: 2.5 grams per 100 pounds of body weight first day followed by 1.25 grams per 100 pounds for the next 4 days in drinking water or as a drench. Chickens: 1.875 grams per gallon for 6 days. Turkeys: Add to drinking water at 0.938 grams per gallon for 6 days.**
Purpose: **Cattle: Treatment of shipping fever complex, calf diphtheria, bacterial pneumonia and foot rot. Chickens, Turkeys: Treatment of coccidiosis, fowl cholera, and in chickens for treatment of infectious coryza.**

FDA File **200-376**
Firm: **Cross Vetpharm Group LTD.**
Use: **Cattle, Chickens, Turkey: Water Soluble Solution**
Dosage: **Cattle: 2.5 grams per 100 pounds of body weight first day followed by 1.25 grams per 100 pounds for the next 4 days in drinking water or as a drench. Chickens: 1.875 grams per gallon for 6 days. Turkeys: Add to drinking water at 0.938 grams per gallon for 6 days.**

Purpose: **Cattle: Treatment of shipping fever complex, calf diphtheria, bacterial pneumonia and foot rot. Chickens, Turkeys: Treatment of coccidiosis, fowl cholera, and in chickens for treatment of infectious coryza.**

SULFAETHOXYPYRIDAZINE

FDA File **013-957**
Firm: **Fort Dodge Animal Health, Div. Of Wyeth**
Use: **Cattle, Swine: Water Soluble Powder**
Dosage: **Cattle: 25 grams per gallon first day followed by 1.9 grams gallon for not less than 3 days nor more than 9 days. Swine: 3.8 grams per gallon for first day, and 1.9 grams per gallon for not less than 3 days nor more than 9 days.**
Purpose: **Cattle: Treatment of respiratory infections, foot rot, and calf scours, and as adjunctive therapy in septicemia accompanying mastitis and metritis. Swine: Treatment of bacterial scours, pneumonia, enteritis, bronchitis and septicemia.**

FDA File **033-653**
Firm: **Fort Dodge Animal Health, Div. Of Wyeth**
Use: **Cattle: Water Soluble Solution**
Dosage: **25 grams per gallon first day followed by 1.9 grams gallon for not less than 3 days nor more than 9 days. Swine: 3.8 grams per gallon for first day, and 1.9 grams per gallon for not less than 3 days nor more than 9 days.**

Purpose: **Treatment of respiratory infections, foot rot, and calf scours, and as adjunctive therapy in septicemia accompanying mastitis and metritis.**

FDA File **033-654**
Firm: **Fort Dodge Animal Health, Div. Of Wyeth**
Use: **Cattle: Oral Bolus**
Dosage: **25 milligrams per 100 pounds of body weight per day for not more than 4 days.**
Purpose: **Treatment of respiratory infections, foot rot, and calf scours, and as adjunctive therapy in septicemia accompanying mastitis and metritis.**

FDA File **033-655**
Firm: **Fort Dodge Animal Health, Div. Of Wyeth**
Use: **Cattle: Injection**
Dosage: **2.5 grams per gallon first day followed by 1.9 grams gallon for not less than 3 days nor more than 9 days. Swine: 3.8 grams per gallon for first day, and 1.9 grams per gallon for not less than 3 days nor more than 9 days.**
Purpose: **Treatment of respiratory infections, foot rot, and calf scours, and as adjunctive therapy in septicemia accompanying mastitis and metritis.**

FDA File **047-033**
Firm: **Fort Dodge Animal Health, Div. Of Wyeth**
Use: **Cattle: Controlled Release Bolus**
Dosage: **100 milligrams per pound of body weight.**

Purpose: **Treatment of respiratory infections, foot rot, and for use prophylactically during periods of stress for reducing losses due to diseases sensitive to the drug.**

SULFAMERAZINE

FDA File **033-950**
Firm: **Alpharma, Inc.**
Use: **Fish: Feed Additive**
Dosage: **10 grams per 100 pounds of fish per day for up to 14 days.**
Purpose: **Control of furunculosis.**

FDA File **100-094**
Firm: **Alpharma, Inc.**
Use: **Chickens, Turkeys: Water Soluble Powder**
Dosage: **Each 195 gram packet contains 78 grams sulfamerazine, 78 grams sulfamethazine, and 39 grams sulfaquinoxaline. Chickens: 0.4 per solution administered for 2 to 3 days, then plain water for 3 days, then medicated water (0.25 percent) for 2 days. If bloody droppings appear, repeat at 0.25 percent level for 2 more days. Turkeys: For coccidiosis administer 0.25 percent solution for 2 days, then plain water for 3 days, then medicated water (0.25 percent) for 2 days, then plain water for 3 days, then medicated water (0.25 percent) for 2 days. For fowl cholera administer 0.4 percent for 2 to 3 days. If disease recurs, repeat treatment.**
Purpose: **Control of coccidiosis and fowl cholera in chickens. Control of coccidiosis and fowl cholera in chickens.**

SULFAMETHAZINE (SODIUM)

FDA File **006-084**
Firm: **Fort Dodge Animal Health, Div. Of Wyeth**
Use: **Cattle, Swine, Chickens, Turkeys: Water Soluble Solution**
Dosage: **112 milligrams per pound of body weight per day on first day and 56.25 milligrams per pound on subsequent days. Chickens: 61 to 89 milligrams per pound of body weight per day. Turkeys: 53 to 130 milligrams per pound of body weight.**
Purpose: **Treatment of bacterial pneumonia, bovine respiratory disease complex, colibacillosis, necrotic pododermatitis, calf diphtheria, acute mastitis, and acute metritis.**

FDA File **008-774**
Firm: **Fort Dodge Animal Health, Div. Of Wyeth**
Use: **Cattle: Injection**
Dosage: **20 milligrams per 50 pounds of body weight initially, 20 milligrams per 100 pounds body weight daily thereafter.**
Purpose: **Treatment of bacterial pneumonia and bovine respiratory disease complex, colibacillosis, necrotic pododermatitis, calf diphtheria, acute mastitis and acute metritis.**

FDA File **035-688**
Firm: **Alpharma, Inc.**
Use: **Swine: Feed Additive**
Dosage: **100 grams per ton of complete feed.**
Purpose: **Reduction in the incidence of cervical abscesses, treatment of bacterial enteritis, maintenance**

of weight gains in the presence of
atrophic rhinitis, increased rate
of weight gain and improved feed
efficiency in swine up to 75 pounds
body weight.

FDA File **035-805**
Firm: **Alpharma, Inc.**
Use: **Cattle: Feed Additive**
Dosage: **350 milligrams per head
per day for 28 days.**
Purpose: **Maintenance of weight
gains in the presence of respirato-
ry diseases such as shipping fever.**

FDA File **041-275**
Firm: **Elanco Animal Health, Div.
Eli Lilly & Co.**
Use: **Swine: Feed Additive**
Dosage: **100 grams per ton of complete feed.**
Purpose: **Maintain rate of weight
gain and feed efficiency in the
presence of atrophic rhinitis, for
prevention of vibrionic swine dysentery, for control of swine pneumonias and to lower the incidence
and severity of *Bordetella bronchiseptica* rhinitis.**

FDA File **041-647**
Firm: **Alpharma, Inc.**
Use: **Cattle: Feed Additive**
Dosage: **350 milligrams per head
per day for 28 days.**
Purpose: **Maintenance of weight
gains in the presence of respirato-
ry diseases such as shipping fever.**

FDA File **041-648**
Firm: **Alpharma, Inc.**
Use: **Cattle: Feed Additive**
Dosage: **350 milligrams per head
per day for 28 days.**

Purpose: **Maintenance of weight
gains in the presence of respiratory diseases such as shipping fever.**

FDA File **041-649**
Firm: **Alpharma, Inc.**
Use: **Cattle: Feed Additive**
Dosage: **350 milligrams per head
per day for 28 days.**
Purpose: **Maintenance of weight
gains in the presence of respirato-
ry diseases such as shipping fever.**

FDA File **041-650**
Firm: **Alpharma, Inc.**
Use: **Cattle: Feed Additive**
Dosage: **350 milligrams per head
per day for 28 days.**
Purpose: **Maintenance of weight
gains in the presence of respirato-
ry diseases such as shipping fever.**

FDA File **041-651**
Firm: **Alpharma, Inc.**
Use: **Cattle: Feed Additive**
Dosage: **350 milligrams per head
per day for 28 days.**
Purpose: **Maintenance of weight
gains in the presence of respirato-
ry diseases such as shipping fever.**

FDA File **041-652**
Firm: **Alpharma, Inc.**
Use: **Cattle: Feed Additive**
Dosage: **350 milligrams per head
per day for 28 days.**
Purpose: **Maintenance of weight
gains in the presence of respirato-
ry diseases such as shipping fever.**

FDA File **041-653**
Firm: **Alpharma, Inc.**
Use: **Cattle: Feed Additive**
Dosage: **350 milligrams per head
per day for 28 days.**

Purpose: **Maintenance of weight gains in the presence of respiratory diseases such as shipping fever.**

FDA File **041-654**
Firm: **Alpharma, Inc.**
Use: **Cattle: Feed Additive**
Dosage: **350 milligrams per head per day for 28 days.**
Purpose: **Maintenance of weight gains in the presence of respiratory diseases such as shipping fever. Feed for 28 days.**

FDA File **042-660**
Firm: **Virbac AH, Inc.**
Use: **Swine: Feed Additive**
Dosage: **100 grams per ton of complete feed for 28 days.**
Purpose: **Maintenance of weight gain and feed efficiency in the presence of atrophic rhinitis, prevention of vibrionic swine dysentery, for control of swine pneumonia and lowering the incidence and severity of rhinitis.**

FDA File **048-892**
Firm: **Fort Dodge Animal Health, Div. Of Wyeth**
Use: **Cattle: Oral Bolus**
Dosage: **27 grams per 150 pounds of body weight as a single dose.**
Purpose: **Treatment of infections such as hemorrhagic septicemia (shipping fever complex) bacterial pneumonia, foot rot and calf diphtheria and as an aid in the control of bacterial diseases usually associated with shipping and handling of cattle.**

FDA File **049-729**
Firm: **Virbac AH, Inc.**

Use: **Cattle, Swine, Chickens, Turkeys: Water Soluble Powder**
Dosage: **Cattle and Swine: 112.5 milligrams per pound of body weight on first day and 56.2 milligrams per pound on subsequent days. Chickens: 61 to 89 milligrams per pound of body weight per day. Turkeys: 53 to 130 milligrams per pound of body weight per day.**
Purpose: **Cattle: Treatment of bacterial pneumonia, bovine respiratory disease complex, colibacillosis, necrotic pododermatitis, calf diphtheria, acute mastitis and acute metritis. Swine: Treatment of colibacillosis and bacterial pneumonia. Chickens: Control of infectious coryza, coccidiosis, acute fowl cholera, and pullorum disease. Turkeys: Control of coccidiosis.**

FDA File **055-012**
Firm: **Fort Dodge Animal Health, Div. Of Wyeth**
Use: **Swine: Water Soluble Powder**
Dosage: **25 milligrams per gallon for not more than 25 days.**
Purpose: **Prevention and treatment of bacterial enteritis, reduction of the incidence of cervical abscesses, and maintenance of weight gains in the presence of atrophic rhinitis and bacterial enteritis.**

FDA File **091-668**
Firm: **Alpharma, Inc.**
Use: **Swine: Feed Additive**
Dosage: **100 grams per ton of complete feed.**
Purpose: **Reduction in the incidence of cervical abscesses, treatment of bacterial enteritis, preven-**

tion of enteritis during stress, maintenance of weight gains in the presence of atrophic rhinitis, increased rate of weight gain and improved feed efficiency in swine up to 75 pounds body weight.

FDA File **091-749**
Firm: **Alpharma, Inc.**
Use: **Swine: Feed Additive**
Dosage: **100 grams per ton of complete feed.**
Purpose: **Maintain weight gains and feed efficiency in the presence of atrophic rhinitis, lowering the incidence and severity of rhinitis, prevent swine dysentery, and control bacterial swine pneumonias.**

FDA File **093-329**
Firm: **Bayer Healthcare LLC, Animal Health Div.**
Use: **Cattle: Oral Bolus**
Dosage: **22.5 grams per 100 pounds of body weight as a single dose.**
Purpose: **Treatment of shipping fever pneumonia, foot rot, mastitis, pneumonia, metritis, bacterial enteritis, calf diphtheria and septicemia. For prolonged treatment of respiratory disease complex and bacterial pneumonia, necrotic pododermatitis and calf diphtheria and acute mastitis and metritis. Treat acutely ill cattle parenterally with a suitable antibacterial.**

FDA File **097-981**
Firm: **Quali-Tech Products, Inc.**
Use: **Swine: Feed Additive**
Dosage: **100 grams per ton of complete feed.**
Purpose: **Maintain weight gains and feed efficiency in the presence**

of atrophic rhinitis, lowering the incidence and severity of rhinitis, prevent swine dysentery, and control bacterial swine pneumonias.

FDA File **098-639**
Firm: **Bioproducts, Inc.**
Use: **Swine: Feed Additive**
Dosage: **100 grams per ton of complete feed.**
Purpose: **Maintain weight gains and feed efficiency in the presence of atrophic rhinitis, lowering the incidence and severity of rhinitis, prevent swine dysentery, and control bacterial swine pneumonias.**

FDA File **097-981**
Firm: **Virbac, Inc.**
Use: **Swine: Feed Additive**
Dosage: **100 grams per ton of complete feed.**
Purpose: **Maintain weight gains and feed efficiency in the presence of atrophic rhinitis, lowering the incidence and severity of rhinitis, prevent swine dysentery, and control bacterial swine pneumonias.**

FDA File **100-094**
Firm: **Alpharma, Inc.**
Use: **Chickens, Turkeys: Water Soluble Powder**
Dosage: **Each 195 gram packet contains 78 grams sulfamerazine, 78 grams sulfamethazine, and 39 grams sulfaquinoxaline. Chickens: 0.4 per solution administered for 2 to 3 days, then plain water for 3 days, then medicated water (0.25 percent) for 2 days. If bloody droppings appear, repeat at 0.25 percent level for 2 more days. Tur-**

keys: For coccidiosis administer 0.25 percent solution for 2 days, then plain water for 3 days, then medicated water (0.25 percent) for 2 days, then plain water for 3 days, then medicated water (0.25 percent) for 2 days. For fowl cholera administer 0.4 percent for 2 to 3 days. If disease recurs, repeat treatment.
Purpose: **Control of coccidiosis and fowl cholera in chickens and turkeys.**

FDA File **101-906**
Firm: **Waterloo Mills Co.**
Use: **Swine: Feed Additive**
Dosage: **100 grams per ton of complete feed.**
Purpose: **Maintain weight gains and feed efficiency in the presence of atrophic rhinitis, lowering the incidence and severity of rhinitis, prevent swine dysentery, and control bacterial swine pneumonias.**

FDA File **107-002**
Firm: **Seeco, Inc.**
Use: **Swine: Feed Additive**
Dosage: **100 grams per ton of complete feed.**
Purpose: **Maintain weight gains and feed efficiency in the presence of atrophic rhinitis, lowering the incidence and severity of rhinitis, prevent swine dysentery, and control bacterial swine pneumonias.**

FDA File **107-957**
Firm: **ADM Animal Health & Nutrition Div.**
Use: **Swine: Feed Additive**

Dosage: **100 grams per ton of complete feed.**
Purpose: **Maintain weight gains and feed efficiency in the presence of atrophic rhinitis, lowering the incidence and severity of rhinitis, prevent swine dysentery, and control bacterial swine pneumonias.**

FDA File **108-484**
Firm: **ADM Animal Health & Nutrition Div.**
Use: **Swine: Feed Additive**
Dosage: **100 grams per ton of complete feed.**
Purpose: **Maintain weight gains and feed efficiency in the presence of atrophic rhinitis, lowering the incidence and severity of rhinitis, prevent swine dysentery, and control bacterial swine pneumonias.**

FDA File **111-069**
Firm: **ADM Animal Health & Nutrition Div.**
Use: **Swine: Feed Additive**
Dosage: **100 grams per ton of complete feed.**
Purpose: **Maintain weight gains and feed efficiency in the presence of atrophic rhinitis, lowering the incidence and severity of rhinitis, prevent swine dysentery, and control bacterial swine pneumonias.**

FDA File **120-614**
Firm: **Webel Feeds, Inc.**
Use: **Swine: Feed Additive**
Dosage: **100 grams per ton of complete feed.**
Purpose: **Maintain weight gains and feed efficiency in the presence of atrophic rhinitis, lowering the**

incidence and severity of rhinitis, prevent swine dysentery, and control bacterial swine pneumonias.

FDA File **120-615**
Firm: **Cross Vetpharm Group LTD.**
Use: **Cattle: Oral Bolus**
Dosage: **Contains 8.02 or 31.2 grams per bolus. Administer two 8.02 g boluses per 100 pounds body weight to calves as a single dose. For mature cattle administer one 32.1 grams bolus per 200 pounds body weight. Two doses are recommended at 72 hour intervals.**
Purpose: **Treatment of bacterial pneumonia, respiratory disease complex, colibacillosis, foot rot, calf diphtheria, acute mastitis, and acute metritis.**

FDA File **122-271**
Firm: **Fort Dodge Animal Health, Div. Of Wyeth**
Use: **Cattle, Horses: Oral Bolus**
Dosage: **Administer 100 milligrams per pound body weight on first day and 50 milligrams per pound body weight on each following day. Continue treatment until 24 to 48 hours after animal is asymptomatic but not to exceed 5 consecutive days.**
Purpose: **Cattle: Treatment of bacterial pneumonia, respiratory disease complex, colibacillosis, foot rot, calf diphtheria, acute mastitis, acute metritis, and coccidiosis. Horses: Treatment of bacterial pneumonia, strangles, and bacterial enteritis. .**

FDA File **122-272**
Firm: **Fort Dodge Animal Health, Div. Of Wyeth**
Use: **Cattle, Swine, Chickens, Turkeys: Water Soluble Powder**
Dosage: **Cattle and Swine: 108 milligrams per pound of body weight on first day and 54 milligrams per pound for 3 more consecutive days. Chickens: 58 to 85 milligrams per pound of body weight per day. Turkeys: 50 to 124 milligrams per pound of body weight per day.**
Purpose: **Cattle: Treatment of bacterial pneumonia, bovine respiratory disease complex, colibacillosis, necrotic pododermatitis, calf diphtheria, acute mastitis and acute metritis. Swine: Treatment of porcine colibacillosis and bacterial pneumonia. Chickens: Control of infectious coryza, coccidiosis, acute fowl cholera and pullorum disease. Turkeys: Control of coccidiosis.**

FDA File **122-522**
Firm: **Custom Feed Blenders Corp.**
Use: **Swine: Feed Additive**
Dosage: **100 grams per ton of complete feed.**
Purpose: **Maintain weight gains and feed efficiency in the presence of atrophic rhinitis, lowering the incidence and severity of rhinitis, prevent swine dysentery, and control bacterial swine pneumonias.**

FDA File **124-391**
Firm: **Ag-Mark, Inc.**
Use: **Swine: Feed Additive**
Dosage: **100 grams per ton of complete feed.**

Purpose: **Maintain weight gains and feed efficiency in the presence of atrophic rhinitis, lowering the incidence and severity of rhinitis, prevent swine dysentery, and control bacterial swine pneumonias.**

FDA File **126-232**
Firm: **Fort Dodge Animal Health, Div. Of Wyeth**
Use: **Cattle: Oral Bolus**
Dosage: **8 grams per 45 pounds of body weight as a single dose.**
Purpose: **Treatment of calves for bacterial pneumonia, colibacillosis, and calf diphtheria.**

FDA File **127-507**
Firm: **Elanco Animal Health, Div. Eli Lilly & Co.**
Use: **Swine: Feed Additive**
Dosage: **100 grams per ton of complete feed.**
Purpose: **Maintain weight gains and feed efficiency in the presence of atrophic rhinitis, lowering the incidence and severity of rhinitis, prevent swine dysentery, and control bacterial swine pneumonias.**

FDA File **128-411**
Firm: **ADM Animal Health & Nutrition Div.**
Use: **Swine: Feed Additive**
Dosage: **100 grams per ton of complete feed.**
Purpose: **Maintain weight gains and feed efficiency in the presence of atrophic rhinitis, lowering the incidence and severity of rhinitis, prevent swine dysentery, and control bacterial swine pneumonias.**

FDA File **129-646**
Firm: **I.M.S., Inc.**

Use: **Swine: Feed Additive**
Dosage: **100 grams per ton of complete feed.**
Purpose: **Maintain weight gains and feed efficiency in the presence of atrophic rhinitis, lowering the incidence and severity of rhinitis, prevent swine dysentery, and control bacterial swine pneumonias.**

FDA File **131-956**
Firm: **ADM Animal Health & Nutrition Div.**
Use: **Swine: Feed Additive**
Dosage: **100 grams per ton of complete feed.**
Purpose: **Maintain weight gains and feed efficiency in the presence of atrophic rhinitis, lowering the incidence and severity of rhinitis, prevent swine dysentery, and control bacterial swine pneumonias.**

FDA File **131-958**
Firm: **Wayne Feed Div., Cont. Grain**
Use: **Swine: Feed Additive**
Dosage: **100 grams per ton of complete feed.**
Purpose: **Maintain weight gains and feed efficiency in the presence of atrophic rhinitis, lowering the incidence and severity of rhinitis, prevent swine dysentery, and control bacterial swine pneumonias.**

FDA File **138-342**
Firm: **Feed Service Co., Inc.**
Use: **Swine: Feed Additive**
Dosage: **100 grams per ton of complete feed.**
Purpose: **Maintain weight gains and feed efficiency in the presence of atrophic rhinitis, lowering the incidence and severity of rhinitis,**

prevent swine dysentery, and control bacterial swine pneumonias.

FDA File **138-934**
Firm: **Pennfield Oil Co.**
Use: **Swine: Feed Additive**
Dosage: **100 grams per ton of complete feed.**
Purpose: **Reduction of the incidence of cervical abscesses; treatment of bacterial enteritis and vibrionic dysentery, and for prevention of these diseases during times of stress; maintenance of weight gains in the presence of atrophic rhinitis; and for growth promotion and increased feed efficiency in swine up to 75 pounds body weight.**

FDA File **140-270**
Firm: **Phoenix Scientific, Inc.**
Use: **Cattle: Oral Bolus**
Dosage: **8 grams per 45 pounds of body weight as a single dose.**
Purpose: **Treatment of respiratory complex (shipping fever), necrotic pododermatitis (foot rot), and acute mastitis and metritis. Treatment of calf diphtheria, colibacillosis, and coccidiosis.**

FDA File **140-681**
Firm: **Pennfield Oil Co.**
Use: **Swine: Feed Additive**
Dosage: **100 grams per ton of complete feed.**
Purpose: **Maintain weight gains and feed efficiency in the presence of atrophic rhinitis, lowering the incidence and severity of rhinitis, prevent swine dysentery, and control bacterial swine pneumonias.**

FDA File **140-820**
Firm: **Furst-Mcness Co.**
Use: **Swine: Feed Additive**
Dosage: **100 grams per ton of complete feed.**
Purpose: **Maintain weight gains and feed efficiency in the presence of atrophic rhinitis, lowering the incidence and severity of rhinitis, prevent swine dysentery, and control bacterial swine pneumonias.**

FDA File **140-908**
Firm: **Lloyd, Inc.**
Use: **Cattle: Oral Bolus**
Dosage: **100 milligrams per pound of body weight first day and 50 milligrams per pound of body weight each following day, not to exceed 5 days.**
Purpose: **Treatment of bacterial pneumonia and bovine respiratory disease complex colibacillosis, necrotic pododermatitis, calf diphtheria, acute mastitis, acute metritis and coccidiosis.**

FDA File **140-909**
Firm: **Fort Dodge Animal Health, Div. Of Wyeth**
Use: **Cattle: Oral Bolus**
Dosage: **10 grams per 100 pounds body weight the first day, then 5 grams per 100 pounds body weight daily for up to 4 additional consecutive days.**
Purpose: **Treatment of bacterial scours, necrotic pododermatitis, calf diphtheria, bacterial pneumonia, and coccidiosis.**

FDA File **200-314**
Firm: **Pennfield Oil Co.**
Use: **Cattle: Feed Additive**

Dosage: **350 milligrams per head per day for 28 days.**
Purpose: **Maintenance of weight gains in the presence of respiratory diseases such as shipping fever.**

FDA File **200-434**
Firm: **Cross Vetpharm Group Ltd.**
Use: **Cattle, Swine, Chickens, Turkeys: Water Additive Powder**
Dosage: **Cattle and Swine: 108 milligrams per pound of body weight on first day and 54 milligrams per pound of body weight for 3 more consecutive days. Chickens: 58 to 85 milligrams per pound of body weight per day. Turkeys: 50 to 124 milligrams per pound of body weight per day.**
Purpose: **Cattle: Treatment of bacterial pneumonia, bovine respiratory disease complex, colibacillosis, necrotic pododermatitis, calf diphtheria, acute mastitis and acute metritis. Swine: Treatment of porcine colibacillisis and bacterial pneumonia. Chickens: Control of infectious coryza, coccidiosis, acute fowl cholera, and pullorum disease. Turkeys: Control of coccidiosis.**

SULFAMETHIZOLE

FDA File **030-416**
Firm: **Fort Dodge Animal Health, Div. Of Wyeth**
Use: **Dogs, Cats:** Rx only **- Oral Tablets**
Dosage: **250 milligrams per 20 pounds body weight three times per day for 10 days after all signs are alleviated.**
Purpose: **Treatment of urinary tract infections and complications arising from surgical manipulation of the urinary tract.**

SULFANITRAN

FDA File **011-141**
Firm: **Fort Dodge Animal Health, Div Of Wyeth**
Use: **Chickens: Feed Additive**
Dosage: **272 grams per ton of complete feed.**
Purpose: **Prevention of coccidiosis.**

FDA File **014-250**
Firm: **Fort Dodge Animal Health, Div Of Wyeth**
Use: **Chickens: Feed Additive**
Dosage: **181.6 grams per ton of complete feed.**
Purpose: **Prevention of coccidiosis.**

FDA File **034-537**
Firm: **Fort Dodge Animal Health, Div Of Wyeth**
Use: **Chickens: Feed Additive**
Dosage: **181.6 grams per ton of complete feed.**
Purpose: **Prevention of coccidiosis.**

FDA File **035-388**
Firm: **Fort Dodge Animal Health, Div Of Wyeth**
Use: **Chickens: Water Additive**
Dosage: **375 milligrams per gallon of drinking water.**
Purpose: **Prevention and treatment of coccidiosis.**

FDA File **039-666**
Firm: **Fort Dodge Animal Health, Div Of Wyeth**
Use: **Chickens: Feed Additive**
Dosage: **272 grams per ton of complete feed.**
Purpose: **Prevention of coccidiosis.**

SULFAQUINOXALINE (SODIUM)

FDA File **006-391**
Firm: **Phoenix Scientific, Inc.**
Use: **Chickens, Turkeys, Rabbits: Feed Additive**
Dosage: **Chickens and Turkeys: 0.015, 0.0175, 0.05 and 0.01 percent in feed.**
Purpose: **Prevention of coccidiosis.**

FDA File **006-677**
Firm: **Phoenix Scientific, Inc.**
Use: **Cattle, Chickens, Turkeys: Water Soluble Solution**
Dosage: **0.015, 0.25 and 0.04 percent in water.**
Purpose: **Cattle: Control of coccidiosis. Chickens and Turkeys: Control of acute fowl cholera and fowl typhoid.**

FDA File **006-707**
Firm: **Fort Dodge Animal Health, Div. Of Wyeth**
Use: **Chickens, Turkeys: Water Soluble Solution**
Dosage: **Chickens: For control of coccidiosis give 0.04 percent in water for 2 to 3 days, skip 3 days then give 0.025 percent for 2 more days. If bloody droppings appear, repeat treatment at 0.025 percent level for 2 more days. Turkeys: For coccidiosis, give 0.025 percent for 2 to 3 days, skip 3 days, give for 2 days, skip 3 days, give for 2 days, skip 3 days, give 2 more days. Chickens and Turkeys: For fowl typhoid and acute fowl cholera, give 0.04 percent for 2 to 3 days.**
Purpose: **Chickens: Control of coccidiosis. Chickens and Turkeys: Control of acute fowl cholera and fowl typhoid.**

FDA File **006-891**
Firm: **Alpharma, Inc.**
Use: **Cattle, Chickens, Turkeys: Water Soluble Solution**
Dosage: **Cattle: 0.015 percent for 3 to 5 days. Chickens: For control of coccidiosis give 0.04 percent in water for 2 to 3 days, skip 3 days then give 0.025 percent for 2 more days. If bloody droppings appear, repeat treatment at 0.025 percent level for 2 more days. Turkeys: For coccidiosis, give 0.025 percent for 2 to 3 days, skip 3 days, give for 2 days, skip 3 days, give for 2 days, skip 3 days, give 2 more days. Chickens and Turkeys: For fowl typhoid and acute fowl cholera, give 0.04 percent for 2 to 3 days.**
Purpose: **Cattle: Treatment and control of coccidiosis. Chickens: Control of coccidiosis. Chickens and Turkeys: Control of acute fowl cholera and fowl typhoid.**

FDA File **007-076**
Firm: **Virbac AH, Inc.**
Use: **Cattle, Chickens, Turkeys: Water Soluble Solution**
Dosage: **Cattle: 0.015 percent for 3 to 5 days. Chickens: For control of coccidiosis give 0.04 percent in water for 2 to 3 days, skip 3 days then give 0.025 percent for 2 more days. If bloody droppings appear, repeat treatment at 0.025 percent level for 2 more days. Turkeys: For coccidiosis, give 0.025 percent for 2 to 3 days, skip 3 days, give for 2 days, skip 3 days, give for 2 days, skip 3 days, give 2 more days. Chickens and Turkeys: For fowl typhoid and acute fowl cholera, give 0.04 percent for 2 to 3 days.**

Purpose: **Cattle: Treatment and control** of coccidiosis. **Chickens: Control of coccidiosis. Chickens and Turkeys: Control of acute fowl cholera and fowl typhoid.**

FDA File **007-087**
Firm: **Phoenix, Inc.**
Use: **Cattle, Chickens, Turkeys: Water Soluble Powder**
Dosage: **Cattle: 6 milligrams per pound of body weight per day. Chickens: 10 to 45 milligrams per pound of body weight per day. Turkeys 3.5 to 5.5 milligrams per pound of body weight per day.**
Purpose: **Cattle: Treatment and control** of coccidiosis. **Chickens: Control of coccidiosis. Chickens and Turkeys: Control of acute fowl cholera and fowl typhoid.**

FDA File **008-244**
Firm: **Virbac AH, Inc.**
Use: **Cattle, Chickens, Turkeys: Water Soluble Solution**
Dosage: **Cattle: 0.015 percent for 3 to 5 days. Chickens: For control of coccidiosis give 0.04 percent in water for 2 to 3 days, skip 3 days then give 0.025 percent for 2 more days. If bloody droppings appear, repeat treatment at 0.025 percent level for 2 more days. Turkeys: For coccidiosis, give 0.025 percent for 2 to 3 days, skip 3 days, give for 2 days, skip 3 days, give for 2 days, skip 3 days, give 2 more days. Chickens and Turkeys: For fowl typhoid and acute fowl cholera, give 0.04 percent for 2 to 3 days.**
Purpose: **Cattle: Treatment and control** of coccidiosis. **Chickens: Control of coccidiosis. Chickens**

and Turkeys: Control of acute fowl cholera and fowl typhoid.

FDA File **100-094**
Firm: **Alpharma, Inc.**
Use: **Chickens, Turkeys: Water Soluble Powder**
Dosage: **Each 195 gram packet contains 78 grams sulfamerazine, 78 grams sulfamethazine, and 39 grams sulfaquinoxaline. Chickens: 0.4 per solution administered for 2 to 3 days, then plain water for 3 days, then medicated water (0.25 percent) for 2 days. If bloody droppings appear, repeat at 0.25 percent level for 2 more days. Turkeys: For coccidiosis administer 0.25 percent solution for 2 days, then plain water for 3 days, then medicated water (0.25 percent) for 2 days, then plain water for 3 days, then medicated water (0.25 percent) for 2 days. For fowl cholera administer 0.4 percent for 2 to 3 days. If disease recurs, repeat treatment.**
Purpose: **Control of coccidiosis and fowl cholera in chickens. Control of coccidiosis and fowl cholera in chickens.**

SULFATHIAZOLE

FDA File **039-077**
Firm: **Alpharma, Inc.**
Use: **Swine: Feed Additive**
Dosage: **100 grams per ton of complete feed from 6 to 16 weeks of age.**
Purpose: **Reduction in the incidence of cervical abscesses, treatment of bacterial enteritis or necrotic**

enteritis and vibrionic dysentery, maintenance of weight gain in the presence of atrophic rhinitis.

FDA File **200-140**
Firm: **Alpharma, Inc.**
Use: **Swine: Feed Additive**
Dosage: **100 grams per ton of complete feed from 6 to 16 weeks of age in swine feed in confinement (dry lot) or limited pasture.**
Purpose: **Reduction in the incidence of cervical abscesses, treatment of bacterial enteritis or necrotic enteritis and vibrionic dysentery, maintenance of weight gain in the presence of atrophic rhinitis.**

FDA File **200-167**
Firm: **Alpharma, Inc.**
Use: **Swine: Feed Additive**
Dosage: **100 grams per ton of complete feed from 6 to 16 weeks of age.**
Purpose: **Reduction in the incidence of cervical abscesses, treatment of bacterial enteritis or necrotic enteritis and vibrionic dysentery, maintenance of weight gain in the presence of atrophic rhinitis.**

SULFISOXAZOLE

FDA File **007-981**
Firm: **Fort Dodge Animal Health, Div. Of Wyeth**
Use: **Dogs, Cats: Oral Tablet**
Dosage: **250 milligrams per 4 pounds of body weight. Repeat dosage at 24 hours intervals until 2 to 3 days after the animal is asymptomatic.**
Purpose: **Treatment of bacterial enteritis and bacterial pneumonia.**

SULFOMYXIN

FDA File **031-944**
Firm: **Pfizer, Inc.**
Use: **Chickens, Turkeys: Injection**
Dosage: **Administer according to the age of the birds: 1 to14 days: 12,500/12,500 units; 15 to 28 days: 25,000/25,000 units; 29 to 63 days: 50,000/50,000 units; over 63 days 50,000/100,000 units.**
Purpose: **Treatment of disease caused or complicated by** *E. coli*, **such as colibacillosis and complicated chronic respiratory disease.**

TETRACYCLINE (HYDROCHLORIDE)

FDA File **011-703**
Firm: **Pharmacia & Upjohn Co.**
Use: **Dog, Cat:** Rx only **- Ophthalmic/Otic Ointment**
Dosage: **1 to 2 drops in the conjunctival sac 3 to 6 times per day, reducing with improvement. Administer 2 to 6 drops in the ear 2 to 3 times per day.**
Purpose: **Treatment of infectious, allergic and traumatic keratitis, conjunctivitis, and acute or chronic otitis externa.**

FDA File **055-073**
Firm: **Pharmacia & Upjohn Co.**
Use: **Dog:** Rx only **- Oral Tablet**
Dosage: **25 milligrams per pound of body weight in divided doses every 6 hours for at least 48 hours after signs of disease have disappeared. Administer for up to 10 days.**
Purpose: **Treatment of acute or infections such as gastroenteritis and urinary tract infections.**

FDA File **055-076**
Firm: **Pharmacia & Upjohn Co.**
Use: **Dogs:** Rx only **- Oral Tablet**
Dosage: **60 milligrams per 6 pounds of body weight every 12 hours for at least 48 hours after signs of disease have disappeared. Treatment not to exceed 10 days.**
Purpose: **Treatment of acute or chronic upper respiratory infections such as tonsillitis, bronchitis, and tracheobronchitis.**

FDA File **065-004**
Firm: **Pharmacia & Upjohn Co.**
Use: **Cattle: Oral Bolus**
Dosage: **10 milligrams per pound of body weight per day in two divided doses for not more than 5 days.**
Purpose: **Treatment of bacterial enteritis and bacterial pneumonia.**

FDA File **065-060**
Firm: **Pharmacia & Upjohn Co.**
Use: **Dog, Cat:** Rx only **- Oral Drops**
Dosage: **25 milligrams per pound of body weight per day in divided doses every six hours. Continue treatment until 48 hours after animal is asymptomatic.**
Purpose: **Treatment of bacterial gastroenteritis and urinary tract infections.**

FDA File **065-061**
Firm: **Pfizer, Inc.**
Use: **Dog:** Rx only **- Oral Drops**
Dosage: **25 milligrams per pound of body weight per day in divided doses every six hours. Continue treatment until 48 hours after animal is asymptomatic.**
Purpose: **Treatment of bacterial gastroenteritis**

FDA File **065-066**
Firm: **Pfizer, Inc.**
Use: **Dog:** Rx only **- Oral Tablet**
Dosage: **25 milligrams per pound of body weight in divided doses every 6 hours for at least 48 hours after signs of disease have disappeared. Administer for up to 10 days.**
Purpose: **Treatment of acute or infections such as gastroenteritis and urinary tract infections.**

FDA File **065-067**
Firm: **Pharmacia & Upjohn Co.**
Use: **Dog:** Rx only **- Oral Tablet**
Dosage: **25 milligrams per pound of body weight in divided doses every 6 hours for at least 48 hours after signs of disease have disappeared. Administer for up to 10 days.**
Purpose: **Treatment of acute or infections such as gastroenteritis and urinary tract infections.**

FDA File **065-069**
Firm: **Pfizer, Inc.**
Use: **Dog:** Rx only **- Oral Capsule**
Dosage: **25 milligrams per pound of body weight in divided doses every 6 hours for at least 48 hours after signs of disease have disappeared. Administer for up to 10 days.**
Purpose: **Treatment of acute or infections such as gastroenteritis and urinary tract infections.**

FDA File **065-090**
Firm: **Pharmacia & Upjohn Co.**
Use: **Dogs:** Rx only **- Oral Tablet**
Dosage: **60 milligrams per 6 pounds of body weight every 12 hours for 48 hours after signs of disease**

have disappeared. Treatment not to exceed 10 days.
Purpose: **Treatment of acute or chronic upper respiratory infections such as tonsillitis, bronchitis, and tracheobronchitis.**

FDA File **065-099**
Firm: **Pharmacia & Upjohn Co.**
Use: **Dog:** Rx only **- Oral Capsule**
Dosage: **25 milligrams per pound of body weight in divided doses every 6 hours for at least 48 hours after signs of disease have disappeared. Administer for up to 10 days.**
Purpose: **Treatment of acute or chronic infections such as gastroenteritis and urinary tract infections.**

FDA File **065-121**
Firm: **Pfizer, Inc.**
Use: **Dog:** Rx only **- Oral Capsule**
Dosage: **25 milligrams per pound of body weight in divided doses every 6 hours for at least 48 hours after signs of disease have disappeared.**
Purpose: **Treatment of acute or chronic infections such as gastroenteritis and urinary tract infections.**

FDA File **065-122**
Firm: **Pfizer, Inc.**
Use: **Dogs:** Rx only **- Ointment**
Dosage: **Apply ointment containing 30 milligrams per gram 2 to 3 times per day and cover with gauze pad.**
Purpose: **Treatment of minor burns, wounds, and abrasions.**

FDA File **065-123**
Firm: **Pfizer, Inc.**
Use: **Chickens, Turkeys: Soluble Powder**
Dosage: **400 to 800 milligrams per gallon of drinking water for 7 to 14 days. For bluecomb in turkeys administer 25 milligrams per pound of body weight per day.**
Purpose: <u>**Chickens: Control of chronic respiratory disease and infectious synovitis. Turkeys: Control of infectious synovitis and bluecomb.**</u>

FDA File **065-125**
Firm: **Premo Pharmaceutical Labs.**
Use: **Dogs, Cats, Horses:** Rx only **- Injection**
Dosage: **Dogs, Cats: 5 milligrams per pound of body weight per day in divided doses. Horses: 1 to 2 milligrams per pound of body weight per day in divided doses.**
Purpose: **Treatment of infections caused by gram-positive and gram-negative bacteria as well as certain rickettsial, protozoan and viral infections.**

FDA File **065-140**
Firm: **Alpharma, Inc.**
Use: **Cattle, Swine, Chickens, Turkeys: Water Soluble Powder**
Dosage: **Calves, Swine: 10 milligrams per pound of body weight per day in drinking water in divided doses. Chickens: 400 to 800 milligrams per gallon of drinking water. For bluecomb in turkeys administer 25 milligrams per pound of body weight per day. Administer for 7 to 14 days.**
Purpose: <u>**Control and**</u> **treatment of bacterial enteritis and bacterial**

pneumonia. Swine: Control and treatment of bacterial enteritis and bacterial pneumonia. Chickens: Control of chronic respiratory diseases, control of infectious synovitis. Turkeys: Control of infectious synovitis and bluecomb disease.

FDA File **065-270**
Firm: **Fort Dodge Animal Health, Div. Of Wyeth**
Use: **Cattle: Oral Tablet**
Dosage: **10 milligrams per pound of body weight per day in divided doses.**
Purpose: **Control and** treatment of **bacterial enteritis and bacterial pneumonia.**

FDA File **065-409**
Firm: **Pharmacia & Upjohn Co.**
Use: **Dog:** Rx only - **Oral Capsule**
Dosage: **25 milligrams per pound of body weight in divided doses every 6 hours for at least 48 hours after signs of disease have disappeared.**
Purpose: **Treatment of acute or infections such as gastroenteritis and urinary tract infections.**

FDA File **065-410**
Firm: **Fort Dodge Animal Health, Div. Of Wyeth**
Use: **Cattle, Swine, Chickens, Turkeys: Water Soluble Powder**
Dosage: **Calves, Swine: 10 milligrams per pound of body weight per day in drinking water in divided doses. Chickens: 100 to 200 milligrams per gallon of drinking water. For bluecomb in turkeys administer 25 milligrams per pound**

of body weight per day. Administer for 7 to 14 days.
Purpose: **Control and** treatment of **bacterial diarrhea and bacterial pneumonia. Swine: Control and treatment of bacterial diarrhea and bacterial pneumonia. Chickens: Control of air sac infection, control of bluecomb, infectious synovitis and sinusitis. Turkeys: Control of infectious synovitis, hexamitiasis, and bluecomb disease.**

FDA File **065-441**
Firm: **Fort Dodge Animal Health, Div. Of Wyeth**
Use: **Cattle: Water Soluble Powder**
Dosage: **Calves: 10 milligrams per pound of body weight per day in drinking water for 3 to 5 days.**
Purpose: **Control and** treatment of **bacterial diarrhea and bacterial pneumonia.**

FDA File **065-496**
Firm: **Boehringer Ingelheim Vetmedica, Inc.**
Use: **Cattle, Swine, Chickens, Turkeys: Water Soluble Powder**
Dosage: **Cattle, Swine: 10 milligrams per pound of body weight per day in drinking water in divided doses. Chickens, Turkeys: 25 milligrams per pound of body weight per day. For bluecomb in turkeys administer 25 milligrams per pound of body weight per day. Administer for 7 to 14 days.**
Purpose: **Calves, Swine: Control and** treatment of **bacterial enteritis and bacterial pneumonia. Swine: Control and treatment of bacterial diarrhea and bacterial pneumonia. Chickens: Control of chronic**

respiratory disease and air sac infection, infectious synovitis. Turkeys: Control of infectious synovitis, and bluecomb disease.

FDA File **140-578**
Firm: **Alpharma, Inc.**
Use: **Chickens: Water Soluble Powder**
Dosage: **25 milligrams per pound of body weight per day for 7 to 14 days.**
Purpose: **Control of chronic respiratory disease, air sac infection and infectious synovitis.**

FDA File **200-049**
Firm: **Agri-Laboratories, Ltd.**
Use: **Cattle, Swine, Chickens, Turkeys: Water Soluble Powder**
Dosage: **Cattle, Swine: 10 milligrams per pound of body weight per day in drinking water in divided doses. Chickens, Turkeys: 25 milligrams per pound of body weight per day. For bluecomb in turkeys administer 25 milligrams per pound of body weight per day. Administer for 7 to 14 days.**
Purpose: **Calves, Swine: Control and treatment of bacterial enteritis and bacterial pneumonia. Swine: Control and treatment of bacterial diarrhea and bacterial pneumonia. Chickens: Control of chronic respiratory disease and air sac infection, infectious synovitis. Turkeys: Control of infectious synovitis, and bluecomb disease.**

FDA File **200-136**
Firm: **Phoenix Scientific, Inc.**

Use: **Cattle, Swine, Chickens, Turkeys: Water Soluble Powder**
Dosage: **Cattle, Swine: 10 milligrams per pound of body weight per day in drinking water in divided doses. Chickens, Turkeys: 25 milligrams per pound of body weight per day. For bluecomb in turkeys administer 25 milligrams per pound of body weight per day. Administer for 7 to 14 days.**
Purpose: **Calves, Swine: Control and treatment of bacterial enteritis and bacterial pneumonia. Swine: Control and treatment of bacterial diarrhea and bacterial pneumonia. Chickens: Control of chronic respiratory disease and air sac infection, infectious synovitis. Turkeys: Control of infectious synovitis, and bluecomb disease.**

FDA File **200-234**
Firm: **Med-Pharmex, Inc.**
Use: **Cattle, Swine, Chickens, Turkeys: Water Soluble Powder**
Dosage: **Cattle, Swine: 10 milligrams per pound of body weight per day in drinking water in divided doses. Chickens, Turkeys: 25 milligrams per pound of body weight per day. For bluecomb in turkeys administer 25 milligrams per pound of body weight per day. Administer for 7 to 14 days.**
Purpose: **Calves, Swine: Control and treatment of bacterial enteritis and bacterial pneumonia. Swine: Control and treatment of bacterial diarrhea and bacterial pneumonia. Chickens: Control of chronic respiratory disease and air sac**

infection, infectious synovitis. Tur-keys: Control of infectious synovi-tis, and bluecomb disease.

FDA File **065-099**
Firm: **Pharmacia & Upjohn Co.**
Use: **Dog:** Rx only - **Oral Capsule**
Dosage: **Dogs 5 to 15 pounds body weight: 60 to 120 milligrams per day; 15 to 30 pounds body weight: 120 to 240 milligrams per day; 30 to 60 pounds body weight: 120 to 240 milligrams per day; greater than 60 pounds body weight: 360 to 480 milligrams per day. Continue treatment 48 hours after animal is asymptomatic.**
Purpose: **Treatment respiratory or gastrointestinal tract infections and other infections.**

TIAMULIN

FDA File **134-644**
Firm: **Novartis Animal Health US, Inc.**
Use: **Swine: Water Soluble Powder**
Dosage: **227 or 677 milligrams per gallon of drinking water. Admin-ister 3.5 milligrams per pound of body weight per day for 5 days for dysentery; 10.5 milligrams per pound of body weight for pneumo-nia.**
Purpose: **Treatment of swine dysen-tery and swine pneumonia.**

FDA File 139-472
Firm: **Novartis Animal Health US, Inc.**
Use: **Swine: Medicated Feed Pre-mix**
Dosage: **35 grams per ton of feed for control of swine dysentery and proliferative enteropathies;** 200 grams per ton for treatment of swine dysentery; 10 grams per ton of feed for increased rate of weight gain and improved feed ef-ficiency.
Purpose: **Treatment and control of swine dysentery and porcine pro-liferative enteropathies (ileitis). For increased rate of weight gain and improved feed efficiency.**

FDA File 140-916
Firm: **Novartis Animal Health US, Inc.**
Use: **Swine: Water Soluble Powder**
Dosage: **227 or 681 milligrams per gallon of drinking water. Admin-ister 3.5 milligrams per pound of body weight per day for 5 days for dysentery; 10.5 milligrams per pound of body weight for pneumo-nia.**
Purpose: **Treatment of swine dysen-tery and swine pneumonia.**

FDA File 141-011
Firm: **Novartis Animal Health US, Inc.**
Use: **Swine: Medicated Feed Pre-mix**
Dosage: **35 grams per ton of feed.**
Purpose: **Control of swine bacterial enteritis, bacterial pneumonia, and swine dysentery.**

FDA File 200-344
Firm: **Ivx Animal Health**
Use: **Swine: Water Soluble Powder**
Dosage: **227 or 677 milligrams per gallon of drinking water. Admin-ister 3.5 milligrams per pound of body weight per day for 5 days for dysentery; 10.5 milligrams per pound of body weight for pneumo-nia.**

Purpose: **Treatment of swine dysentery and swine pneumonia.**

FDA File 200-356
Firm: **Pennfield Oil Co.**
Use: **Swine: Medicated Feed Premix**
Dosage: **35 grams per ton of feed.**
Purpose: **Control of swine bacterial enteritis, bacterial pneumonia, and swine dysentery.**

FDA File 200-360
Firm: **Ivx Animal Health**
Use: **Swine: Water Soluble Powder**
Dosage: **227 or 681 milligrams per gallon of drinking water. Administer 3.5 milligrams per pound of body weight per day for 5 days for dysentery; 10.5 milligrams per pound of body weight for pneumonia.**
Purpose: **Treatment of swine dysentery and swine pneumonia.**

TICARCILLIN (SODIUM)

FDA File **055-095**
Firm: **Pfizer, Inc.**
Use: **Horses:** Rx only **- Intrauterine Infusion**
Dosage: **6 grams per day for 3 consecutive days during estrus.**
Purpose: **Treatment of endometritis caused by beta-hemolytic streptococci.**

TILMICOSIN (PHOSPHATE)

FDA File **140-929**
Firm: **Elanco Animal Health, Div. Eli Lilly & Co.**
Use: **Cattle, Sheep:** Rx only **- Injection**

Dosage: **10 milligrams per kilogram of body weight by subcutaneous injection only.**
Purpose: **Cattle: Treatment of bovine respiratory disease associated with *Mannheimia (Pasteurella) haemolytica*. For control of respiratory disease in cattle at high risk of developing respiratory disease with the same pathogen.** Sheep: Treatment of ovine respiratory disease associated with the same pathogen.

FDA File **141-064**
Firm: **Elanco Animal Health, Div. Eli Lilly & Co.**
Use: **Swine:** Rx only **- Feed Additive**
Dosage: **181 to 363 grams per ton for up to 21 days during each phase of production.**
Purpose: **Control of swine respiratory disease associated with *Actinobacillus pleuropneumoniae* and *Pasteurella multocida.***

TRIMETHOPRIM

FDA File **095-614**
Firm: **Schering-Plough Animal Health**
Use: **Dog:** Rx only **- Oral Tablet**
Dosage: **14 milligrams per pound of body weight until 2 to 3 days after animal is asymptomatic but not to exceed 14 consecutive days.**
Purpose: **Treatment of bacterial infections where potent systemic antibacterial action is required, either alone or as an adjunct to surgery or debridement with associated infection; also in acute infections of the urinary, respiratory, or alimentary tracts or ab-**

scesses, or acute bacterial complications of distemper.

FDA File **105-093**
Firm: **Schering-Plough Animal Health**
Use: **Dog:** Rx only **- Injection**
Dosage: **40 milligrams per 20 pounds of body weight for 3 to 5 days. Not to exceed 14 consecutive days.**
Purpose: **Treatment of acute urinary tract infections, bacterial complications of distemper, respiratory tract, alimentary tract infections, wounds and abscesses, and acute septicemia due to *Streptococcus zooepidemicus*.**

FDA File **106-965**
Firm: **Schering-Plough Animal Health**
Use: **Horse:** Rx only **- Injection**
Dosage: **160 milligrams per 100 pounds of body weight for 5 to 7 days. Continue for 2 to 3 days after clinical signs have subsided.**
Purpose: **Treatment of acute strangles, respiratory tract infections, acute urogenital infections, and wound infections and abscesses.**

FDA File **115-578**
Firm: **Fort Dodge Animal Health, Div. Of Wyeth**
Use: **Dog:** Rx only **- Oral Tablet**
Dosage: **14 milligrams per pound of body weight per day and continue for 2 to 3 days after clinical signs have subsided. Not to exceed 14 consecutive days.**
Purpose: **Treatment of acute bacterial infections of the urinary,**

respiratory and alimentary tracts, of wounds and abscesses, and of complications of distemper.

FDA File **131-918**
Firm: **Schering-Plough Animal Health**
Use: **Horse:** Rx only **- Oral Paste**
Dosage: **5 milligrams per kilogram of body weight per day as a single dose for 5 to 7 days. Continue for 2 to 3 days after clinical signs have subsided.**
Purpose: **Treatment of acute strangles, respiratory tract infections, acute urogenital infections, and wound infections and abscesses.**

FDA File **132-486**
Firm: **Fort Dodge Animal Health, Div. Of Wyeth**
Use: **Dog:** Rx only **- Injection**
Dosage: **1 milliliter containing 40 milligrams per 20 pounds of body weight per day. For severe infections, after the initial dose subsequent doses may be halved and given every 12 hours. Continue for 2 to 3 days after clinical signs have subsided. Not to be used for more than 14 consecutive days.**
Purpose: **Treatment of acute urinary tract infections, acute bacterial complications of distemper, acute respiratory tract infections, acute alimentary tract infections, and acute septicemia due to *Streptococcus zooepidemicus*.**

FDA File **134-778**
Firm: **Fort Dodge Animal Health, Div. Of Wyeth**
Use: **Horse:** Rx only **- Injection**
Dosage: **160 milligrams per 100 pounds of body weight per day**

and continue for 5 to 7 days after clinical signs have subsided.
Purpose: **Control of bacterial infections during treatment of acute strangles, respiratory tract infections, acute urogenital tract infections, and wound infections and abscesses.**

FDA File **136-342**
Firm: **Fort Dodge Animal Health, Div. Of Wyeth**
Use: **Horse: Oral Paste**
Dosage: **335 milligrams per 500 pounds of body weight per day and continue for 5 to 7 days after clinical signs have subsided. Dosage may be halved and given morning and evening.**
Purpose: **Control of bacterial infections during treatment of acute strangles, respiratory tract infections, acute urogenital tract infections, and wound infections and abscesses.**

FDA File **136-741**
Firm: **Schering-Plough Animal Health**
Use: **Dog:** Rx only - **Oral Suspension**
Dosage: **10 milligrams per 5 pounds of body weight per day as a single dose or one-half daily dose every 12 hours. Continue for 2 to 3 days after clinical signs have subsided but not to exceed 14 consecutive days.**
Purpose: **Control of bacterial infections during the treatment of acute urinary, respiratory or alimentary tract infections, acute bacterial complications of distemper and for wound infections and abscesses.**

FDA File **200-033**
Firm: **Macleod Pharmaceuticals**
Use: **Horse:** Rx only - **Feed Additive**
Dosage: **Each gram of powder contains 67 milligrams trimethoprim. Administer 3.75 grams per 110 pounds of body weight per day in a small amount of feed, as a single daily dose for 5 to 7 days. Continue for 2 to 3 days after clinical signs have subsided.**
Purpose: **Control of bacterial infections during treatment of acute strangles, respiratory tract infections, acute urogenital infections, wound infections and abscesses.**

FDA File **200-244**
Firm: **Pharmacia & Upjohn Co.**
Use: **Horse:** Rx only - **Feed Additive**
Dosage: **Each gram of powder contains 67 milligrams trimethoprim. Administer 3.75 grams per 110 pounds of body weight per day in a small amount of feed, as a single daily dose for 5 to 7 days. Continue for 2 to 3 days after clinical signs have subsided.**
Purpose: **Control of bacterial infections during treatment of acute strangles, respiratory tract infections, acute urogenital infections, wound infections and abscesses.**

TULATHROMYCIN

FDA File **141-244**
Firm: **Pfizer, Inc.**
Use: **Cattle, Swine:** Rx only - **Injection**
Dosage: **Cattle: 2.5 milligrams per kilogram of body weight as a single subcutaneous injection in the neck. Swine: Same dose**

administered imtramuscularly in the neck.

Purpose: **Cattle: Treatment of bovine respiratory disease; <u>control of respiratory disease in cattle at high risk of developing respiratory disease</u>. Treatment of infectious bovine keratoconjunctivitis associated with *Moraxella bovis* and for treatment of bovine foot rot (interdigital necrobacillosis) in beef and non-lactating dairy cattle. Swine: For treatment of respiratory disease.**

TYLOSIN (PHOSPHATE, TARTRATE)

FDA File **012-491**
Firm: **Elanco Animal Health, Div. Eli Lilly & Co.**
Use: **Cattle, Swine: Feed Additive**
Dosage: **60 to 100 grams per ton of complete feed.**
Purpose: **Cattle, Swine: <u>Reduce the incidence of certain liver diseases; to prevent swine dysentery, to increase rate of weight gains and feed efficiency. Control of porcine proliferative enteropathies associated with *Lawsonia intracellularis*.</u> Treatment <u>and control</u> of swine dysentery associated with *Brachyspira <u>hyodysenteriae</u>. <u>In swine this medicated feed may be used following the use of tylosin in water for 3 to 10 days.</u>***

FDA File **012-548**
Firm: **Elanco Animal Health Div. Eli Lilly & Co.**
Use: **Swine: Feed Additive**
Dosage: **10 to 100 grams per ton of complete feed.**
Purpose: **<u>Increased rate of weight gain and feed efficiency.</u>**

FDA File **012-965**
Firm: **Elanco Animal Health Div. Eli Lilly & Co.**
Use: **Dogs, Cats:** Rx only **- Cattle, Swine:** OTC**: Injection**
Dosage: **Cattle: 8 milligrams per pound of body weight twice per day for not more than 5 consecutive days. Swine: 4 milligrams per pound of body weight twice per day for not more than 3 consecutive days. Dogs, Cats: 3 to 5 milligrams per pound of body weight at 12 to 24 hour intervals.**
Purpose: **Cattle: Treatment of contagious calf pneumonia, diphtheria, foot rot, metritis and pneumonia. Swine: Treatment of erysipelas, pneumonia, dysentery, and arthritis due to PPLO organisms. Dogs: Treatment of upper respiratory infections. Cats: Treatment of feline pneumonitis.**

FDA File **013-076**
Firm: **Pharmacia & Upjohn Co.**
Use: **Swine, Chickens, Turkeys, Bees: Water Additive**
Dosage: **Swine: 50 grams in 200 gallons of water. Chickens and Turkeys: 100 grams in 50 gallons of drinking water. Bees: 200 milligrams in 20 grams confectioners powdered sugar and dust over top bars of the brood chamber once weekly for 3 weeks in early spring or fall and assure consumption 4 weeks before the main honey flow begins.**
Purpose: **<u>Control</u> and treatment of swine dysentery in swine. In swine use of this water additive for 3 to 10 days may be followed by use of tylosin medicated feed. Increased rate of weight gain, improved feed efficiency and control**

of chronic respiratory disease in chickens. Control of American foulbrood in bees.

FDA File **013-162**
Firm: **Elanco Animal Health Div. Eli Lilly & Co.**
Use: **Chickens: Feed Additive**
Dosage: **20 to 50 or 1,000 grams per ton of complete feed.**
Purpose: **Increased rate of weight gain and feed efficiency and control of chronic respiratory disease.**

FDA File **013-388**
Firm: **Elanco Animal Health Div. Eli Lilly & Co.**
Use: **Chickens: Feed Additive**
Dosage: **4 to 50 grams per ton of complete feed.**
Purpose: **Increased rate of weight gain and feed efficiency.**

FDA File **015-166**
Firm: **Elanco Animal Health Div. Eli Lilly & Co.**
Use: **Chickens: Feed Additive**
Dosage: **4 to 50 grams or 800 to 1000 grams per ton of complete feed.**
Purpose: **Increased rate of weight gain and feed efficiency at low levels and control of chronic respiratory disease at high levels.**

FDA File **041-275**
Firm: **Elanco Animal Health Div. Eli Lilly & Co.**
Use: **Swine: Feed Additive**
Dosage: **100 grams per ton of complete feed.**
Purpose: **Maintain rate of weight gain and feed efficiency in the presence of atrophic rhinitis; prevention of vibrionic dysentery, con-**

trol of swine pneumonias, and to lower the incidence and severity of *Bordetella bronchiseptica* rhinitis.

FDA File **042-650**
Firm: **Virbac AH, Inc.**
Use: **Swine: Feed Additive**
Dosage: **100 grams per ton of complete feed.**
Purpose: **Maintain rate of weight gain and feed efficiency in the presence of atrophic rhinitis; prevention of vibrionic dysentery, control of swine pneumonias, and to lower the incidence and severity of *Bordetella bronchiseptica* rhinitis.**

FDA File **043-387**
Firm: **Virbac AH, Inc.**
Use: **Cattle, Swine, Chickens: Feed Additive**
Dosage: **Cattle: 8 to 10 grams per ton of complete feed. Swine: 1 to 1000 grams per ton of complete feed. Chickens: 4 to 1000 grams per ton of complete feed.**
Purpose: **Cattle: Reduction of the incidence of certain liver abscesses. Swine: Increased rate of weight gain, improved feed efficiency, prevention, treatment and control of swine dysentery and for maintaining weight gain and feed efficiency in the presence of atrophic rhinitis. Chickens: Increased rate of weight gain, improved feed efficiency and control of chronic respiratory disease.**

FDA File **046-415**
Firm: **Farmland Industries**
Use: **Cattle, Swine, Chickens: Feed Additive**
Dosage: **Cattle: 8 to 10 grams per ton of complete feed. Swine: 1 to**

100 grams per ton of complete feed. Chickens: 4 to 1000 grams per ton of complete feed.
Purpose: **Cattle: Reduction of the incidence of certain liver abscesses. Swine: Increased rate of weight gain, improved feed efficiency, prevention, treatment and control of swine dysentery and for maintaining weight gain and feed efficiency in the presence of atrophic rhinitis. Chickens: Increased rate of weight gain, improved feed efficiency and control of chronic respiratory disease.**

FDA File **046-190**
Firm: **Purina Mills, Inc.**
Use: **Swine: Feed Additive**
Dosage: **1 to 100 grams per ton of complete feed.**
Purpose: **Increased rate of weight gain, improved feed efficiency, prevention, treatment and control of swine dysentery and for maintaining weight gain and feed efficiency in the presence of atrophic rhinitis.**

FDA File **049-890**
Firm: **Norfolk Feed Mills Co.**
Use: **Swine: Feed Additive**
Dosage: **10 to 100 grams per ton of complete feed.**
Purpose: **Increased rate of weight gain and feed efficiency, maintain rate of weight gain and feed efficiency in the presence of atrophic rhinitis, and prevention of swine dysentery.**

FDA File **091-582**
Firm: **ADM Animal Health & Nutrition Div.**

Use: **Cattle, Swine, Chickens: Feed Additive**
Dosage: **Cattle: 8 to 10 grams per ton of complete feed. Swine: 10 to 1000 grams per ton of complete feed. Chickens: 4 to 1000 grams per ton of complete feed.**
Purpose: **Cattle: Reduction of the incidence of certain liver abscesses. Swine: Increased rate of weight gain, improved feed efficiency, prevention, treatment and control of swine dysentery and for maintaining weight gain and feed efficiency in the presence of atrophic rhinitis. Chickens: Increased rate of weight gain, improved feed efficiency and control of chronic respiratory disease.**

FDA File **091-738**
Firm: **Land O Lakes, Inc.**
Use: **Swine: Feed Additive**
Dosage: **10 to 40 grams per ton of complete feed.**
Purpose: **Increased rate of weight gain and feed efficiency.**

FDA File **091-749**
Firm: **Alpharma, Inc.**
Use: **Swine: Feed Additive**
Dosage: **100 grams per ton of complete feed.**
Purpose: **Increased rate of weight gain and feed efficiency, maintain rate of weight gain and feed efficiency in the presence of atrophic rhinitis, and prevention of swine dysentery.**

FDA File **095-550**
Firm: **ADM Animal Health & Nutrition Div.**
Use: **Cattle, Swine, Chickens: Feed Additive**

Dosage: **Cattle: 8 to 10 grams per ton of complete feed. Swine: 10 to 1000 grams per ton of complete feed. Chickens: 4 to 1000 grams per ton of complete feed.**
Purpose: **Cattle: <u>Reduction of the incidence of certain liver abscesses. Swine: Increased rate of weight gain and improved feed efficiency, prevention, treatment and control of vibrionic dysentery, to maintain weight gains and feed efficiency in the presence of atrophic rhinitis. Chickens: Improved feed efficiency, increased rate of weight gain and control of chronic respiratory disease.</u>**

FDA File **095-953**
Firm: **ADM Alliance Nutrition, Inc.**
Use: **Cattle, Swine, Chickens: Feed Additive**
Dosage: **Cattle: 8 to 10 grams per ton of complete feed. Swine: 10 to 1000 grams per ton of complete feed. Chickens: 4 to 1000 grams per ton of complete feed.**
Purpose: **Cattle: <u>Reduction of the incidence of certain liver abscesses. Swine: Increased rate of weight gain and improved feed efficiency, prevention, treatment and control of vibrionic dysentery, to maintain weight gains and feed efficiency in the presence of atrophic rhinitis. Chickens: Improved feed efficiency, increased rate of weight gain and control of chronic respiratory disease.</u>**

FDA File **096-161**
Firm: **Yoder Feed**
Use: **Cattle, Swine, Chickens: Feed Additive**

Dosage: **Cattle: 8 to 10 grams per ton of complete feed. Swine: 10 to 1000 grams per ton of complete feed. Chickens: 4 to 1000 grams per ton of complete feed.**
Purpose: **Cattle: <u>Reduction of the incidence of certain liver abscesses. Swine: Increased rate of weight gain and improved feed efficiency, prevention, treatment and control of vibrionic dysentery, to maintain weight gains and feed efficiency in the presence of atrophic rhinitis. Chickens: Improved feed efficiency, increased rate of weight gain and control of chronic respiratory disease.</u>**

FDA File **096-273**
Firm: **Protein Blenders, Inc.**
Use: **Cattle, Swine, Chickens: Feed Additive**
Dosage: **Cattle: 8 to 10 grams per ton of complete feed. Swine: 10 to 1000 grams per ton of complete feed. Chickens: 4 to 1000 grams per ton of complete feed.**
Purpose: **Cattle: <u>Reduction of the incidence of certain liver abscesses. Swine: Increased rate of weight gain and improved feed efficiency, prevention, treatment and control of vibrionic dysentery, to maintain weight gains and feed efficiency in the presence of atrophic rhinitis. Chickens: Improved feed efficiency, increased rate of weight gain and control of chronic respiratory disease.</u>**

FDA File **096-843**
Firm: **Purina Mills, Inc.**
Use: **Cattle: Feed Additive**
Dosage: **Cattle: 8 to 10 grams per ton of complete feed.**

Purpose: **Reduction of the incidence of certain liver abscesses.**

FDA File **097-980**
Firm: **Quali-Tech Products, Inc.**
Use: **Cattle, Swine, Chickens: Feed Additive**
Dosage: **Cattle: 8 to 10 grams per ton of complete feed. Swine: 10 to 1000 grams per ton of complete feed. Chickens: 4 to 1000 grams per ton of complete feed.**
Purpose: **Cattle: Reduction of the incidence of certain liver abscesses. Swine: Increased rate of weight gain and improved feed efficiency, prevention, treatment and control of vibrionic dysentery, to maintain weight gains and feed efficiency in the presence of atrophic rhinitis. Chickens: Improved feed efficiency, increased rate of weight gain and control of chronic respiratory disease.**

FDA File **097-981**
Firm: **Quali-Tech Products, Inc.**
Use: **Swine: Feed Additive**
Dosage: **100 grams per ton of complete feed.**
Purpose: **Maintain weight gains and feed efficiency in the presence of atrophic rhinitis, prevent swine dysentery and control swine pneumonias.**

FDA File **098-429**
Firm: **J.C. Feed Mills**
Use: **Swine: Feed Additive**
Dosage: **10 to 100 grams per ton of complete feed.**
Purpose: **Increased rate of weight gain and feed efficiency.**

FDA File **098-431**
Firm: **Phibro Animal Health, Inc.**
Use: **Cattle, Swine, Chickens: Feed Additive**
Dosage: **Cattle: 8 to 10 grams per ton of complete feed. Swine: 10 to 1000 grams per ton of complete feed. Chickens: 4 to 1000 grams per ton of complete feed.**
Purpose: **Cattle: Reduction of the incidence of certain liver abscesses. Swine: Increased rate of weight gain and improved feed efficiency, prevention, treatment and control of vibrionic dysentery, to maintain weight gains and feed efficiency in the presence of atrophic rhinitis. Chickens: Improved feed efficiency, increased rate of weight gain.**

FDA File **098-639**
Firm: **Bioproducts, Inc.**
Use: **Swine: Feed Additive**
Dosage: **100 grams per ton of complete feed.**
Purpose: **Maintain rate of weight gain and feed efficiency in the presence of atrophic rhinitis; prevention of swine dysentery, control of pneumonias, and to lower the incidence and severity of *Bordetella bronchiseptica* rhinitis.**

FDA File **098-970**
Firm: **Rath Packing Co.**
Use: **Swine: Feed Additive**
Dosage: **10 to 100 grams per ton of complete feed.**
Purpose: **Increased rate of weight gain and feed efficiency.**

FDA File **099-468**
Firm: **Wayne Feed Div., Cont. Grain**
Use: **Cattle, Swine, Chickens: Feed Additive**

Dosage: **Cattle: 8 to 10 grams per ton of complete feed. Swine: 10 to 100 grams per ton of complete feed. Chickens: 4 to 1000 grams per ton of complete feed.**
Purpose: **Cattle: <u>Reduction of the incidence of certain liver abscesses. Swine: Increased rate of weight gain, improved feed efficiency, prevention, treatment and control</u> of swine dysentery <u>and for maintaining weight gain and feed efficiency in the presence of atrophic rhinitis. Chickens: Increased rate of weight gain, improved feed efficiency and control of chronic respiratory disease.</u>**

FDA File **099-767**
Firm: **Virbac AH, Inc.**
Use: **Swine: Feed Additive**
Dosage: **100 grams per ton of complete feed.**
Purpose: **<u>Maintain rate of weight gain and feed efficiency in the presence of atrophic rhinitis; prevention of swine dysentery, control of pneumonias, and to lower the incidence and severity of *Bordetella bronchiseptica* rhinitis.</u>**

FDA File **100-128**
Firm: **Cross Vetpharm Group Ltd.**
Use: **Swine: Feed Additive**
Dosage: **10 to 100 grams per ton of complete feed.**
Purpose: **<u>Maintain rate of weight gain and feed efficiency in the presence of atrophic rhinitis; prevention of swine dysentery, control of pneumonias, and to lower the incidence and severity of *Bordetella bronchiseptica* rhinitis.</u>**

FDA File **100-352**
Firm: **Nutri Basics Co.**
Use: **Cattle, Swine, Chickens: Feed Additive**
Dosage: **Cattle: 8 to 10 grams per ton of complete feed. Swine: 10 to 100 grams per ton of complete feed. Chickens: 4 to 1000 grams per ton of complete feed.**
Purpose: **Cattle: <u>Reduction of the incidence of certain liver abscesses. Swine: Increased rate of weight gain, improved feed efficiency, prevention, treatment and control</u> of swine dysentery <u>and for maintaining weight gain and feed efficiency in the presence of atrophic rhinitis. Chickens: Increased rate of weight gain, improved feed efficiency and control of chronic respiratory disease.</u>**

FDA File **100-556**
Firm: **Springfield Milling Corp.**
Use: **Swine: Feed Additive**
Dosage: **10 to 100 grams per ton of complete feed.**
Purpose: **<u>Maintain rate of weight gain and feed efficiency.</u>**

FDA File **100-991**
Firm: **Furst-Mcness Co.**
Use: **Cattle, Swine, Chickens: Feed Additive**
Dosage: **Cattle: 8 to 10 grams per ton of complete feed. Swine: 10 to 100 grams per ton of complete feed. Chickens: 4 to 1000 grams per ton of complete feed.**
Purpose: **Cattle: <u>Reduction of the incidence of certain liver abscesses. Swine: Increased rate of weight gain, improved feed efficiency, prevention, treatment and control</u> of swine dysentery <u>and for</u>**

maintaining weight gain and feed efficiency in the presence of atrophic rhinitis. Chickens: Increased rate of weight gain, improved feed efficiency and control of chronic respiratory disease.

FDA File **101-905**
Firm: **Waterloo Mills Co.**
Use: **Swine: Feed Additive**
Dosage: **10 to 100 grams per ton of complete feed.**
Purpose: **Increased rate of weight gain and feed efficiency.**

FDA File **101-906**
Firm: **Waterloo Mills Co.**
Use: **Swine: Feed Additive**
Dosage: **100 grams per ton of complete feed.**
Purpose: **Maintain rate of weight gain and feed efficiency in presence of atopic rhinitis, lower the incidence and severity of rhinitis, prevention of vibrionic dysentery, and control of pneumonia.**

FDA File **103-089**
Firm: **North American Nutrition Companies, Inc.**
Use: **Cattle, Swine, Chickens: Feed Additive**
Dosage: **Cattle: 8 to 10 grams per ton of complete feed. Swine: 10 to 100 grams per ton of complete feed. Chickens: 4 to 1000 grams per ton of complete feed.**
Purpose: **Cattle: Reduction of the incidence of certain liver abscesses. Swine: Increased rate of weight gain, improved feed efficiency, prevention, treatment and control of swine dysentery and for maintaining weight gain and feed efficiency in the presence of atro-**

phic rhinitis. Chickens: Increased rate of weight gain, improved feed efficiency and control of chronic respiratory disease.

FDA File **104-646**
Firm: **Elanco Animal Health, Div. Eli Lilly & Co.**
Use: **Cattle: Feed Additive**
Dosage: **8 to 100 grams per ton of complete feed.**
Purpose: **Cattle: Reduction of the incidence of certain liver abscesses and for improvement of feed efficiency in cattle fed in confinement for slaughter.**

FDA File **100-991**
Firm: **Furst-Mcness Co.**
Use: **Cattle, Swine, Chickens: Feed Additive**
Dosage: **Cattle: 8 to 10 grams per ton of complete feed. Swine: 10 to 100 grams per ton of complete feed. Chickens: 4 to 1000 grams per ton of complete feed.**
Purpose: **Cattle: Reduction of the incidence of certain liver abscesses. Swine: Increased rate of weight gain, improved feed efficiency, prevention, treatment and control of swine dysentery and for maintaining weight gain and feed efficiency in the presence of atrophic rhinitis. Chickens: Increased rate of weight gain, improved feed efficiency and control of chronic respiratory disease.**

FDA File **106-507**
Firm: **Custom Feed Blenders Corp.**
Use: **Cattle, Swine, Chickens: Feed Additive**

Dosage: **Cattle: 8 to 10 grams per ton of complete feed. Swine: 10 to 100 grams per ton of complete feed. Chickens: 4 to 1000 grams per ton of complete feed.**
Purpose: **Cattle: <u>Reduction of the incidence of certain liver abscesses. Swine: Increased rate of weight gain, improved feed efficiency, prevention</u>, treatment <u>and control</u> of swine dysentery <u>and for maintaining weight gain and feed efficiency in the presence of atrophic rhinitis. Chickens: Increased rate of weight gain, improved feed efficiency and control of chronic respiratory disease.</u>**

FDA File **107-002**
Firm: **Seeco, Inc.**
Use: **Swine: Feed Additive**
Dosage: **100 grams per ton of complete feed.**
Purpose: **<u>Maintain rate of weight gain and feed efficiency in presence of atropic rhinitis, lower the incidence and severity of rhinitis, prevention of vibrionic dysentery, and control of pneumonia.</u>**

FDA File **107-057**
Firm: **ADM Animal Health & Nutrition Div.**
Use: **Swine: Feed Additive**
Dosage: **100 grams per ton of complete feed.**
Purpose: **<u>Maintain rate of weight gain and feed efficiency in presence of atrophic rhinitis, lower the incidence and severity of rhinitis, prevention of vibrionic dysentery, and control of pneumonia.</u>**

FDA File **108-484**
Firm: **ADM Animal Health & Nutrition Div.**

Use: **Swine: Feed Additive**
Dosage: **100 grams per ton of complete feed.**
Purpose: **<u>Maintain rate of weight gain and feed efficiency in presence of atrophic rhinitis, lower the incidence and severity of rhinitis, prevention of vibrionic dysentery, and control of pneumonia.</u>**

FDA File **110-044**
Firm: **Peavy Co.**
Use: **Swine: Feed Additive**
Dosage: **10 to 100 grams per ton of complete feed.**
Purpose: **<u>Increased rate of weight gain and feed efficiency.</u>**

FDA File **110-045**
Firm: **ADM Animal Health & Nutrition Div.**
Use: **Cattle, Swine, Chickens: Feed Additive**
Dosage: **Cattle: 8 to 10 grams per ton of complete feed. Swine: 10 to 100 grams per ton of complete feed. Chickens: 4 to 1000 grams per ton of complete feed.**
Purpose: **Cattle: <u>Reduction of the incidence of certain liver abscesses. Swine: Increased rate of weight gain, improved feed efficiency, prevention</u>, treatment <u>and control</u> of swine dysentery <u>and for maintaining weight gain and feed efficiency in the presence of atrophic rhinitis. Chickens: Increased rate of weight gain, improved feed efficiency and control of chronic respiratory disease.</u>**

FDA File **110-047**
Firm: **Phibro Animal Health, Inc.**
Use: **Swine: Feed Additive**

Dosage: **40 to 100 grams per ton of feed for at least 3 weeks followed by 40 grams per ton until market weight.**
Purpose: **Prevention or treatment and control of swine dysentery.**

FDA File **110-315**
Firm: **Ivy Laboratories, Div. of Ivy A.H., Inc.**
Use: **Cattle: Ear Implant**
Dosage: **Nine pellets, one containing 29 milligrams tylosin tartrate.**
Purpose: **Local antibacterial.**

FDA File **111-069**
Firm: **ADM Alliance Nutrition, Inc.**
Use: **Swine: Feed Additive**
Dosage: **100 grams per ton of complete feed**
Purpose: **Maintain weight gains and feed efficiency in the presence of atrophic rhinitis, lowering the incidence and severity of rhinitis, prevention of swine dysentery, and control of swine pneumonias.**

FDA File **120-614**
Firm: **Webel Feeds, Inc.**
Use: **Swine: Feed Additive**
Dosage: **100 grams per ton of complete feed**
Purpose: **Maintain weight gains and feed efficiency in the presence of atrophic rhinitis, lowering the incidence and severity of rhinitis, prevention of swine dysentery, and control of swine pneumonias.**

FDA File **121-147**
Firm: **Ag-Mark, Inc.**
Use: **Cattle, Swine, Chickens: Feed Additive**
Dosage: **Cattle: 8 to 10 grams per ton of complete feed. Swine: 10 to 100 grams per ton of complete feed. Chickens: 4 to 1000 grams per ton of complete feed.**
Purpose: **Cattle: Reduction of the incidence of certain liver abscesses. Swine: Increased rate of weight gain, improved feed efficiency, prevention, treatment and control of swine dysentery and for maintaining weight gain and feed efficiency in the presence of atrophic rhinitis. Chickens: Increased rate of weight gain, improved feed efficiency and control of chronic respiratory disease.**

FDA File **121-147**
Firm: **Ag-Mark, Inc.**
Use: **Cattle, Swine, Chickens: Feed Additive**
Dosage: **Cattle: 8 to 10 grams per ton of complete feed. Swine: 10 to 100 grams per ton of complete feed. Chickens: 4 to 1000 grams per ton of complete feed.**
Purpose: **Cattle: Reduction of the incidence of certain liver abscesses. Swine: Increased rate of weight gain, improved feed efficiency, prevention, treatment and control of swine dysentery and for maintaining weight gain and feed efficiency in the presence of atrophic rhinitis. Chickens: Increased rate of weight gain, improved feed efficiency and control of chronic respiratory disease.**

FDA File **122-522**
Firm: **Custom Feed Blenders Corp.**
Use: **Swine: Feed Additive**
Dosage: **100 grams per ton of complete feed.**
Purpose: **Maintain rate of weight gain and feed efficiency in pres-**

ence of atrophic rhinitis, lower the incidence and severity of rhinitis, prevention of vibrionic dysentery, and control of pneumonia.

FDA File **124-391**
Firm: **Ag-Mark, Inc.**
Use: **Swine: Feed Additive**
Dosage: **100 grams per ton of complete feed.**
Purpose: **Maintain rate of weight gain and feed efficiency in presence of atrophic rhinitis, lower the incidence and severity of rhinitis, prevention of vibrionic dysentery, and control of pneumonia.**

FDA File **127-195**
Firm: **L.M.S., Inc.**
Use: **Cattle, Swine, Chickens: Feed Additive**
Dosage: **Cattle: 8 to 10 grams per ton of complete feed. Swine: 10 to 100 grams per ton of complete feed. Chickens: 4 to 1000 grams per ton of complete feed.**
Purpose: **Cattle: Reduction of the incidence of certain liver abscesses. Swine: Increased rate of weight gain, improved feed efficiency, prevention, treatment and control of swine dysentery and for maintaining weight gain and feed efficiency in the presence of atrophic rhinitis. Chickens: Increased rate of weight gain, improved feed efficiency and control of chronic respiratory disease.**

FDA File **127-507**
Firm: **Elanco Animal Health, Div. Eli Lilly & Co.**
Use: **Swine: Feed Additive**

Dosage: **100 grams per ton of complete feed.**
Purpose: **Maintain rate of weight gain and feed efficiency in presence of atrophic rhinitis, lower the incidence and severity of rhinitis, prevention of vibrionic dysentery, and control of pneumonia.**

FDA File **128-411**
Firm: **ADM Animal Health & Nutrition Div.**
Use: **Swine: Feed Additive**
Dosage: **100 grams per ton of complete feed.**
Purpose: **Maintain rate of weight gain and feed efficiency in presence of atrophic rhinitis, lower the incidence and severity of rhinitis, prevention of vibrionic dysentery, and control of pneumonia.**

FDA File **131-537**
Firm: **Gossett Nutrition, Inc.**
Use: **Swine: Feed Additive**
Dosage: **10 to 100 grams per ton of complete feed.**
Purpose: **Increased rate of weight gain and feed efficiency, prevention of swine dysentery and maintaining weight gains in the presence of atrophic rhinitis.**

FDA File **131-956**
Firm: **ADM Animal Health & Nutrition Div.**
Use: **Swine: Feed Additive**
Dosage: **100 grams per ton of complete feed.**
Purpose: **Maintaining weight gains in the presence of atrophic rhinitis lowering the incidence and severity of rhinitis, preventing swine**

dysentery, and controlling swine pneumonias.

FDA File **131-957**
Firm: **ADM Animal Health :& Nutrition Div.**
Use: **Cattle, Swine, Chickens: Feed Additive**
Dosage: **Cattle: 8 to 10 grams per ton of complete feed. Swine: 10 to 100 grams per ton of complete feed. Chickens: 4 to 1000 grams per ton of complete feed.**
Purpose: **Cattle: Reduction of the incidence of certain liver abscesses. Swine: Increased rate of weight gain, improved feed efficiency, prevention, treatment and control of swine dysentery and for maintaining weight gain and feed efficiency in the presence of atrophic rhinitis. Chickens: Increased rate of weight gain, improved feed efficiency and control of chronic respiratory disease.**

FDA File **131-958**
Firm: **Wayne Feed Div., Cont. Grain**
Use: **Swine: Feed Additive**
Dosage: **100 grams per ton of complete feed.**
Purpose: **Maintaining weight gains in the presence of atrophic rhinitis lowering the incidence and severity of rhinitis, preventing swine dysentery, and controlling swine pneumonias.**

FDA File **133-833**
Firm: **Southern Micro-Blenders**
Use: **Cattle, Swine, Chickens: Feed Additive**
Dosage: **Cattle: 8 to 10 grams per ton of complete feed. Swine: 10 to 100 grams per ton of complete feed. Chickens: 4 to 1000 grams per ton of complete feed.**
Purpose: **Cattle: Reduction of the incidence of certain liver abscesses. Swine: Increased rate of weight gain, improved feed efficiency, prevention, treatment and control of swine dysentery and for maintaining weight gain and feed efficiency in the presence of atrophic rhinitis. Chickens: Increased rate of weight gain, improved feed efficiency and control of chronic respiratory disease.**

FDA File **135-906**
Firm: **Ivy Laboratories, Div. of Ivy A.H., Inc.**
Use: **Cattle: Ear Implant**
Dosage: **Product consists of nine pellets with one pellet containing 29 milligrams tylosin tartrate.**
Purpose: **Local antibacterial.**

FDA File **138-187**
Firm: **Micro Chemical, Inc.**
Use: **Cattle, Swine, Chickens: Feed Additive**
Dosage: **Cattle: 8 to 10 grams per ton of complete feed. Swine: 10 to 100 grams per ton of complete feed. Chickens: 4 to 1000 grams per ton of complete feed.**
Purpose: **Cattle: Reduction of the incidence of certain liver abscesses. Swine: Increased rate of weight gain, improved feed efficiency, prevention, treatment and control of swine dysentery and for maintaining weight gain and feed efficiency in the presence of atrophic rhinitis. Chickens: Increased rate of weight gain, improved feed**

efficiency and control of chronic
respiratory disease.

FDA File **138-192**
Firm: **Pharmacia & Upjohn Co.**
Use: **Cattle: Feed Additive**
Dosage: **8 to 10 grams per ton of
complete feed.**
Purpose: **Increased rate of weight
gain, improved feed efficiency, and
reduction of the incidence of liver
abscesses in heifers being fed in
confinement for slaughter.**

FDA File **138-342**
Firm: **Feed Service Co., Inc.**
Use: **Swine: Feed Additive**
Dosage: **100 grams per ton of complete feed.**
Purpose: **Maintain rate of weight
gain and feed efficiency in presence of atrophic rhinitis, lower the
incidence and severity of rhinitis,
prevention of vibrionic dysentery,
and control of pneumonia.**

FDA File **138-792**
Firm: **Pharmacia & Upjohn Co.**
Use: **Cattle: Feed Additive**
Dosage: **90 milligrams per head per
day.**
Purpose: **Increased rate of weight
gain, improved feed efficiency, and
reduction of the incidence of liver
abscesses in heifers being fed in
confinement for slaughter.**

FDA File **138-870**
Firm: **Pharmacia & Upjohn Co.**
Use: **Cattle: Feed Additive**
Dosage: **90 milligrams per head per
day.**

Purpose: **Increased rate of weight
gain, improved feed efficiency, and
reduction of the incidence of liver
abscesses in heifers being fed in
confinement for slaughter.**

FDA File **138-904**
Firm: **Pharmacia & Upjohn Co.**
Use: **Cattle: Feed Additive**
Dosage: **8 to 10 grams per ton of
complete feed.**
Purpose: **Increased rate of weight
gain, improved feed efficiency, and
reduction of the incidence of liver
abscesses in heifers being fed in
confinement for slaughter.**

FDA File **138-955**
Firm: **Boehringer Ingelheim Vetmedica, Inc.**
Use: **Cattle, Swine: Injection**
Dosage: **Cattle: 8 milligrams per
pound of body weight once per day
for not more than 5 consecutive
days. Continue treatment 24 hours
after animal is asymptomatic.
Swine: 4 milligrams per pound
of body weight twice per day for
not more than 3 consecutive days.
Continue treatment for 24 hours
after animal is asymptomatic.**
Purpose: **Cattle: Treatment of bovine respiratory complex, necrotic
pododermatitis, and calf diphtheria. Swine: Treatment of swine
arthritis, swine pneumonia, swine
erysipelas, and swine dysentery.**

FDA File **138-995**
Firm: **Pharmacia & Upjohn Co.**
Use: **Cattle: Feed Additive**
Dosage: **90 milligrams per head per
day.**
Purpose: **Increased rate of weight
gain, improved feed efficiency, and**

reduction of the incidence of liver abscesses in heifers being fed in confinement for slaughter.

FDA File **139-192**
Firm: **Pharmacia & Upjohn Co.**
Use: **Cattle: Feed Additive**
Dosage: **90 milligrams per head per day.**
Purpose: **Increased rate of weight gain, improved feed efficiency, and reduction of the incidence of liver abscesses in heifers being fed in confinement for slaughter.**

FDA File **140-681**
Firm: **Pennfield Oil Co.**
Use: **Swine: Feed Additive**
Dosage: **100 grams per ton of complete feed.**
Purpose: **Maintaining weight gains in the presence of atrophic rhinitis lowering the incidence and severity of rhinitis, preventing swine dysentery, and controlling swine pneumonias.**

FDA File **140-820**
Firm: **Furst-Mcness Co.**
Use: **Swine: Feed Additive**
Dosage: **100 grams per ton of complete feed.**
Purpose: **Maintaining weight gains in the presence of atrophic rhinitis lowering the incidence and severity of rhinitis, preventing swine dysentery, and controlling swine pneumonias.**

FDA File **140-939**
Firm: **Elanco Animal Health, Div. Eli Lilly & Co.**
Use: **Cattle: Feed Additive**

Dosage: **90 milligrams per head per day.**
Purpose: **Improved feed efficiency and reduction of the incidence of liver abscesses in cattle being fed in confinement for slaughter.**

FDA File **141-276**
Firm: **Intervet, Inc.**
Use: **Cattle: Feed Additive**
Dosage: **8 to 10 grams per ton of feed.**
Purpose: **Improved feed efficiency and reduction of the incidence of liver abscesses in cattle being fed in confinement for slaughter during the last 20 to 40 days on feed.**

FDA File **141-280**
Firm: **Intervet, Inc.**
Use: **Cattle: Feed Additive**
Dosage: **8 to 10 grams per ton of feed.**
Purpose: **Increased rate of weight gain, improved feed efficiency, and reduction of the incidence of liver abscesses in cattle being fed in confinement for slaughter during the last 20 to 40 days on feed.**

FDA File **200-346**
Firm: **Ivy Laboratories, Div. of Ivy A.H., Inc.**
Use: **Cattle: Ear Implant**
Dosage: **Five pellets, one containing 29 milligrams tylosin tartrate.**
Purpose: **Local antibacterial.**

FDA File **141-149**
Firm: **Alpharma, Inc.**
Use: **Cattle: Feed Additive**
Dosage: **8 to 10 grams per ton of complete feed (60 to 90 milligrams**

per head per day) for cattle being fed in confinement for slaughter.
Purpose: **Reduction of the incidence of certain liver abscesses and improved feed efficiency.**

FDA File **141-164**
Firm: **Elanco Animal Health, Div. Eli Lilly & Co.**
Use: **Chickens: Feed Additive**
Dosage: **4 to 50 grams per ton of complete feed.**
Purpose: **Increased rate of weight gain and improved feed efficiency.**

FDA File **141-170**
Firm: **Elanco Animal Health, Div. Eli Lilly & Co.**
Use: **Chickens: Feed Additive**
Dosage: **4 to 50 grams per ton of complete feed.**
Purpose: **Increased rate of weight gain and improved feed efficiency.**

FDA File **141-172**
Firm: **Elanco Animal Health, Div. Eli Lilly & Co.**
Use: **Swine: Feed Additive**
Dosage: **40 or 100 grams per ton of complete feed.**
Purpose: **Increased rate of weight gain, improved feed efficiency, prevention and/or control of porcine proliferative enteropathies and for prevention of swine dysentery.**

FDA File **141-198**
Firm: **Elanco Animal Health, Div. Eli Lilly & Co.**
Use: **Chickens: Feed Additive**
Dosage: **4 to 50 grams per ton of complete feed for broiler chickens.**
Purpose: **Increased rate of weight gain and improved feed efficiency.**

FDA File **141-224**
Firm: **Elanco Animal Health, Div. Eli Lilly & Co.**
Use: **Cattle: Feed Additive**
Dosage: **8 to 10 grams per ton of complete feed.**
Purpose: **Increased rate of weight gain, improved feed efficiency, and reduction of the incidence of liver abscesses in cattle being fed in confinement for slaughter.**

FDA File **141-233**
Firm: **Elanco Animal Health, Div. Eli Lilly & Co.**
Use: **Cattle: Feed Additive**
Dosage: **8 to 10 grams per ton of complete feed.**
Purpose: **Increased rate of weight gain, improved feed efficiency, and reduction of the incidence of liver abscesses in heifers being fed in confinement for slaughter during the last 28 to 42 days on feed.**

FDA File **200-221**
Firm: **Ivy Laboratories, Div. of Ivy A.H., Inc.**
Use: **Cattle: Ear Implant**
Dosage: **Five pellets, one containing 29 milligrams tylosin tartrate.**
Purpose: **Local antibacterial.**

FDA File **200-224**
Firm: **Ivy Laboratories, Div. of Ivy A.H., Inc.**
Use: **Cattle: Ear Implant**
Dosage: **Eight pellets, one containing 29 milligrams tylosin tartrate.**
Purpose: **Local antibacterial.**

FDA File **200-346**
Firm: **Ivy Laboratories, Div. of Ivy A.H., Inc.**
Use: **Cattle: Ear Implant**

Dosage: **Several pellets, one containing 29 milligrams tylosin tartrate.**
Purpose: **Local antibacterial.**

FDA File **200-424**
Firm: **Ivy Laboratories, Div. of Ivy A.H., Inc.**
Use: **Cattle: Feed Additive**
Dosage: **8 to 10 grams per ton of complete feed.**
Purpose: **Increased rate of weight gain, improved feed efficiency, and reduction of the incidence of liver abscesses in heifers being fed in confinement for slaughter during the last 28 to 42 days on feed.**

FDA File **200-427**
Firm: **Ivy Laboratories, Div. of Ivy A.H., Inc.**
Use: **Cattle: Feed Additive**
Dosage: **90 milligrams per head per day for heifers being fed in confinement for slaughter.**
Purpose: **Increased rate of weight gain, improved feed efficiency, and reduction of the incidence of liver abscesses in heifers being fed in confinement for slaughter.**

FDA File **139-192**
Firm: **Ivy Laboratories, Div. of Ivy A.H., Inc.**
Use: **Cattle: Feed Additive- Liquid Feed**
Dosage: **90 milligrams per head per day.**
Purpose: **Increased rate of weight gain, improved feed efficiency, and reduction of the incidence of liver abscesses in heifers being fed in confinement for slaughter.**

VIRGINIAMYCIN

FDA File **091-467**
Firm: **Phibro Animal Health, Inc.**
Use: **Swine, Chickens, Turkeys: Feed Additive**
Dosage: **Swine: 10 to 100 grams per ton of complete feed. Chickens: 5 to 20 grams per ton of complete feed. Turkeys: 10 to 20 grams per ton of complete feed.**
Purpose: **Swine: Treatment and control of swine dysentery and increased rate of weight gain and improved feed efficiency. Chickens: Prevention of necrotic enteritis and increased rate of weight gain and improved feed efficiency. Turkeys: Increased rate of weight gain and improved feed efficiency in growers.**

FDA File **091-513**
Firm: **Phibro Animal Health, Inc.**
Use: **Swine, Chickens: Feed Additive**
Dosage: **Swine: 10 to 100 grams per ton of complete feed. Chickens: 5 to 20 grams per ton of complete feed.**
Purpose: **Swine: Treatment and control of swine dysentery and increased rate of weight gain and improved feed efficiency. Chickens: Prevention of necrotic enteritis and increased rate of weight gain and improved feed efficiency.**

FDA File **095-513**
Firm: **Pfizer, Inc.**
Use: **Swine: Feed Additive**
Dosage: **5 to 100 grams per ton of complete feed.**
Purpose: **Treatment and control of swine dysentery and increased**

rate of weight gain and improved
feed efficiency.

FDA File **120-724**
Firm: **Phibro Animal Health, Inc.**
Use: **Chickens: Feed Additive**
Dosage: **5 to 15 grams per ton of
complete feed.**
Purpose: **Increased rate of weight
gain and improved feed efficiency.**

FDA File **122-481**
Firm: **Phibro Animal Health, Inc.**
Use: **Chickens: Feed Additive**
Dosage: **5 to 15 grams per ton of
complete feed.**
Purpose: **Increased rate of weight
gain and improved feed efficiency.**

FDA File **122-608**
Firm: **Phibro Animal Health, Inc.**
Use: **Chickens: Feed Additive**
Dosage: **5 to 15 grams per ton of
complete feed.**
Purpose: **Increased rate of weight
gain and improved feed efficiency.**

FDA File **122-822**
Firm: **Phibro Animal Health, Inc.**
Use: **Chickens: Feed Additive**
Dosage: **5 to 15 grams per ton of
complete feed.**
Purpose: **Increased rate of weight
gain and improved feed efficiency.**

FDA File **133-333**
Firm: **North American Nutrition
Companies, Inc.**
Use: **Swine: Feed Additive**
Dosage: **5 to 100 grams per ton of
complete feed.**
Purpose: **Treatment and control of
swine dysentery and increased
rate of weight gain and improved
feed efficiency.**

FDA File **133-334**
Firm: **Alpharma, Inc.**
Use: **Swine: Feed Additive**
Dosage: **5 to 100 grams per ton of
complete feed.**
Purpose: **Treatment and control of
swine dysentery and increased
rate of weight gain and improved
feed efficiency.**

FDA File **133-335**
Firm: **Quali-Tech Products, Inc.**
Use: **Swine: Feed Additive**
Dosage: **5 to 100 grams per ton of
complete feed.**
Purpose: **Treatment and control of
swine dysentery and increased
rate of weight gain and improved
feed efficiency.**

FDA File **138-828**
Firm: **Phibro Animal Health, Inc.**
Use: **Chickens: Feed Additive**
Dosage: **5 to 15 grams per ton of
complete feed.**
Purpose: **Increased rate of weight
gain and improved feed efficiency.**

FDA File **138-953**
Firm: **Phibro Animal Health, Inc.**
Use: **Chickens: Feed Additive**
Dosage: **5 grams per ton of com-
plete feed.**
Purpose: **Increased rate of weight
gain and improved feed efficiency.**

FDA File **139-473**
Firm: **Intervet, Inc.**
Use: **Chickens: Feed Additive**
Dosage: **5 to 15 grams per ton of
complete feed.**
Purpose: **Increased rate of weight
gain and improved feed efficiency.**

FDA File **140-998**
Firm: **Phibro Animal Health, Inc.**
Use: **Cattle: Feed Additive**
Dosage: **11 to 22.5 grams per ton of complete feed.**
Purpose: **Increased rate of weight gain and improved feed efficiency and reduction in the incidence of liver abscesses in cattle fed in confinement for slaughter.**

FDA File **141-090**
Firm: **Huvepharma AD**
Use: **Chickens: Feed Additive**
Dosage: **5 to 15 grams per ton of complete feed.**
Purpose: **Increased rate of weight gain and improved feed efficiency.**

FDA File **141-110**
Firm: **Elanco Animal Health, Div. Eli Lilly & Co.**
Use: **Turkeys: Feed Additive**
Dosage: **10 to 20 grams per ton of complete feed.**
Purpose: **Increased rate of weight gain and improved feed efficiency.**

FDA File **141-114**
Firm: **Phibro Animal Health, Inc.**
Use: **Chickens: Feed Additive**
Dosage: **5 to 20 grams per ton of complete feed.**
Purpose: **Increased rate of weight gain and improved feed efficiency and prevention of necrotic enteritis.**

FDA File **141-150**
Firm: **Alpharma, Inc.**
Use: **Turkeys: Feed Additive**
Dosage: **10 to 20 grams per ton of complete feed.**
Purpose: **Increased rate of weight gain and improved feed efficiency.**

FDA File **141-226**
Firm: **Phibro Animal Health, Inc.**
Use: **Chickens: Feed Additive**
Dosage: **20 grams per ton of complete feed.**
Purpose: **Increased rate of weight gain and improved feed efficiency and prevention of necrotic enteritis.**

FDA File **200-092**
Firm: **Intervet, Inc.**
Use: **Chickens: Feed Additive**
Dosage: **5 to 15 grams per ton of complete feed.**
Purpose: **Increased rate of weight gain and improved feed efficiency.**

FDA File **200-094**
Firm: **Intervet, Inc.**
Use: **Chickens: Feed Additive**
Dosage: **5 grams per ton of complete feed.**
Purpose: **Improved feed efficiency.**

ZOALENE

FDA File **011-116**
Firm: **Alpharma, Inc.**
Use: **Chickens, Turkeys: Feed Additive**
Dosage: **Chickens: 0.004 to 0.0125 percent in complete feed. Turkeys: 0.0125 to 0.01875 percent in complete feed.**
Purpose: **Prevention of coccidiosis.**

FDA File **013-747**
Firm: **Alpharma, Inc.**
Use: **Chickens, Turkeys: Feed Additive**
Dosage: **Chickens: 0.0083 to 0.0125 percent in complete feed. Turkeys: 0.0125 to 0.01875 percent in complete feed.**

Purpose: **Prevention and control of coccidiosis. Aid in development of active immunity under severe, moderate and light exposure to coccidiosis, depending on dosage.**

FDA File **038-241**
Firm: **Cross Vetpharm Group Ltd.**
Use: **Chickens: Feed Additive**
Dosage: **0.004 to 0.0125 percent in complete feed.**
Purpose: **Prevention and control of coccidiosis.**

FDA File **038-879**
Firm: **Alpharma, Inc.**
Use: **Turkeys: Feed Additive**
Dosage: **113.4 to 170.3 grams per ton of complete feed.**
Purpose: **Prevention and control of coccidiosis.**

FDA File **048-954**
Firm: **Pharmacia & Upjohn Co.**
Use: **Chickens: Feed Additive**
Dosage: **113.5 grams per ton of complete feed.**
Purpose: **Prevention and control of coccidiosis.**

FDA File **094-295**
Firm: **ADM Animal Health & Nutrition Div.**
Use: **Chickens: Feed Additive**
Dosage: **36.3 to 113.5 grams per ton of complete feed.**
Purpose: **Prevention and control of coccidiosis. Development of immunity against coccidiosis.**

FDA File **101-628**
Firm: **Intervet, Inc.**
Use: **Chickens: Feed Additive**

Dosage: **113.5 grams per ton of complete feed.**
Purpose: **Prevention of coccidiosis.**

FDA File **101-629**
Firm: **Intervet, Inc.**
Use: **Chickens: Feed Additive**
Dosage: **113.5 grams per ton of complete feed.**
Purpose: **Prevention of coccidiosis.**

FDA File **141-085**
Firm: **Alpharma, Inc.**
Use: **Chickens, Turkeys: Feed Additive**
Dosage: **Chickens: 36.3 to 112.5 grams per ton of complete feed up to 14 weeks of age. Turkeys: 113.5 to 170.3 grams per ton of complete feed until 14 to 16 weeks of age.**
Purpose: **Chickens: Aid in development of active immunity to coccidiosis, depending on dosage. Turkeys: Prevention and control of coccidiosis.**

FDA File **141-130**
Firm: **Alpharma, Inc.**
Use: **Chickens: Feed Additive**
Dosage: **36.3 to 113.5 grams per ton of complete feed.**
Purpose: **Prevention of coccidiosis.**

FDA File **141-131**
Firm: **Alpharma, Inc.**
Use: **Chickens: Feed Additive**
Dosage: **36.3 to 113.5 grams per ton of complete feed.**
Purpose: **Development of active immunity to coccidiosis.**

FURTHER READING

Persons who desire to further explore the grandeur of the bacterial world and the phenomenon of antibiotic resistance will find some additional references useful:

Internet Resources

Google searching for "antibiotic resistance" on March 5, 2008, produced 130,000 hits and the same search performed on August 24, 2008, produced 215,000 hits--an indication of the explosive amount of attention being given to the subject, however some of the increase may be due to enhancements in Google's search engine as well as to older documents being placed on the internet for the first time. Many of the hits are government agencies or consumer activist groups, and a large number are scientific papers. There are also the many predictable emotionally charged commentaries. The following are web sites recommended to provide a general overview of the issues surrounding antibiotic resistance.

The US National Institute of Allergy and Infectious Diseases provides an Internet site with scientific presentations and a discussion forum to promote communication between researchers at www.narsa.net. The organization also co-chairs the Federal government's Task Force on Antimicrobial Resistance in cooperation with the Center for Disease Control, the Food and Drug Administration, the Agency for Healthcare Research and Quality, the Department of Agriculture, the Department of Defense, the Department of Veterans Affairs, the Environmental Protection Agency, the Center for Medicaid and Medicare Services, and the Health Resources and Services. Their antimicrobial resistance action plan that reflects a broad consensus of these agencies with input from a variety of constituents and collaborators is available online at www.cdc.gov/drugresistance/actionplan/index.htm.

The US Centers for Disease Control and Prevention maintains an Internet site at www.cdc.gov/drugresistance/community/.

The US Food and Drug Administration maintains an Internet site on antibiotic resistance at www.FDA.gov/oc/opacom/hottopics/anti_resist.html.

The US National Library of Medicine database on antibiotic resistance may be accessed at http://www.nlm.nih/gov/medlineplus/antibiotics.html.

The Alliance for the Prudent Use of Antibiotics, headed up by Stuart B. Levy, the author of the book, *The Antibiotic Paradox*, maintains a website at www.tufts.edu/med/apua and at www.apua.org.

The Union of Concerned Scientists website regarding antibiotic resistance may be accessed at www.ucsusa.org/food_and_environment/antibiotic_resistance/index.cfm.

The Sierra Club position on antibiotic resistance may be seen at www.sierraclub.org/factoryfarms.

The group known as Keep Antibiotics Working is "a coalition of health, consumer, agricultural, environmental and other advocacy groups with more than nine million members dedicated to eliminating a major cause of antibiotic resistance—the inappropriate use of antibiotics in animals". Their position is set forth in some detail at www.keepantibioticsworking.com.

The U.S. Institute of Food Technologists maintains a web site that includes a link to their June 2006 expert report on antibiotic resistance at www.ift.org.

The US Animal Health Institute maintains a web site at www.ahi.org which includes links to the antibiotics debate.

Consumers Union has a website on how to get involved in the anti-infection movement at www.stophospitalinfections.org.

The US American Association of Retired Persons provides tips for patients on safer surgery at www.aarp.org/bulletin/yourhealth/surgery_safer.html.

The Heritage Foundation Lecture # 818 regarding the perils of "The Precautionary Principle" may be accessed at http://www.heritage.orgResearch/Regulation/h1818.cfm.

Books

Surprisingly few books have been published about antibiotic resistance. The following are suggested as general reading.

Brownlee, Shanon. 2007. *Overtreated: Why too much medicine is making us sicker and poorer.* New York: Bloomsbury USA.

Diamond, Jared. 1997. *Guns, germs, and steel: The fates of human societies.* New York: W.W. Norton & Company.

Drexler, Madeline. 2005. *Secret agents: The menace of emerging infections.* New York: The Penguin Group.

Fagerberg, Diane J. and Carey L. Quarles. 1979. *Antibiotic feeding, antibiotic resistance & alternatives.* New Jersey: American Hoechst.

Garrett, Laurie. 1995. *The coming plague.* New York: The Penguin Group.

Hager, Thomas. 2006. *The demon under the microscope.* New York: Harmony Books.

Institute of Medicine. 1999. *The use of drugs in food animals: Benefits and risks.* Washington, D.C.: National Academy Press.

Lax, Eric. 2004. *The mold in Dr. Florey's coat.* New York: Henry Holt and Company

Sachs, Jessica Snyder. 2007. *Good germs, bad Germs.* New York: Hill and Wang.

Levy, Stuart B. 1992. *The antibiotic paradox: How miracle drugs are destroying the miracle.* Cambridge, MA: Plenum Press.

Levy, Stuart B. 2002. *The antibiotic paradox: How the misuse of antibiotics destroys their curative powers.* Cambridge, MA.: Perseus Publishing.

McKeown, Thomas. 1998. *The origins of human disease.* New York: Basil Blackwell.

Mullany, Peter, (Editor). 2005. *The dynamic bacterial genome.* London: Cambridge University Press.

Ratcliff, J.D. 1945. *Yellow magic.* New York: Random House.

Regan, Tom. 1983. *The case for animal rights.* Berkeley, Los Angeles: University of California Press.

Ridley, Matt. 2003. *The agile gene: How nature turns on nuture.* New York: Harper Collins.

Salyers, Abigail A. and Dixie D. Whitt. 2005. *Revenge of the microbes: How bacterial resistance is undermining the antibiotic miracle.* Washington, D.C.: ASM Press, 2005.

Shnayerson, Michael and Mark J. Plotkin. 2002. *The killers within: The deadly rise of drug-resistant bacteria.* New York: Little, Brown and Company.

Singer, Peter. 1990. *Animal liberation,* Second Edition, New York: Random House.

White, David G., Alecshun, Michael N., and Patrick F. McDermott. (Editors). 2005. *Frontiers in antimicrobial resistance: A tribute to Stuart B. Levy.* Washington, D.C.: ASM Press.

Governmental Reports

United States General Accounting Office. Antibiotic resistance: Federal agencies need to better focus efforts to address risk to humans from antibiotic use in animals, *Publication GAO-04-490*, April 2004. Available at http://www.gao.gov/cgi-bin/getrpt?GAO-04-490.

Important Papers Published

Bassler, B.L. and R. Losick. 2006. Bacterially speaking. *Cell* 125 (2) 237–46.

D'Costa, Vanessa M., Katherin M. McGrann, Donald W. Hughes, and Gerard D. Wright. 2006. Sampling the antibiotic resistome, *Science* 311:374–377.

Denamur, Erick and Ivan Matic. 2006. Evolution of mutation rates in bacteria. *Molecular Microbiology* 60:(4) 820–827.

Guardabassi, Stephan Schwarz and David H. Lloyd. 2004. Pet animals as reservoirs of antimicrobial-resistant bacteria. *Journal of Antimicrobial Chemotherapy* 54:321–332.

Hardin, Garrett. 1968. The tragedy of the commons. *Science* 162:1243–1248.

Hecker, Michelle T., et.al. 2003. Unnecessary use of antimicrobials in hospitalized patients: current patterns of misuse with an emphasis on the antianaerobic spectrum of activity. *Archives of Internal Medicine* 163:972–978.

Holloway, Marguerite. 2004. Talking bacteria. *Scientific American* February 34–35.

Jones, F.T. and S.C. Ricke. 2003. Observations on the history of the development of antimicrobials and their use in poultry feeds. *Poultry Science* 82:613–17.

Kingsland, James. 2007. Superbugs bite back. *New Scientist* 29:37–39.

Phillips, Ian, Mark Casewell, Tony Cox, Brad De Groot, Christian Friis, Ron Jones, and Charles Nightingale. 2004. Does the use of antibiotics in food animals pose a risk to human health? A critical review of published data. *Journal of Antimicrobial Chemotherapy* 53:28–52.

Steinman, Michael A., et al. 2003. Changing use of antibiotics in community-based outpatient practice 1991–1999. *Annals of Internal Medicine* 138:525–533.

Yari, Donna. 2006. Animals as kin: The religious significance of Marc Bekoff"s work. *Zygon* 41:(1)21–28.

INDEX